MOLECULAR
BIOLOGY
INTELLIGENCE
UNIT

THE TH1/TH2 PARADIGM IN DISEASE

Sergio Romagnani, M.D.

Institute of Internal Medicine and Immunoallergology
University of Florence
Florence, Italy

Springer
New York Berlin Heidelberg London Paris
Tokyo Hong Kong Barcelona Budapest

R.G. LANDES COMPANY
AUSTIN

MOLECULAR BIOLOGY INTELLIGENCE UNIT
THE TH1/TH2 PARADIGM IN DISEASE

R.G. LANDES COMPANY
Austin, Texas, U.S.A.

International Copyright © 1997 Springer-Verlag, Heidelberg, Germany

Please address all inquiries to the Publishers:
R.G. Landes Company, 810 S. Church Street, Georgetown, Texas, U.S.A. 78626
Phone: 512/ 863 7762; FAX: 512/ 863 0081

International distributor (except North America):

Springer-Verlag GmbH & Co. KG
Tiergartenstrasse 17, D-69121 Heidelberg, Germany

 Springer

International ISBN: 3-540-61949-6

Library of Congress Cataloging-in-Publication Data

Romagnani, S. (Sergio)
    The Th1-Th2 paradigm in disease/ Sergio Romagnani
        p. cm. — (Molecular biology intelligence unit)
    Includes bibliographical references and index.
    ISBN 0-57059-409-0 (alk. paper)
    1. Th1 cells. 2. Th2 cells. 3. Immune response—Regulation.
        4. Immunopathology. I. Title II. Series.
QR185.8.T24R66 1996
616.07'9—dc20
                                                96-43792
                                                CIP

Publisher's Note

R.G. Landes Company publishes six book series: *Medical Intelligence Unit, Molecular Biology Intelligence Unit, Neuroscience Intelligence Unit, Tissue Engineering Intelligence Unit, Biotechnology Intelligence Unit* and *Environmental Intelligence Unit.* The authors of our books are acknowledged leaders in their fields and the topics are unique. Almost without exception, no other similar books exist on these topics.

Our goal is to publish books in important and rapidly changing areas of bioscience and environment for sophisticated researchers and clinicians. To achieve this goal, we have accelerated our publishing program to conform to the fast pace in which information grows in bioscience. Most of our books are published within 90 to 120 days of receipt of the manuscript. We would like to thank our readers for their continuing interest and welcome any comments or suggestions they may have for future books.

Shyamali Ghosh
Publications Director
R.G. Landes Company

CONTENTS

ACKNOWLEDGMENTS

I thank all my co-workers: Gianfranco Del Prete, Enrico Maggi, Fabio Almerigogna, Paola Parronchi, Roberto Manetti, Francesco Annunziato, Maria-Grazia Giudizi, Roberta Biagiotti, Marco De Carli, Marie-Pierre Piccinni, Lucio Beloni, Salvatore Sampognaro, Loretta Giannarini, Valeria Giannò, Liliana Tomasevic, Grazia Galli, Patrizia Germano, Lorenzo Cosmi, Kurt Daniel, Adriana Ravina, Marcello Mazzetti, Mario D'Elios, Maria Manghetti, Carmelo Mavilia, Cinzia Manueli, Cristina Scaletti and Lorenzo Emmi for their valuable collaboration. I would like to mention the extramural collaborations with G. Trinchieri (Wistar Institute, Philadelphia), L. Moretta and M-C. Mingari (University of Genova), G. Pizzolo and M. Chilosi (University of Verona), P. Romagnani, C. Pupilli, C. Livi, G. Scarselli and F. Tonelli (University of Florence), the Immunex Corporation (Seattle) and the Ares-Serono (Geneve), who also gave important contributions. I would like to thank Prof. A. B. Kay (London), M. Chilosi (Verona), M. D'Elios (Florence), F. Annunziato (Florence) and P. Romagnani (Florence) for their kindness in providing some of the photographic material. The experiments here reported have been performed with funds from AIRC, Istituto Superiore di Sanità (AIDS Project), European Comunity and the Italian National Research Council.

CHAPTER 1

INTRODUCTION

Infectious agents present their hosts with enormous immunological problems. Most infectious agents are antigenically complex, and some have complicated life cycles in which the various stages, often occupying different sites, differ antigenically from one another. Added to this, all infectious agents, although capable of eliciting an immunological response, have evolved numerous ways of evading the consequences of immune attack. Therefore, teleologically, attempts at colonizing by microorganisms were continually held at bay by the process of natural selection, which in humans and other higher organisms continuously shaped and refined the mechanisms used by the immune system to defend against infection. The 'first line of defense' is provided by cells and molecules of the so-called 'innate' or 'natural' immunity, which include phagocytic cells, T cell receptor (TCR) $\gamma\delta^+$ T cells, natural killer (NK) cells, mast cells and eosinophils, as well as complement components and pro-inflammatory cytokines, such as interferons (IFNs), interleukin (IL)-1, IL-6, IL-12 and tumor necrosis factor (TNF)-α. When this 'first line of defense' is overcome, the more specialized TCR $\alpha\beta^+$ T lymphocytes are involved. These cells provide the basis of the so-called 'specific or adaptive immunity.' Specialized types of specific immune responses have evolved in response to different microrganisms that allow vertebrates to recognize and eliminate, or at least control, infectious microorganisms that colonize different body compartments. For example, viruses, which grow within the cytoplasm and the nucleus of the infected cell, can be eliminated only by killing their host cells. To enable this to happen, viral antigens are synthesized within infected cells and presented on the surface of the cells in association with class I major histocompatibility complex (MHC) molecules, leading to the stimulation of $CD8^+$ class I MHC-restricted cytotoxic T lymphocytes. The majority of microbial antigens, however, are endocytosed by antigen-presenting cells (APC), which include macrophages, dendritic cells and B lymphocytes, processed and presented preferentially in association with class II MHC molecules to $CD4^+$ class II MHC-restricted T helper (Th) cells. $CD4^+$ T cells collaborate with B lymphocytes for the production of antibodies which are able, with or without the collaboration of serum complement proteins, to challenge microbes living outside cells or neutralize their soluble toxic products (exotoxins). This branch of the specific Th cell-mediated immune response is known as 'humoral immunity' (Fig. 1.1a). On the other side, other microbes such as mycobacteria can survive and multiply within macrophages despite the unfavorable life conditions provided by the activity of proteolytic enzymes and other toxic substances produced by these cells. CD4[+] Th cells, activated by mycobacterial soluble antigens, can in turn activate macrophages. Reactive oxygen intermediates, reactive nitrogen intermediates, such as nitric oxide (NO) and TNF-α, produced by activated macrophages, then lead to microbes' destruction. This branch of the specific Th cell-mediated immune response is called 'cellular or cell-mediated immunity' (CMI) (Fig. 1.1b). Since the occurrence of CMI can be easily revealed by the demonstration of an indurative skin reaction, due to the accumulation of mononuclear cells, which appears 24-96 hours after the intradermal injection of antigen, it is also commonly defined as delayed type hypersensitivity (DTH) reaction. Most immune responses involve both branches of the immune system (humoral immunity and DTH) acting in concert. However, in some conditions the two types of effector reactions may also be mutually exclusive. More importantly, in certain experimental models suppression of DTH may be associated with increased levels of antibody production. This phenomenon is known as "split tolerance" or "immune deviation." Using chemically modified *Salmonella* flagellin as an antigen, Parish and Liew[2] showed that antibody production and DTH could be reciprocally expressed. Very low concentrations of antigen yielded responses in which DTH reactions were dominant. As the antigen dose was increased, antibody responses increased and DTH responses diminished. Finally at high doses of antigen, DTH again dominated. The mechanisms by which CD4[+] Th cells may be responsible for this dichotomy in the specific immune response remained unclear until 1986, when Mosmann and his co-workers[3] provided evidence that repeated stimulation of murine CD4[+] Th lymphocytes in vitro with given antigens results in the development of restricted and stereotyped pattern of lymphokine production (type 1 or Th1 and type 2 or Th2) that could account for effector reactions characterized by prevalent DTH or antibody response, respectively.

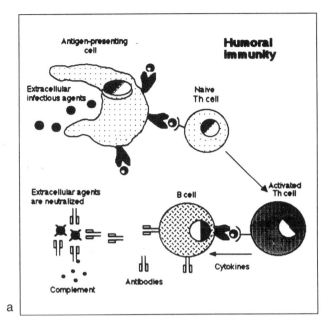

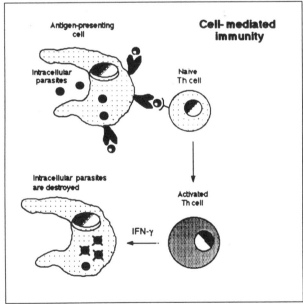

Fig. 1.1. The humoral and cell-mediated arms of the specific effector immune response. Protection against extracellular infectious agents is mainly provided by soluble antibodies which are produced by B cells via the collaboration with activated CD4⁺ Th cells, which can neutralize the infectious agents in every part of the body (humoral immunity). Protection against infectious agents living within the cells (where they cannot be challenged by antibodies) is mainly due to toxic products (NO, O_2^-) released by macrophages activated via cytokines (mainly IFN-γ) produced by the activated CD4⁺ Th cells (cell-mediated or cellular immunity). Reprinted with permission from Romagnani S, Science & Medicine 1994; 69.[1]

CHAPTER 2

TYPE 1 AND TYPE 2 LYMPHOKINES: POLARIZED FORMS OF THE SPECIFIC IMMUNE RESPONSE

DEFINITION AND FUNCTIONS OF MURINE CD4+ TH1 AND TH2 CELLS

Murine Th1 cells produce IFN-γ, IL-2 and TNF-β and promote the production of IgG2a opsonizing and complement-fixing antibodies, activation of macrophages, antibody-dependent cell cytotoxicity (ADCC) and DTH[4] (Table 2.1). For these reasons, Th1 cells can be considered responsible for the phagocyte-dependent host response[5,6] (Fig. 2.1a). On the other side, Th2 cells produce IL-4, IL-5, IL-6, IL-9, IL-10 and IL-13 and provide optimal help for humoral immune responses, including IgE and IgG1 isotype switching, and mucosal immunity, through production of mast cell and eosinophil growth and differentiation and facilitation to IgA synthesis. Moreover, some Th2-derived cytokines, such as IL-4, IL-10 and IL-13 inhibit several macrophage functions.[4] Therefore, it is possible to refer to Th2 cells as responsible for the phagocyte-independent host response[5,6] (Fig. 2.1b). Other cytokines, such as IL-3, granulocyte/macrophage colony-stimulating factor (GM-CSF), and TNF-α are produced by both Th1 and Th2 cells[4] (Table 2.1). Th1 and Th2 are not the only cytokine patterns possible. T cells expressing cytokines of both patterns have been designated Th0, that usually mediate intermediate effects depending upon the ratio of lymphokines produced and the nature of the responding cells.[7-9] T cells producing high amounts of transforming growth factor (TGF)-β have been termed Th3,[10] and additional patterns have been described among long-term clones.[11] Th0 cells probably represent a heterogenous population of partially differentiated effector cells consisting of multiple discrete subsets which can secrete both Th1 and

Table 2.1. Main functional properties of murine Th1 and Th2 cells

Property	Th1	Th2
Cytokine production		
IL-2	++	–
IFN-γ	++	–
TNF-β	++	–
TNF-α	++	+
GM-CSF	++	+
IL-3	++	++
IL-4	–	++
IL-5	–	++
IL-6	–	+
IL-9	–	++
IL-10	–	++
IL-13	–	++
B cell help		
IgM	++	++
IgG1	+	++
IgG2a	++	+
IgE	–	++
Macrophage activation	++	–
DTH	++	–
Cytotoxicity	++	–
ADCC	++	–
Inhibition of macrophage function	–	++
Eosinophil differentiation and activation	–	++
Mast cell growth	–	++

Th2 cytokines. The cytokine response at effector level can remain mixed or can be induced to further differentiate into Th1 or the Th2 pathway under the influence of signals received from the microenvironment[12] (see below). Some studies, however, have demonstrated heterogeneity of cytokine synthesis at the single-cell level even in polarized Th1 and Th2 responses.[13,14] Moreover, each of the cytokine genes seems to be under unique control, with distinct tendencies for concordance (e.g., IL-4 and IL-5) or discordance (e.g., IL-4 and IFN-γ).[15] Thus, another possibility is that cytokine profiles are largely random at the clonal level and that the exogenous signals which appear to direct T cells to differentiate into Th1 or Th2 cells (see below) act by increasing the probability of expression of certain cytokine genes at the population level, rather than by activating the expression of a cassette of transcriptionally linked genes in the individual cell.[14]

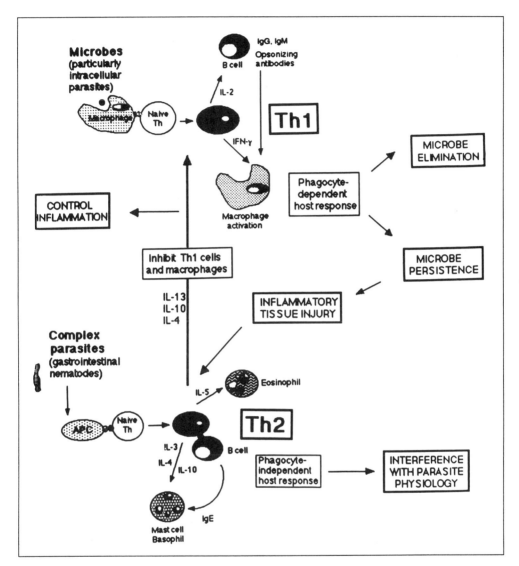

Fig. 2.1. Schematic representation of the role of Th1 and Th2 cells. Microbes and especially intracellular parasites are challenged by Th1 cells, since they are able to promote both the activation of macrophages (via the production of IFN-γ) and the production of opsonizing antibodies (via the production of IL-2). This "phagocyte-dependent response" usually results in microbe elimination. However, if despite this response the microbe persists, the chronic and intense inflammatory reaction triggered by Th1 cells results in severe tissue injury.

Large and complex parasites, such as gastrointestinal nematodes, which cannot be rapidly eliminated by Th1 cells because of their size, are better challenged by Th2 cells which interfere with their physiology, without trying to kill them. Rather, to avoid the effects of concomitant Th1 responses, the Th2 cells inhibit several macrophage functions (via the release of IL-4, IL-10 and IL-13). This "phagocyte-independent response" may also occur as a result of a "switch" during infections sustained by microbes which are not rapidly cleared by Th1 cells, thus resulting in the control of dangerous inflammation.

Regardless of whether the variation in T cell cytokine synthesis represents a continuum or discrete subsets, there is no doubt that many T cell clones and in vivo immune responses show a dramatic Th1 or Th2 polarization. Thus, although Th1 and Th2 cells are certainly not the result of a preexisting functional dichotomy of CD4+ T cells, they can be regarded as polarized forms of the specific immune response that frequently occur under the combined action of genetic and environmental conditions. It should also be remembered that we currently speak of CD4+ T cells that have been differentiated to produce IL-4 but not IFN-γ as Th2 (or Th2-like) cells and of cells that produce IFN-γ but not IL-4 as Th1 (or Th1-like) cells without considering the other set of Th1 or Th2 cytokines. Bearing all these points in mind, the Th1/Th2 paradigm may provide a useful model for understanding the pathogenesis of several pathophysiologic conditions and, possibly, for the development of novel immunotherapeutic strategies.

PROPERTIES AND FUNCTIONS
OF HUMAN TH1 AND TH2 CELLS

Evidence for the existence of human Th1 and Th2 cells similar to those described in mice was provided by establishing CD4+ T cell clones specific for peculiar antigens. CD4+ T lymphocytes that produce IL-4, but low or no IFN-γ, were found to occur in high frequencies in the allergen-specific repertoires of atopic donors.[16,17] However, the first clear-cut demonstration on the existence of human Th1 and Th2 cells was provided by establishing T cell clones specific for *Toxocara canis* excretory/secretory (TES) antigens and purified protein derivative (PPD) of *Mycobacterium tuberculosis* from normal donors. TES-specific clones exhibited a Th2-like profile of cytokine secretion (production of IL-4 and IL-5, but no or low IFN-γ and IL-2), whereas the great majority of PPD-specific T cell clones derived from the same donors showed a clear-cut Th1 profile (production of IL-2 and IFN-γ, but no IL-4 and IL-5).[18,19] Additional evidence in favor of the existence of Th1 cells specific for mycobacterial antigens or heat shock proteins was contemporarily provided in other laboratories.[20-22] More importantly, T cell clones with opposite Th1-like or Th2-like cytokine profile were generated from the target organs of patients affected by Hashimoto's thyroiditis[19,23] or children with vernal conjunctivitis,[24] respectively.

In general, however, human T cell clones exhibit a less restricted cytokine profile than murine T cells. IL-2, IL-6, IL-10 and IL-13 tend to segregate less clearly among human CD4+ subsets than in the mouse[25-27] (Table 2.2). In addition, unlike mouse IL-10,[28] human IL-10 inhibits the proliferative response and lymphokine production not only by Th1 but also by Th2 cells.[25] Human Th1 and Th2 cells also show different responsiveness to lymphokines. Both Th1 and Th2 cells proliferate in response to IL-2, but Th2 are much more responsive to IL-4 than Th1. IFN-γ plays a selective inhibitory effect on the proliferative response of Th2 cells.[25] Moreover, human Th1 and Th2 cells clearly differ for their cytolytic potential and mode of help for B cell antibody synthesis. In fact, Th2 clones, that usually had no cytolytic potential, induced IgM, IgG, IgA and IgE synthesis by autologous B cells in the presence of the specific antigen with a response proportional to the number of Th2 cells added to B cells.[29] In contrast, Th1 clones (of which the majority were cytolytic) provided B cell help for IgM, IgG, IgA (but not IgE) synthesis at low T cell:B cell ratios. At T cell:B cell ratios higher than 1:1 there was a decline in B cell help, that appeared to be related to their lytic activity against autologous antigen-presenting B cell targets.[29] This may represent an important mechanism for the downregulation of antibody responses in vivo.[19,29] Finally, in agreement with the results previously reported in the murine system,[4] human Th1 and Th2 cells exhibit different ability to activate monocytic cells.[30] Th1, but not Th2, cells can help tissue factor (TF) production and procoagulant activity by monocytes (Table 2.2). Indeed, both cell-to-cell contacts with activated T cells and Th1 cytokines, in particular IFN-γ, were required for optimal TF synthesis, whereas Th2-derived cytokines (IL-4, IL-10 and IL-13) were inhibitory.[30]

Table 2.2. Main functional properties of human Th1 and Th2 cells

FunctionTh1	Th2	
Cytokine secretion		
IFN-γ	+++	–
TNF-β	+++	–
IL-2	+++	+
TNF-α	+++	+
GM-CSF	++	++
IL-3	++	+++
IL-10	+	++
IL-13	++	+++
IL-4	–	+++
IL-5	–	+++
Cytolytic potential	+++	–
B cell help for Ig synthesis		
IgE	–	+++
IgM, IgG, IgA		
at low T/B ratios	+++	++
at high T/B ratios	–	+++
Macrophage activation		
Induction of PCA	+++	–
TF production	+++	–

METHODS FOR DETECTING TH1 AND TH2 CELLS

The possibility to detect the presence of Th1- or Th2-dominated responses in normal and pathological conditions is limited by serious methodological problems. First, all cytokines are produced by T cells in small amounts and some of them are not released in the microenvironment, but are directly transmitted from one cell to another during cell-to-cell contact. Therefore, it is virtually impossible to measure or even detect spontaneously secreted cytokines in biological fluids or even in supernatants of T cell suspensions. Secondly, some cytokines, such as IL-4, are practically undetectable even in supernatants of T cells activated in short-term cultures, since repeated in vitro stimulation is required to obtain the production of measurable IL-4 amounts. In order to characterize the cytokine profile of Th-cell-mediated effector responses, different methodological approaches have been proposed.

CLONING PROCEDURES

As mentioned above, the initial demonstration of Th1 and Th2 cells in both mice and humans was provided by the use of cloning techniques.[1,18] These methods are based on the expansion of single T cells stimulated with polyclonal activators, superantigens or antigens, in the presence of both feeder cells and T cell growth factors, such as IL-2 and/or IL-4. In the case of polyclonal stimulators or superantigens, single T cells can be plated from the beginning under limiting dilution conditions.[31] In the case of antigens, in order to enhance the cloning efficiency, heterogenous cell suspensions are stimulated with the antigen for some days and then single T cells are distributed under limiting dilution conditions and expanded by the use of polyclonal activators plus IL-2[17,18] (Fig. 2.2). When cells present in tissue fragments have to be expanded, the fragment is cultured for some days in medium containing IL-2 to get an initial number of cells sufficient for distribution in the wells.[32]

The main advantage of cloning techniques rests on the possibility to have the same cytokine produced by high numbers of cells belonging to the same clone, so that nanogram values can be quantitated by appropriate ELISAs or biological assays. To this end, 10^5-10^6 clonal T cells are stimulated for 24-36 hours with the specific antigen in the presence of irradiated MHC-restricted APCs or with polyclonal activators, such as phytohemagglutinin (PHA), phorbol-myristate-acetate (PMA) or insolubilized anti-CD3 antibody. The maximum stimulation is provided by the combined use of PMA and PHA, PMA and anti-CD3 antibody, or PMA and ionomycin. The disadvantages of cloning techniques are: (1) the hard-working and long-lasting procedure and (2) the fact that they reflect the potential rather than current cytokine profile of a given T cell or T cell suspension.

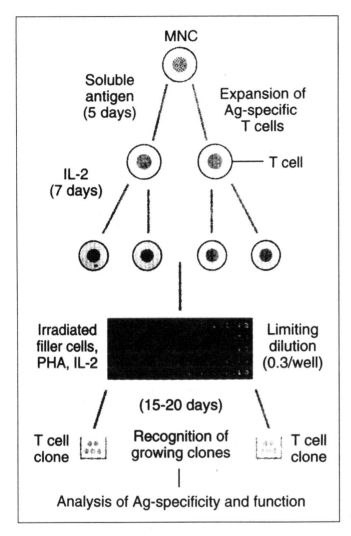

Fig. 2.2. Cloning procedure. Mononuclear cells (MNC) are stimulated with a given antigen (Ag) for 5 days, followed by the addition of IL-2 for subsequent 7 days, to expand Ag-specific T cells. These cells are then cloned under limiting dilution conditions (0.3-0.5 cell/well) and single T cells are stimulated with PHA in the presence of irradiated filler (or feeder) cells and IL-2. The resulting progenies from each cell is expanded for 2-3 weeks by repeated additions of IL-2 until the size of clone is sufficient to allow the execution of phenotypic and functional studies. To establish the cytokine profile of each clone, 10^6 clonal T cell blasts are usually stimulated for 24-72 hours with the specific Ag under MHC-restriced conditions or with PMA and ionomycin, and cytokines released into cell-free supernatant are quantitated by appropriate ELISAs. Reprinted with permission from Romagnani S, Science & Medicine 1994; 1:68-77.[1]

2. **REVERSE TRANSCRIPTASE-POLYMERASE CHAIN REACTION (RT-PCR) ASSAY**

RT-PCR is a very sensitive technique (1000- to 10,000-fold more sensitive than the traditional RNA blotting techniques) that makes it possible to detect mRNAs of extremely rare abundance, mRNAs in small numbers of cells or small amounts of tissue, and mRNAs expressed in mixed cell populations where the cells expressing the mRNA are rare. RT-PCR also allows to determine the expression of multiple mRNAs simultaneously, which is difficult to achieve by traditional methods. Depending upon available quantities as source of RNA, total RNA or poly(A)⁺ RNA can be used. The direct mRNA extraction provides a fast and simple way to isolate poly(A)⁺ RNA from less than 100 cells to up to 10^8 cells, or less than 10 mg to up to 1 g of tissue, or from 50 ml of blood. Once mRNA is extracted, cDNA can be synthesized by reverse transcription, using AMV or MMLV RT. Then, cDNA is amplified by PCR, a very simple technique consisting of subsequent cycles of denaturing, annealing and extension of DNA. After denaturing, the single-stranded DNA (ssDNA) preparation is annealed with two short primer sequences (e.g., 20 bases each) that are complementary to sites on the opposite strands on either side of the target region. DNA polymerase is used to synthesize a single strand from the 3'-OH end of each primer. The entire cycle can then be repeated by denaturing the preparation and starting again so that 30 cycles should result in a 270 million-fold amplification of the product.[33] Finally, the PCR product is visualized on gel (Fig. 2.3).

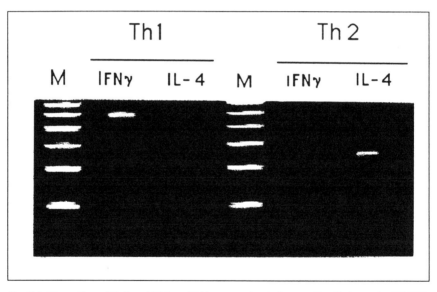

Fig. 2.3. *Detection of IL-4 and IFN-γ mRNA expression in human T cell clones by RT-PCR. After stimulation of one Th1 and one Th2 CD4⁺ T cell clone for 18 hours with PMA plus anti-CD3 antibody, mRNA was extracted by mRNA direct isolation kit (Qiagen Gmbh, Hilden, Germany) and converted into cDNA by the oligo-dT method. Samples were amplified under equal conditions by a 30 cycle PCR and visalized on gel.*
    IFN-γ specific primers were:
        sense ATGAAATATACAAGTTATATCTTGGCTTT;
        antisense GATGCTCTTCGACCTCGAAACAGCAT;
    IL-4 specific primers were:
        sense AACACAACTGAGAAGGAAACCTCCTGC;
        antisense CTCTCTCATGATCGTCTTTAGCCTTTC.
Courtesy of Dr. M. M. D'Elios, Institute of Internal Medicine and Immunoallergology, University of Florence.

The advantages of RT-PCR are the elevated sensitivity of the assay and the possibility to examine not only cell suspensions but also tissue specimens. The disadvantages include: (1) the high risk for nonspecific reactions; (2) the possibility that a given cytokine is transcribed, but not secreted, and (3) the impossibility to characterize the cell type responsible for cytokine gene transcription.

IN SITU HYBRIDIZATION

In situ hybridization allows the demonstration of nucleic acid sequences in their morphologically preserved cellular environment. Together with immunohistochemistry, in situ hybridization is capable of relating microscopic topological information to gene activity at the DNA, mRNA and protein level. The principle of the technique is simple and involves three steps: (1) pretreatment of the cellular preparations to unmask target nucleic acids (denaturation); (2) hybridization of a nucleic acid probe, of complementary base sequence, to the target (hybridization) and (3) detection of the label attached to the probe and hence the visualization of the target. At the time when the technique was first introduced, radioisotopes were the only labels available for nucleic acids, and autoradiography was the only way of detecting hybridized sequences. Moreover, as molecular cloning was not yet possible, in situ hybridization was restricted to those sequences that could be purified and isolated by conventional biochemical methods (e.g., mouse satellite DNA, viral DNA and ribosomal RNAs). Molecular cloning of nucleic acids and improved radiolabeling techniques have dramatically improved the technique, inasmuch as radioactive in situ detection of low copy number mRNA molecules, e.g., cytokine mRNA, in individual cells is now possible. More recently, the use of fluorocromes to label and to detect the probes, which provide highly sensitive detection, good spatial resolution of signal, and the potential for simultaneous multicolor analysis with different probes, is becoming increasingly popular. The signal is observed directly using a conventional fluorescence microscope or, for greater resolution, a confocal laser microscope or CCD camera. According to the probe preparation, three types of nucleic acid are used for in situ hybridization: DNA cloned sequences, RNA cloned sequences and oligonucleotides. Each of them has some advantages and other disadvantages. With cloned DNA, long sequences can be produced but with low hybridization efficiency, whereas RNA probes have high efficiency of hybridization, but they are difficult to produce; finally, oligonucleotide probes have high hybridization efficiency but they are insensitive unless used as "cocktails" of several labeled sequences. Besides radioactive labeling, two types of hybridization methods can be distinguished: (1) the direct and (2) the indirect procedure. In the direct method, the detectable reporter molecule is bound directly to the nucleic acid probe so that formed hybrids can be visualized microscopically immediately after their hybridization to the target nucleic acid. Indirect procedures require that the probe contains a reporter molecule introduced chemically or enzymatically that renders it detectable by affinity cytochemistry, hence the term indirect. A number of such hapten modifications have been described: one of the most used is surely the biotin-streptavidin system; an alternative method is the digoxigenin-system.[34] Although in situ hybridization is a more hard-working procedure than RT-PCR, it has the advantage of allowing the identification of the cell type responsible for the production of a given cytokine (Fig. 2.4).

ELIspot Assay

In this assay, wells from nitrocellulose-backed microtiter plates are coated with a monoclonal anti-cytokine antibody and incubated with serial dilutions of a single cell suspension, starting with 10^5-10^6 cells/

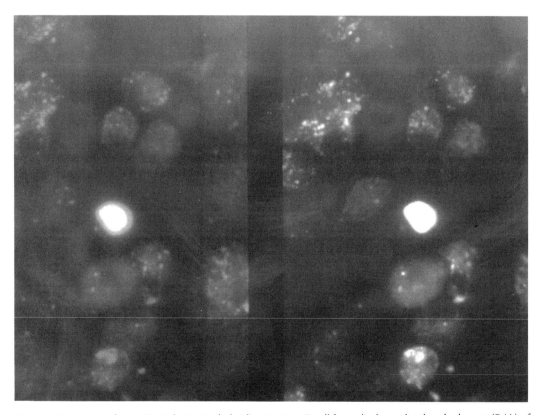

Fig. 2.4. Detection of IL-4 mRNA by in situ hybridization in a T cell from the bronchoalveolar lavage (BAL) of an asthmatic patient. In situ hybridization of IL-4 mRNA expression was performed by using a biotinylated probe developed with Texas Red (left) and characterization of the T cell by using cell immunohistochemistry with FITC-labeled monoclonal antibody to CD3 (right). Background autofluorescence is from alveolar macrophages. Courtesy of Dr. A. B. Kay, Department of Allergy and Clinical Immunology, National Heart and Lung Institute, London.

well. The plates are then washed and overlaid with biotinylated anti-cytokine antibody, followed by avidin-conjugated alkaline phosphatase.[35] The cytokine secreted by single cells is visualized by the addition of a solution of BCIP/NBT, which yields a purple precipitate in the presence of phosphatase. The colorimetric reaction is halted by washing, and spots are enumerated under magnification. This technique is relatively simple, but it has recently been overcome by the intracellular cytokine staining method based on the use of cytofluorimetry.

FLOW CYTOMETRIC ANALYSIS OF INTRACELLULAR CYTOKINE

The assay for intracellular staining of cytokines is a sensitive technique that allows to measure the percentage of cells capable of producing a given cytokine.[36,37] In this assay, cells are stimulated in the presence of substances which cause intracellular accumulation of newly synthesized proteins. In general, monensin, which arrests protein transport principally in the Golgi complex, or brefaldin A, which disrupts the Golgi apparatus, are used. After stimulation in the presence of protein transport blocker, cells are fixed with 4% formaldehyde and then permeabilized with 0.1-0.5% saponin before staining with labeled anti-cytokine antibody (or isotype control), followed by analysis on a cytofluorimeter. It has been shown that following stimulation with PMA plus ionomycin in both murine and human T cell clones intracellular synthesis of IFN-γ is sustained throughout several hours, whereas IL-4 synthesis is very early and relatively transient, since it declines rapidly straight after a synthesis peak at 4 hours (Fig. 2.5).

IMMUNOHISTOCHEMISTRY

The presence of cytokines in tissue cells has also been assessed by immunohistochemistry. To this end, freshly frozen or formalin-fixed, paraffin-embedded tissue sections are stained with anti-cytokine monoclonal antibodies, followed by incubation with standard avidin biotin complex-alkaline phosphatase or horseradish peroxidase conjugate. The sections are then counterstained with haematoxilin, and positive cells visualized and counted under light microscopy.[38] By using this method, several cytokines have been detected in different tissues (Fig. 2.6). However, while it is possible to detect all types of cytokines in cells, such as mast cells, where they are stored preformed, the possibility to detect some cytokines, especially IL-4, in T cells has been questioned.[38] This is probably due to the fact that IL-4 is rapidly transported from the cell (see also Fig. 2.5) and therefore does not accumulate in sufficient concentrations to be detected by the immunohistochemical method.

SURFACE MOLECULES PREFERENTIALLY ASSOCIATED WITH TH1 OR TH2 CELLS

The possibility that the Th1 or Th2 polarization of the effector response associates with expression of distinctive molecules on the cell

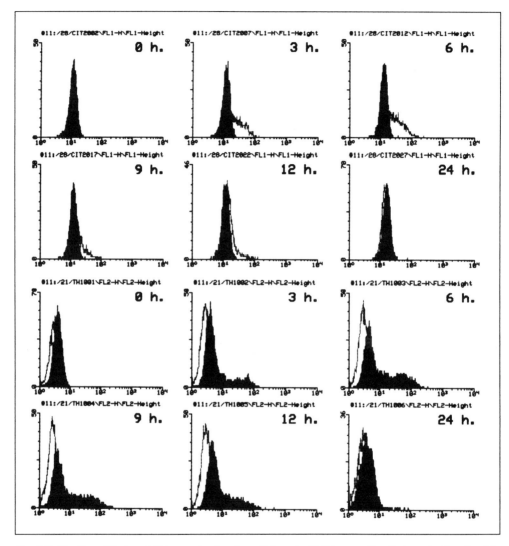

Fig. 2.5. Kinetics of IL-4 and IFN-γ production by a Th1 and a Th2 human T cell clone by fluorimetric intracellular assay. One Th1 clone (top) and one Th2 clone (bottom) were stimulated with PMA and ionomycin and assessed at different times (0, 3, 6, 9, 12 and 24 hours) for intracellular expression of IFN-γ(open) and IL-4 (shaded) by cytofluorimetry, according to the method described by Assenmacher et al (1994).[37] Courtesy of Dr. F. Annunziato, Institute of Internal Medicine and Immunoallergology, University of Florence.

surface has also been investigated (Table 2.3). Differential expression of CD45 family antigens was found in murine Th1 and Th2 cell lines. In Th2-like T cell lines the prevalent phenotype was CD45R[high], whereas in their Th1-like counterparts most of the cells were CD45R[low],[39,40] but this conclusion has been questioned.[41] Different expression by Th1 and Th2 murine cell lines and clones of disialogangliosides has also

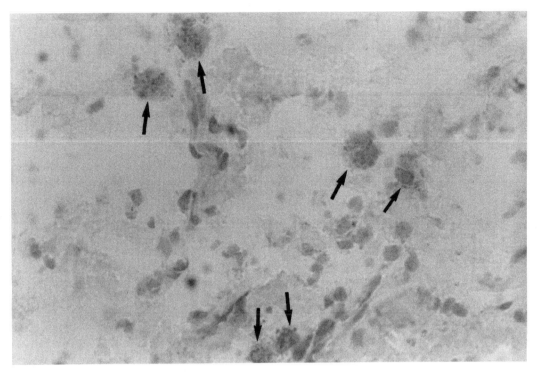

Fig. 2.6. Detection by immunohistochemistry of cells producing IFN-γ in the intestinal lamina propria of a patient with Crohn's disease. Immunohistochemical staining was performed on 4% paraformaldehyde fixed sections by an anti-IFN-γ mouse monoclonal antibody, followed by biotinylated anti-mouse IgG antibody and the avidin-biotin-peroxidase complex. Sections were then counterstained with Gill's hematoxylin. Arrows indicate IFN-γ expressing cells. Courtesy of Dr. P. Romagnani, Department of Physiopathology, Endocrinology Unit, University of Florence.

been reported. GD1a was detected only in Th2 cells, whereas GD1α was preferentially, but not exclusively, expressed by Th1 lymphocytes.[42] The selective expression on murine Th2 cells of the IFN-γ receptor β chain (IFN-γRβ) has been described.[43] However, whether detection of IFN-γRβ could be a critical diagnostic tool for determining whether a prevalent Th1 or Th2 immune response has been mounted is still unclear.

Some surface molecules preferentially associated with the Th1 or the Th2 phenotype have also been described in human T cells (Table 2.3). For example, the expression of CD26, an ectopeptidase present in a wide range of tissues, has been reported to correlate with Th1-like reactions in granulomatous diseases.[44] In contrast, L-selectin (CD62L)-positive memory CD4+ T cells produce mainly Th2-type cytokines, whereas L-selectin-negative CD4+ T cells produce mainly IFN-γ.[45] Moreover, by means of a highly sophisticated cytofluorimetric technique, it has been shown that detection of surface membrane IFN-γ

Table 2.3. Surface molecules preferentially expressed on Th1 or Th2 cells

Molecule	Th1	Th2
Mouse		
CD45R[high]		+
CD45R[low]	+	
GD1a		+
GD1α	+	
IFN-γ R β chain		+
membrane IFN-γ	+	
Man		
CD26	+	
CD30		+
LAG-3	+	
membrane IFN-γ	+	
L-selectin (CD62L)		+

(IFN-γ is expressed on the cell surface before to be secreted) may be a useful marker for Th1 cells in both mouse and man.[46] Other molecules that have been shown to be preferentially associated with human Th2 and Th1 clones are CD30 and lymphocyte activation gene (LAG)-3, respectively.

CD30, a member of the TNF receptor family,[47] was found to be consistently expressed, and its soluble form (sCD30) released by Th2 and Th0 clones, whereas Th1 clones usually showed poor and transient or no CD30 expression.[48] CD30 expression by Th0/Th2 clones was not constitutive, but required T cell activation and the presence in culture of IL-2. Although the possibility that CD30 expression may discriminate Th1 and Th2 cells has been questioned,[49-51] additional in vitro and in vivo observations support the view that CD30 expression and production of Th2 cytokines are significantly associated. First, costimulation of antigen-specific Th0 or Th2 clones with an agonistic anti-CD30 monoclonal antibody resulted in increased proliferation and cytokine production, whereas it had no significant effects on both proliferative response and cytokine production by Th1 clones.[52] Accordingly, CD30 ligation induced activation of NFκB transcription factors in Th0 and Th2, but not in Th1, clones.[53] The preferential association of CD30 with T cells producing Th2 cytokines was not limited to T cell clones established in vitro, but was also supported by some findings in vivo. Very small numbers of CD4+CD30+ T cells were detected in the circulation of atopic grass pollen-sensitive donors during the seasonal exposure to grass pollens. When sorted and IL-2 expanded in vitro, these cells developed into T cell lines able to proliferate in response to grass-pollen allergens and to produce IL-4 and IL-5, but not IFN-γ and TNF-β in response to polyclonal stimulation. In contrast, T cell lines generated from the CD4⁺CD30⁻ cells of the same donors developed into T cell lines that did not react to grass-pollen allergens and produced high IFN-γ and TNF-β, but low IL-4 and IL-5, in response to polyclonal activators.[48] Moreover, high serum levels of sCD30 were found in the majority of patients with atopic dermatitis.[54] More importantly, high numbers of CD30⁺ T cells were detected in the lymph node and skin biopsies of three children with Omenn's syndrome (OS) and in the lymph node and peripheral blood of one child with Omenn's-like syndrome.[55] When circulating CD30⁺ T cells from this child were separated from the CD30⁻ T cells by cell sorting and the two cell fractions were cloned under limiting dilution conditions and single T cells stimulated with PHA, a clear-cut difference in the cytokine profile of T cell clones was found. Most CD30⁺ T cells developed into Th0/Th2 clones, whereas the majority of CD30⁻ T cells differentiated into Th1-like clones. Furthermore, high levels of sCD30 were found in the serum of all four children and in one of them such a level was dramatically decreased after successful bone marrow transplantation.[55] As is known, OS is a rare congenital form of severe combined immunodeficiency syndrome (SCID), in which a polyclonal activation of Th2 cells has been suggested to play a pathogenic role.[56] More recently, high proportions of CD30⁺ (CD4⁺) T cells were found in the skin biopsy specimens of patients with systemic sclerosis (SSc), another Th2-dominated disorder (see below). On the other hand, no accumulation of CD30⁺ cells was found by performing immunohistochemical staining in bronchial biopsy specimens from patients with allergic asthma or in conjunctival biopsies from patients with vernal conjunctivitis, which are also considered disorders associated with a Th2-type immune response. Likewise, very few CD30⁺ T cells were detected in the skin lesions of patients with the lepromatous form of leprosy (LL),[51] a Th2-like reaction,[22] and there was no difference in the accumulation of CD30⁺ cells between tuberculoid leprosy (TL), a Th1 reaction,[22] and LL.[51] From these results we conclude that high numbers of CD30⁺ T cells can be detected only under conditions of polyclonal and persistent Th2 activation such as in the OS and SSc; in diseases sustained by antigen-specific oligoclonal activation of Th2 cells, CD30⁺ cells can probably be detected in discrete numbers at lymph node level during clonal expansion, but they cannot be expected to accumulate in target organs where they usually act as effector cells without remarkable proliferation. It is noteworthy however, that neither CD30 mRNA expression nor accumulation of CD30⁺ T cells was found in biopsy specimens of gastric antrum mucosa from *Helicobacter pilori*-infected patients, as well as of gut from patients with Crohn's disease, that are both characterized by the presence of activated T cells showing high expression of IFN-γ, but not IL-4 (see below). Recently, the association of CD30 expression with production of Th2 cytokines has also been observed in a model of TCR-transgenic mice (R. Flavell, personal communication).

LAG-3, a member of the immunoglobulin superfamily,[57] showed a different behavior in comparison with CD30. First, surface LAG-3 expression correlated with IFN-γ, but not IL-4, production in antigen-stimulated T cells. For example, T cells from atopic donors that produced high IL-4 and low IFN-γ in response to *Dermatophagoides pteronyssinus* group 1 (Der p 1) showed poor expression of LAG-3. T cells from nonatopic donors exhibited high IFN-γ production and LAG-3 expression in response to Der p 1, as well as high IFN-γ production and LAG-3 expression, but neither IL-4 production nor CD30 expression in response to streptokinase.[58] Secondly, LAG-3 expression was strongly upregulated by IL-12,[58] a powerful Th1-inducing agent (see below). Finally, following activation with PHA and IL-2, most CD4+ T cell clones with established Th1 profile of cytokine secretion expressed LAG-3 (but not CD30) on their surface, whereas the great majority of Th2 clones showed CD30 expression, but neither surface LAG-3 nor LAG-3 mRNA.[58] In contrast, under the same activation conditions, many Th0 clones expressed both CD30 and LAG-3 on their surface membrane.[58] The majority of CD4+ T cell clones also released soluble LAG-3-related peptide(s) (sLAG-3) and sLAG-3 concentrations in T cell clone supernatants correlated positively with the concentrations of IFN-γ, but inversely with those of IL-4.[58] Thus, CD30 and LAG-3 expression by activated CD4+ human T cells appear to be preferentially, even if not exclusively, associated with the differentiation/activation pathway leading to the prevalent production of Th2-type or Th1-type cytokines, respectively.

CD8+ AND γδ+ TYPE 1 AND TYPE 2 CELLS AND THEIR FUNCTIONS

The demonstration that long-term CD4+ T cell clones could be segregated into subsets producing distinct types of cytokines formed the basis of similar studies with CD8+ T cells. Although the great majority of CD8+ T cells produce IFN-γ, but no IL-4,[59] CD8+ T cell clones producing IL-4 can be obtained by stimulation of murine CD8+ T cells with anti-CD3 antibody,[60] mitogen or allostimulation[61,62] and antigen[63,64] in the presence of IL-4. Based on these findings the names Tc1 and Tc2 for cytotoxic CD8+ T cells secreting Th1-like and Th2-like cytokines were proposed.[62] CD8+ T cell clones that produce IL-4 have also been generated from the skin of immunologically unresponsive individuals with leprosy,[22] the Kaposi's sarcoma skin lesions of HIV-infected patients,[65] the peripheral blood of HIV-infected patients,[66,67] and more recently, from the gengiva of subjects with chronic adult periodontitis[68] and from normal human peritoneum.[69] The generation of Tc2 clones from HIV-infected patients did not require T cell conditioning with exogenous IL-4, suggesting that in these specific patients there is an in vivo operating condition which favors the conversion of CD8⁺ T cells from the Tc1 to the Tc2 functional phenotype. More recently, we have found that when CD8⁺ T cells from HIV-infected individuals are cloned in the presence of autologous feeder cells, most of them develop into clear-cut Tc2 clones and such a tendency can be corrected by addition in bulk culture of IL-12 and/or anti-IL-4 antibody (Maggi et al, submitted).

While the functional role of CD8⁺ Tc1 cells is well established, the in vivo functional meaning of CD8⁺ TC2 cells is still unclear. A possible IL-4-mediated suppressive effect has been suggested;[22] however, IL-4 alone is not able to induce the suppression.[68] Murine CD8⁺ Tc2 clones generated in the presence of IL-4 exhibited normal cytolytic potential and failed to provide cognate help for B cell antibody production.[62] However, at least some of them can express the CD40 ligand (CD40L),[67] may have reduced cytolytic activity[66] and favor eosinophil activation and accumulation via the production of IL-5.[62] Likewise, CD8⁺ Tc2 clones generated from HIV-infected individuals showed reduced cytolytic activity, expressed the CD40L and provided optimal polyclonal B cell helper activity for production of immunoglobulin,

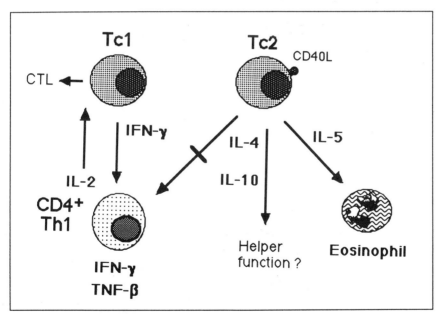

Fig. 2.7. Possible functional activities of Tc1- and Tc2-type CD8⁺ T cells. Tc1 cells act as CTL (cytotoxic T lymphocytes) and also contribute to the preferential development of Th cells into the Th1 profile (via the production of IFN-γ). Tc2 cells, which may have or may not have reduced CTL activity, promote the differentiation and activation of eosinophils (via the production of IL-5), help B cells to produce antibodies, including IgE (via the expression of CD40L and the production of IL-4), and inhibit the development of Th1 cells (via the production of IL-4 and IL-10).

including IgE.[66,67,70] It is also of interest that IL-4 in the absence of antigenic stimulation induces an anergy-like state in differentiated CD8[+] Tc1 cells (loss of IL-2 synthesis and autonomous proliferation).[71] Thus, one possible explanation is that CD8[+] Tc2 cells act as suppressor or anti-inflammatory cells through the production of "helper" cytokines[72] (Fig. 2.7). It is of note that, as for CD4[+] T cell clones, CD30 and sCD30 are usually not detectable in CD8[+] Tc1 clones, but are consistently found in CD8[+] Tc2 clones generated from HIV-infected individuals.[73] In contrast, LAG-3 was apparently expressed by both Tc1 and Tc2 clones (unpublished results).

T cells bearing γδ receptors (Tγδ[+] cells) can also show opposite patterns of cytokine production (Th1-like and Th2-like) in response to pathogens, such as *Listeria monocytogenes* (*L. Monocytogenes*) and *Nippostrongylus brasiliensis* (*N. brasiliensis*), that promote prevalent Th1 or Th2 responses, respectively.[74] Since several data suggest a 'first line of defense' for γδ T cells in protection, it is possible that these cells may not only aid in the direct elimination of certain pathogens, but also contribute to the cytokine milieu that influences the differentiation of antigen-specific CD4[+] T cells into either Th1 or Th2 cells (see below). Of interest is that activation of Th2-type cells in BALB/c mice infected by *Leishmania major* (*L. major*), as well as in mice treated with anti-immunoglobulin D antibodies or infected with *N. brasiliensis*, results in expansion of γδ[+] T cells.[75]

═══ CHAPTER 3 ═══

NATURE OF T1/T2-
POLARIZING SIGNALS

Although, theoretically, Th1 and Th2 cells might arise from distinct precursors, experiments using limiting dilution analysis,[76] immunization with oligopeptides,[77] and bulk culture experiments with homogenous population of cells from T cell receptor (TCR) transgenic mice[78,79] have confirmed the ability of a single precursor to differentiate to either a Th1 or Th2 phenotype.[80] Using transgenic mice in which IL-4-producing cells expressed herpes simplex virus (HSV) type 1 thymidine kinase and could therefore be eliminated by ganciclovir, it was shown that activation of transgenic T cells in the presence of ganciclovir eliminates IL-4 and IFN-γ production.[81] This very elegant experiment demonstrated that effector cells producing either IL-4 or IFN-γ have a common precursor, which expresses the IL-4 gene. The realization that Th1 and Th2 cells differentiate from a common pool of precursors allows questions to be asked about the factors that affect these differentiation pathways (Table 3.1).

SITE OF ANTIGEN PENETRATION

The site of antigen presentation may play some role in determining the type of effector response. Inhaled ovalbumin (OVA) has a greater propensity than parenterally injected OVA to stimulate a Th2 response.[82] Likewise, oral immunization with OVA or tetanus toxoid also selectively induces Th2 cells in mucosa associated tissues.[83,84] When enterocoated OVA is administered with anti-IL-4 antibody a shift to the Th1 phenotype occurs, suggesting that the dominance of the Th2 cell phenotype in oral immunity is strongly influenced by the production and presence of IL-4.[85] Moreover, when administered orally, antigens that stimulate a strong systemic antibody response can induce tolerance that is associated with T cell production of TGF-β.[86] In particular, low-dose feeding induced prominent secretion of IL-4, IL-10 and TGF, whereas minimal secretion of these cytokines was observed with high dose feeding.[87] Finally, epicutaneous exposure of protein antigen

Table 3.1. *Factors involved in the differentiation of CD4$^+$ T cells into Th1 or Th2 cells*

Factors	Th1	Th2
Cytokines		
IL-12 + IFN-γ (or IFN-α)	+++	
TGF-β	+	
IL-4		+++
IL-1, IL-10		+
Hormones		
glucocorticoids		+
androgen steroids	+	
25(OH) D3		+
progesteron		+
relaxin	+	
APCs		
professional APC (macrophages, dendritic cells, B cells)	+	+
keratinocytes		+
Adjuvants		
CFA	+	
oxidized mannan	+	
alum		+
pertussis toxin		+
colera toxin		+
Costimulatory interactions		
B7.1-CD28	+	+
B7.2-CD28		+(?)
CD40-CD40L	+(?)	
CD30L-CD30		+
ICAM-1-LFA-1		+
MHC class II-CD4	+	
Physical form of the immunogen		
corpuscolate	+	
soluble	+	+
Dose of antigen		
high		+
medium-low	+	
very low		+
Peptide density		
high	+	
low		+
Peptide affinity to MHC		
high	+	
low		+

CFA = complete Freund's adjuvant; (?) = conflicting results. Reprinted with permission from Romagnani S, Clin Immunol Immunopathol 1996; 80:225-235.[54]

also induces a predominant Th2-like response with high IgE production.[88] These results my reflect unique populations of T cells or APCs in the skin, lung or gut, the influence of cytokines that are expressed at these sites, or other uncharacterized factors.

TYPE OF ANTIGEN-PRESENTING CELL

Attention has also been focused on the possibility that the type of response is dependent upon the nature of antigen-presenting cell (APC). Some differences in the response of Th1 and Th2 cells to different APC have been reported.[89] Murine hepatic accessory cells were found to support the proliferation of Th1 but not Th2 clones.[90] Moreover, adherent cells stimulated optimal proliferation of Th1 clones, whereas purified B cells stimulated optimal proliferation of Th2 clones.[91,92] Accordingly, when antigen was presented by macrophages normal resting Th cells differentiated into Th1 cells, whereas presentation by B cells generated Th cells producing IL-2, which could differentiate into Th2 cells upon re-stimulation.[93] B cells seem to play an essential role in the induction of IL-4 gene expression by the T cells that provided helper activity for antibody synthesis.[94] Finally, murin brain microvessel endothelial cells preferentially activated Th2 clones, whereas smooth muscle/pericytes selectively activated Th1 clones.[95] However, no independent relationship between the type of APC and cytokine response has been definitely established. Mice immunized with antibodies that are focused onto B cells (anti-IgD), macrophages (anti-CD11b) or dendritic cells (aggregated 33D1 antibody) all generate predominantly IgG1 responses, and macrophages, dendritic cells and B cells can all induce either a Th1 or a Th2 response, given the proper cytokine environment.[96]

COSTIMULATORY MOLECULES

Several costimulatory molecules present on the surface of APCs are involved in the T cell activation and function (Table 3.2). Costimulatory molecules that have received considerable attention as possible regulatory signals for Th1/Th2 development are B7/CD28/CTLA-4, CD4/MHC, CD40L/CD40, CD30L/CD30, LFA-1/ICAM-1.

Interactions Between B7 and CD28/CTLA-4

It was initially suggested that at least in vitro CD28 signaling may be required for Th1 but not for Th2 cells. Indeed, Th1 clones and fresh T cells needed CD28 signaling in addition to TCR signaling for activation and IL-2 production, whereas in the absence of such costimulation, Th1 cells were anergized.[97] Moreover, soluble recombinant CTLA-4 inhibited alloantigen-specific responses and IL-2 and IFN-γ gene expression in mixed leukocyte cultures (MLCs), but increased IL-4 gene expression and some proliferation persisted.[98] However, the injection in vivo of soluble CTLA-4 in mice infected with *Heligmosomoides*

Table 3.2. Receptor-ligand pairs involved in delivering costimulatory signals

Ligand	Receptor
B7-1 (CD80)	CD28/CTLA-4
B7-2 (CD86)	CD28/CTLA-4
ICAM-1 (CD54)/	
ICAM-2/ICAM-3	LFA-1 (CD11a/CD18)
LFA-3 (CD58)	CD2
VCAM-1	VLA-4 (α4b1)
CD40L	CD40
OX40L	OX40
CD30L	CD30
HSA (CD24)	HSA (CD24)

polygyrus (*H. polygyrus*) completely inhibited the Th2 response against this nematode parasite.[99] Likewise, both soluble CD28 and CTLA-4 inhibited the IL-4 dominant in vivo immune response induced by goat anti-mouse IgD antibody, whereas IL-10 expression was unaffected.[100] Finally, injection of soluble CTLA-4 also abrogated progressive disease in *L. major*-infected susceptible BALB/c mice, without having any effect on the protective immune response developed by resistant C57BL/6 mice (see below).[101] Taken together, these data suggest that, with the notable exception of IL-10, interaction of B7 with its ligands is required for elevated Th2 cytokine gene expression and secretion during primary Th2 responses. Similar conclusions were drawn in humans by using an in vitro system in which adult and neonatal CD4+ T cells were stimulated in the absence or presence of anti-CD28 antibody.[102,103] Stimulation with anti-CD28 antibody in the absence of TCR-CD3 stimulation primed human naive T cells to develop into Th2 cells.[95] Other findings, however, indicate that the regulation of costimulation mediated by the B7-CD28/CTLA-4 system is far more complex than previously appreciated. First, under certain circumstances, T cell activation can be CD28-independent as a result of engagement of alternative costimulatory pathways or high potency TCR ligation. Second, the CD28 homologue, CTLA-4, functions to downregulate immunity by binding with high affinity to B7. Finally, B7 consists of three different molecules (B7-1; B7-2; B7-3), at least two of which can act as costimulatory molecules for CD28. Interestingly, B7-1 (CD80) and B7-2 (CD86) ligands are differently expressed and regulated on

APCs.[105,106] For example, both IFN-γ and IL-10 are able to selectively suppress B7.1 expression in Langerhans cells (LC), thus inhibiting their APC ability.[107] More importantly, B7.1 and B7.2 were found to deliver different costimulatory signals. B7-1 appeared to be a neutral differentiative signal, whereas B7-2 provided an initial signal to induce naive T cells to become IL-4 producers.[108] In the experimental allergic enecephalomyelitis (EAE) model, a classic Th1-mediated disorder (see below), neutralization of B7-1 reduced disease severity and increased the production of IL-4, whereas neutralization of B7-2 increased both disease severity and IFN-γ production,[109] suggesting that interaction of B7-1 and B7-2 with their counterreceptors can influence the commitment of precursors to the Th1 or the Th2 pathway. This may be possible because B7-1 and B7-2 molecules bind distinct regions of, and have distinct kinetics of binding to, CTLA-4 molecule.[110] Thus, such differential binding may have unique signaling properties that affect T cell activation and subsequent Th1/Th2 development. Other findings do not agree, however, with this possibility. First, B7-2 neutralization very efficiently blocks both DTH and humoral immunity, as well as the development of insulin-dependent diabetes mellitus (IDDM) in nonobese diabetic (NOD) mice (another Th1-dependent autoimmune disorder).[111] More importantly, stimulation of murine and human T cells with B7-1 or B7-2 transfectants can induce similar levels of Th1-type and Th2-type cytokines.[112,113] Thus, factors other than involvement of B7-1 or B7-2 costimulatory molecules may also be involved.

CD4 MOLECULE

Evidence that negative, as well as positive, signals can be delivered to the CD4+ T cell through the CD4 molecule itself has come from studies on the binding of the CD4 ligand, HIV-gp120.[114] In vitro experiments using rat CD4+ T cells showed that a mouse anti-rat CD4 antibody, which completely prevents the development of paralysis associated with EAE,[115] completely inhibited the synthesis of IFN-γ in a primary MLC, whereas after secondary stimulation the synthesis of both IL-4 and IL-13 was greatly enhanced.[116] Accordingly, it was found that in human T cells IFN-γ production is more susceptible than production of IL-4 to the inhibitory effects of anti-CD4 antibody. Interestingly, anti-CD4-mediated downregulation of IFN-γ production may occur without inhibition of antigen-dependent proliferation.[117]

INTERACTION BETWEEN CD40L AND CD40

In an experimental model for a Th1-mediated disease, the hapten reagent (2,4,6-trinitrobenzene sulfonic acid)-induced colitis, the administration of anti-CD40L antibodies during the induction phase of the Th1 response prevented IFN-γ production by *lamina propria* CD4+

T cells and also clinical and histological evidence of disease, whereas the secretion of IL-4 was increased after anti-CD40L treatment. As demonstrated by immunohistochemistry, the prevention of disease activity was caused by an inhibition of IL-12 secretion.[118] IL-12 production by murine macrophages is indeed critically dependent on CD40L expression by activated T cells.[119] Thus, a CD40L-CD40 interaction seems to be crucial for the in vivo priming of Th1 cells via the stimulation of IL-12 secretion by APC (see also below). However, crosslinking of the CD40 ligand on human CD4+ T cells generates a costimulatory signal that upregulates IL-4 synthesis.[120]

INTERACTION BETWEEN CD30L AND CD30

CD30 is a member of the TNF receptor family which is expressed by a subset of activated CD4+ and CD8+ T cells and by established T cell clones showing a Th0/Th2 profile (see above). The ligand for CD30 (CD30L) is a member of TNF family which is expressed by activated macrophages, activated T cells and B cells.[47] Recently, we have shown that costimulation of human peripheral blood mononuclear cells (PBMC) with an agonistic anti-CD30 antibody resulted in the preferential development of antigen-specific T cell lines and clones showing a Th2-like profile of cytokine secretion. In contrast, early blockade in bulk culture of CD30L/CD30 interaction by a CD30-binding but nonagonistic antibody, an anti-CD30L antibody or a CD30-Ig fusion protein shifted the development of antigen-specific T cells towards the opposite (Th1-like) phenotype.[52] The shifting effect was comparable to that obtained by the addition in bulk culture of an anti-IL-4 antibody.[121] Taken together, these data suggest that, at least in humans, CD30 triggering of activated Th cells by CD30L-expressing APCs may represent an important costimulatory signaling for the development of Th2-type responses.

INTERACTIONS BETWEEN LFA-1 AND ICAM-1/ICAM-2

The β2-integrin LFA-1 (CD11a/CD18) is present on T cells and contributes to their activation and proliferation. The counter receptors for LFA-1 are members of the immunoglobulin superfamily: ICAM-1 (CD54) is expressed on a variety of tissues including PBMC, vascular endothelium and epithelial cells; ICAM-2 is the predominant binding ligand on resting endothelium; ICAM-3 is strongly expressed on all leukocytes but absent from endothelial cells.[122,123] Human Th2 cells seem to be more susceptible to the abrogation of interactions between LFA-1 and ICAM-1 than Th1 clones. Moreover, costimulatory activity through LFA-1 could be provided to a Th2, but not to a Th1, clone.[124] These data suggest that human Th2 cells may have a greater requirement for the costimulatory activity of LFA-1 than cells of the Th1 phenotype.

PROPERTIES OF THE IMMUNOGEN

PHYSICAL FORM OF IMMUNOGEN AND TYPE OF ADJUVANT

In general, it appears that corpuscolate immunogens more easily promote Th1 responses than soluble antigens. The Th1-inducing activity of corpuscolate immunogens is probably related to their greater ability to induce IL-12 production by macrophages that are responsible for phagocytosis (see below). However, IL-12 is also produced by dendritic cells and Langerhans cells;[125,126] moreover, some animal strains, due to a particular genetic background, as well as some human strains, mount prevalent Th2 responses even in response to intracellular parasites that usually evoke Th1 responses. Antigen polymerization also preferentially evokes Th1-type responses in comparison to the unmodified antigen. Following administration of high molecular weight OVA polymers, there was a marked inhibition of OVA-specific IgE and strong increase of IgG2a production.[127,128] This was due to marked upregulation of IFN-γ and downregulation of IL-10 production, whereas the frequency of IL-4-producing cells was unchanged in response to the polymerized form of antigen.[129] The type of adjuvant is also important in determining the profile of cytokine secretion. Complete Freund's adjuvant (CFA) evokes Th1 responses,[130] probably because the components of the mycobacterial cell wall induce high IL-12 production by macrophages, with subsequent upregulation of IFN-γ production (see below), whereas incomplete Freund's adjuvant (IFA), alum, acellular *Bordetella pertussis* (*B. pertussis*) toxin and cholera toxin expand prevalent Th2 responses.[4,83,84,131] Moreover, influenza virus envelope proteins incorporated in immunostimulating complexes stimulate a prevalent Th1 response, whereas the same antigens in a micelle induce a more prominent Th2 response.[132] Of interest is the recent finding indicating that conjugation of recombinant antigens to the polysaccharide mannan (polymannose) under reducing conditions favors predominant type 2 responses. By contrast, the same antigen coupled to oxidized mannan selectively promotes type 1 responses.[133]

DOSE OF ANTIGEN

It is now over 20 years that it was shown that the dose of antigen administered to an animal could determine the class of immune response towards either cell-mediated or humoral immunity.[2] More recent studies suggest that differentiated effector CD4$^+$ T cells may produce different cytokines depending on the dose of antigen used. Low doses promoted DTH by stimulating the development of Th1 cells, whereas higher doses induced antibody production because of the predominant production of Th2-type cytokines. The normal susceptibility of BALB/c mice to infection with *L. major* could be reversed by initially injecting the mice with small numbers of parasites. Not only were the mice resistant to the small inoculum of *L. major*, but they were resistant when challenged 4 months later with a dose of parasites that would normally have been lethal. These mice developed a protective CMI characterized by predominant IFN-γ rather than the IL-4-dominated response that normally mounts.[134] However, these studies involved priming with complex antigens, so that different peptides might be presented at varying densities depending on the antigen dose. Exposure of CD4+ T cells from naive mice transgenic for a TCR recognizing moth cytochrome c bound to Eβ^b:Eα^k to high antigen doses led to differentiation into Th1-like cells producing abundant IFN-γ, while low doses of the same peptide induced cells with the same TCR to differentiate into Th2-like cells producing abundant IL-4.[135] On the other hand, by using naive CD4+ T cells from the TCR-transgenic D011.10 mice, at doses of antigen that induced seemingly similar levels of T cell proliferation, low to medium doses of antigen promoted the development of Th1 cells producing IFN-γ and undetectable levels of IL-4, whereas increasing the dose of antigen resulted in the disappearance of IFN-γ cells and the development of IL-4 producing cells.[136] Coincidental with this disappearance of IFN-γ producing cells was the observation of massive cell death in the cultures. The differential trend of IFN-γ versus IL-4-producing Th cell development was still observed even when antigen dose was varied in primary cultures of high density CD4+LECAM-1+ T cells. This suggests that it is not due to a small contaminating population of IL-4 producing cells which will be evident at higher doses of antigen, although this cannot be completely ruled out.[13] The development of Th2 cells resulting from high antigen doses was completely abrogated by the addition of neutralizing anti-IL-4 antibodies. At extremely low doses of antigen, when there was a poor recovery of T cells after culture of high density CD4+, LECAM-1+ T cells, IL-4 production was dominant over IFN-γ, again suggesting possible contamination with a subset of CD4+ T cells with enhanced viability. This effect of antigen dose in directly inducing the development of Th1 or Th2-type T cells could be observed regardless of the APCs used.[13] However, it is likely that in normal antigen-specific T cells, where a much lower frequency of cells recognizes the same antigen, there will be a fine balance between APCs producing cytokines such as IL-12 and CD4+ T cells producing IL-4, and that the dose of antigen will be critical in determining the development of IFN-γ versus IL-4-producing cells.

PEPTIDE DENSITY AND BINDING AFFINITY

Although it is clearly proved that different antigens can preferentially expand the two extreme patterns of lymphokine secretion in both mice and humans, characterization of the TCR expressed by Th1 and Th2 cells, direct sequencing of antigen-specific Th1 and Th2 clones, and analysis of mRNA and genomic TCR expression demonstrated usage of the same receptors by both subsets of CD4$^+$ cells, suggesting that the same peptide can underlie both responses.[77,137] Nevertheless, it also appears that certain epitopes can preferentially induce one of the two subsets of Th cells. A repetitive peptide of *L. major* selectively activated Th2 cells and enhanced disease progression.[138] In contrast, a recombinant 403 AA protein from *L. braziliensis*, homologous to ribosomal protein eIF-4A (LeIF) preferentially stimulated human PBMC to express a Th1-type cytokine profile and to produce IL-12.[139] Changes as little as those concerning single aminoacid residues greatly deviated the ability of the immunodominant CD4 T cell epitope of the bacteriophage λ cI repressor protein to induce IL-4 production and immediate-type hypersensitivity.[140] Likewise, a peptide differing from its wildtype in a single residue failed to evoke a proliferative response by a Th2 clone, but retained the ability to induce IL-4 production.[77] A similar observation was made by Racioppi et al.[141] On the other hand, it has also been shown that mice primed with human collagen IV developed either IL-4-secreting Th2 cells or IFN-γ-secreting Th1 cells, depending on their genotype at MHC class II.[142] More recently, it was reported that varying either the antigenic peptide or the MHC class II molecules could determine whether Th1-like or Th2-like responses are obtained. High MHC class II-peptide density on the APC surface favored Th1-like responses, while low ligand densities favored Th2-like responses.[143] Likewise, by using a set of ligands with various class binding affinities, but unchanged T cell specificity, it was shown that stimulation with the highest affinity ligand resulted in IFN-γ production. In contrast, ligands that demonstrated relatively lower MHC class II binding induced only IL-4 secretion.[144] A single MHC polymorphism may dictate Th1/Th2 selection by determining the level of peptide presented to a given TCR on APC.[145] Taken all together, these findings suggest that the MHC binding affinity of antigenic determinants, leading to differential interactions at the T cell-APC interface, can be crucial for the differential development of cytokine patterns in T cells.

CYTOKINES

There is general consensus that cytokines themselves are the major factors determining the differentiation of naive, and probably even memory, Th cells into the polarized Th1 or Th2 phenotype. There is also complete agreement that in both mice and humans IL-12 and IL-4 are the most important cytokines in directing the development of Th1 and Th2 cells, respectively (Fig. 3.1).

IL-12 DIRECTS TH1 DEVELOPMENT

IL-12, a heterodimeric cytokine produced primarily by phagocytic cells, with multiple activities on NK cells and T cells, including augmentation of IFN-γ production,[146] is the dominant factor in directing the development of Th1 cells. The Th1-inducing effect of IL-12 was

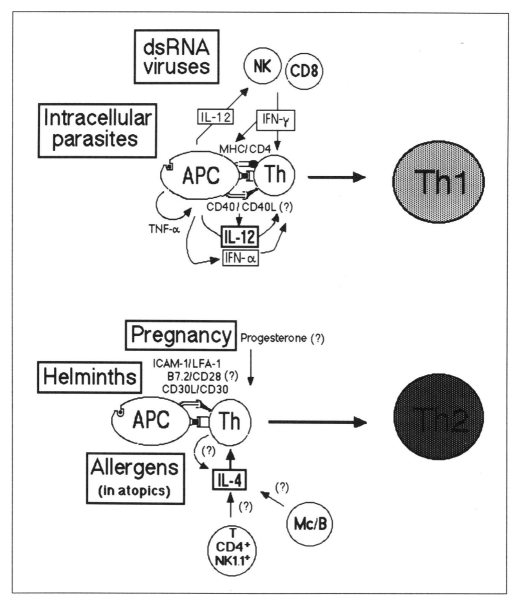

Fig. 3.1. Schematic representation of some mechanisms responsible for Th1 or Th2 polarization. Intracellular parasites and dsRNA viruses induce the production of IL-12 and IFN-α by APC and of IFN-γ by NK cells and CD8⁺ T cells. The presence of these cytokines favors the development of Th1 cells.

Helminths and allergens (the latter only in atopic individuals) induce early IL-4 production, which favors the Th2-cell development. IL-4 may be produced by cells of the mast cell/basophil lineage, by the CD4⁺NK1.1⁺ T cell subset, or by the naive Th cell itself. The Th2 predominance at the fetus-placenta interface during pregnancy may be favored by high local progesterone levels.

Costimulatory molecules seem also to be involved in the process of Th1/Th2 polarization. CD30L/CD30 and LFA-1/ICAM-1 interactions favor Th2 responses (humans), whereas MHC/CD4 interaction favors Th1 responses (rats). The role of B7.1 or B7.2/CD28 and CD40L/CD40 interactions in favoring Th1 or Th2 responses is controversial (mice).

contemporarily and independently demonstrated in both mice and humans. In mice expressing an OVA-specific transgenic TCR, dendritic cells induced strong antigen-specific proliferation of CD4⁺ T cells, but addition of *L. monocytogenes*-activated macrophages, producing high levels of IL-12, were essential for the development of Th1 cells producing high levels of IFN-γ.[147] In subsequent studies, it was found that dendritic cells themselves drive Th1 development by their production of IL-12 provided that IL-4 was removed with the use of neutralizing antibodies, or depletion of IL-4-producing CD4⁺, LECAM-1⁻ T cells from primary cultures.[125,148] Thus, it was concluded that the relative levels of T cell derived IL-4 versus APC (macrophage or dendritic cell)-derived IL-12 strictly control whether Th1 cells responsible for CMI develop in response to antigen. In contrast to dendritic cells, B cells, even when highly activated so that they can induce similar levels of proliferation as dendritic cells, still drive a Th0-type response with low levels of IFN-γ, and IL-4 produced, even upon neutralization of IL-4 or removal of CD4⁺, LECAM-1⁻ cells. The low levels of IFN-γ produced by the Th0 cells developing from CD4⁺ T cells stimulated with antigen and B cell as APC in primary cultures was not IL-12-dependent,[136] suggesting that B cells do not produce this cytokine. Likewise, keratinocytes, which show a specific ability to induce Th2 responses, were found to produce little if any mRNA and no protein for IL-12 compared with professional APCs.[149] The ability of IL-12 to promote the development of murine Th1 cells was then confirmed by other studies utilizing different models.[150,151] More recently, by using immunofluorescent detection of intracellular IFN-γ and IL-4, it was found that in TCR transgenic DO11.10 mice (which have a genetic facility to develop Th2 cells) many T cells in the absence of exogenous stimuli developed into IL-4-producing cells. The presence of exogenous IL-4 together with IL-12 during repeated stimulation gave rise to cells synthesizing both IFN-γ and IL-4, whereas in the presence of IL-12 alone the frequency of both cells producing only IFN-γ and cells producing both cytokines was increased.[12] Although required, IL-12 is not essential for a Th1 response. Recent in vivo data from IL-12-deficient mice show that Th1 responses can be generated, although the magnitude of DTH is substantially decreased and secretion of IL-4 is enhanced.[152]

In humans, the addition in PBMC bulk culture of IL-12 shifted the development of Der p I-specific T cells from the Th0/Th2 to the Th1 profile. Conversely, the addition in PBMC bulk culture of anti-IL-12 antibody shifted the development of PPD-specific T cells from the Th1 to the Th0 profile. Therefore, not only did IL-12 appear to be a factor able to favor Th1 differentiation, but the development of Th1 cells in the PBMC cultures stimulated with PPD was shown to depend at least in part on the production of endogenous IL-12 in cultures. In this in vitro system, IL-12 not only induced strong augmentation in IFN-γ production, but also inhibited the development of

IL-4-producing T cells.[153] Subsequently, using culture conditions with high T cell clonal efficiency, it was demonstrated that IL-12 directly affects at the single cell level the differentiation of both CD4+ and CD8+ human T cells, by inducing a stable priming effect for high IFN-γ production, if present during the first few days of culture of the T cell clones. The net production of IFN-γ by CD4+ and CD8+ T cells seems to be dependent on the relative contribution of IL-12 (upregulatory) and prostaglandin E_2 (PGE$_2$) (downregulatory).[154] When added to established T cell clones, IL-12 did not have a stable priming effect, but only induced, in the presence of other costimuli, a transient increase in IFN-γ production in Th2 clones.[155] Because the priming was observed on all T cells present in PBMC preparations, it is likely that this differentiation effect of IL-12 is effective on both naive and memory T cells. This raises the possibility that, regardless of prior commitment, memory CD4+ cells may retain the capacity to be further influenced by IL-4, IFN-γ or IL-12 during effector cell development in order to become subsets that are at least temporarily polarized to have a particular pattern of cytokine secretion. This possibility has recently been substantiated even by studies performed in the murine system.[156,157] Whereas the priming effect of IL-12 on IFN-γ production reflects a direct action on the Th cell, its inhibitory activity on the development of IL-4-producing cells is due to a mechanism that involves APCs, since it occurs even when APCs are preincubated with IL-12.[158] More recently, it was found that IL-12 primes T cells not only to IFN-γ production, but also to the production of IL-10.[159–161]

ROLE OF OTHER CYTOKINES IN DIRECTING TH1 DEVELOPMENT

IL-12-driven development of murine Th1 cells is dependent on another cytokine, IFN-γ.[162] The requirement for this factor in the Th1 development has been controversial. Using a priming model, in which T cells were derived from a BALB/c background, an addition of anti-IFN-γ antibody to priming cultures resulted in diminished priming for IFN-γ, suggesting a role for endogenous IFN-γ.[147] Moreover, an addition of anti-IFN-γ antibody to cultures containing IL-12 also diminished the ability of IL-12 to enhance the response demonstrating that the effects of IL-12 on augmenting IFN-γ production are not direct.[163] In the murine *Mycobacterium bovis* (*M. bovis*) model, it was demonstrated that IL-12 production was not initially induced in macrophages, but was dependent on IFN-γ and TNF-α.[164] Finally, IFN-γ deficient animals display a default to the Th2 phenotype when challenged with *L. major*, suggesting that IFN-γ is required for Th1 induction.[165] Likewise, T cells activated in the presence of IFN-γ unresponsive APCs failed to develop towards the Th1 phenotype.[166] By contrast, in the system of transgenic T cells from mice on a B10.A background, neutralization of endogenous IFN-γ had little effect on the IL-12-induced increase in IFN-γ priming.[150] Accordingly, in three separate in vivo models, the ability of IL-12 to augment IFN-γ production was not affected by coadministration of anti-IFN-γ antibody.[159,167,168] Moreover, IFN-γ receptor deficient mice, infected with either *Pseudorabies virus*[169] or *L. major*,[170] were able to mount vigorous Th1 responses. These contrasting results may now in part be explained by the observation that IFN-α can replace the requirement for IFN-γ. Interestingly, in this study, naive T cells were found to require IFN-γ during primary activation for maximal IL-12-induced Th1 development, whereas memory T cells were not. When the endogenous IFN-γ present in primary T cell cultures was neutralized, IFN-α treatment augmented IL-12-induced effects on inhibition of subsequent IL-4 production, even if it failed to significantly enhance IL-12 priming for subsequent IFN-γ production.[171] In addition to the dominant effect of IL-12 and IFN-γ/IFN-α in driving Th1 development, the role of other cofactors, including IL-1 and TNF-α, for development of Th1 cells producing maximal levels of IFN-γ was suggested.[13] It has also been demonstrated that TGF-β may play a role in the development of Th1 cells,[172-174] but thus far its mechanism of action remains unclear, particularly since this factor may also inhibit an ongoing effector Th1-type cell-mediated immune response.[175] Moreover, it has been shown that TGF-β may have opposing effects on the Th1 cell development of naive CD4+ T cells isolated from different mouse strains.[176]

The role of IFN-γ, IFN-α and TGF-β in favoring the in vitro development of Th1 cells has been demonstrated in humans, as well.[121,177-179] The addition in PBMC bulk cultures of either IFN-γ or anti-IL-4 antibody markedly inhibited the development of Der p 1-specific T cells into IL-4- and IL-5-producing T cell lines. Accordingly, the development into Der p 1-specific Th2-like T cell clones was significantly reduced by the addition of IFN-γ in bulk culture and was virtually suppressed by the presence of both IFN-γ and anti-IL-4 antibody.[121] The addition in bulk culture before cloning of either IFN-γ or IFN-α favored the development of TES- or Poa pratensis group 9 (Poa p 9)-specific T cell clones showing a Th1-like profile and displaying strong cytolytic activity, whereas both TES- and Poa p 9-specific T cell clones generated from the same donors under the same experimental conditions except the presence of IFN-γ or IFN-α in bulk culture showed a Th0/Th2 profile and were devoid of cytolytic potential.[177] Additional evidence on the role of IFN-α in promoting the development of human Th1 cells was provided by testing the activity of polyinosinic-polycytidilic acid (poly I-poly C). Poly I-poly C was able to shift the differentiation of Der p 1-specific T cells into the Th1 profile and such an effect was prevented only by the simultaneous addition in bulk culture of both anti-IL-12 and anti-IFN-α antibody, but not by anti-IL-12 or anti-IFN-α antibody alone.[180]

Recently, a new cytokine named IFN-γ-inducing factor (IGIF), that induces IFN-γ production by both NK cells and T cells more potently than does IL-12 has been cloned.[181] IGIF may be involved in the development of Th1 cells, as well as in mechanisms of tissue injury in inflammatory reaction.

IL-4 DIRECTS TH2 DEVELOPMENT

The addition of exogenous IL-4 to in vitro culture of naive, CD4+ murine T cells in the presence of mitogens or antigen directs the naive CD4+ T cells to develop into a population of effectors, which on restimulation produce high levels of IL-4, IL-5, IL-10, as well as IL-3 and GM-CSF (Th2 pattern). The effects of IL-4 include suppression of the development of IL-2 and IFN-γ secreting effectors, as well as the promotion of those with Th2 pattern.[182-184] Studies in TCR transgenic mice have then confirmed that the presence of IL-4 during primary stimulation of naive CD4+ T cells with mitogen or specific antigen plus APC results in the development of T cell populations that can secrete high levels of IL-4 upon restimulation.[79,185] Another important model suggestive for the IL-4-directed Th2 development is represented by the *L. major* infection. When BALB/c mice, which normally develop a T cell response to infection with *L. major* in which IL-4-producing T cells dominate, were treated with anti-IL-4 antibodies at the time of priming, they developed an immune response in which IFN-γ was the dominant product of CD4+ T cells and they cleared the parasites rather than developing a progressive infection and dying.[186,187] These experiments were extended by studies demonstrating that injection of anti-IL-4 antibody at the time of immunization strikingly diminished the magnitude of IL-4 production even in response to a conventional nonliving antigen.[188] Finally, nematode infection of mice lacking the IL-4 gene, as a result of functional inactivation of the gene by homologous recombination, resulted in much more reduced levels of Th2 cytokines IL-5, IL-9 and IL-10 from CD4+ T cells than of wildtype control mice.[189] However, even in IL-4-knockout mice the Th2 response was not completely absent,[189] suggesting that, in spite of IL-4's dominant role, factors other than IL-4 may also direct the Th2 development.

CD4+ populations producing high amounts of IL-4 and IL-5 in addition to IFN-γ and IL-2 (Th0 cells) or even IL-4 and/or IL-5 alone (Th2 cells) were also found to develop from PB human T cells stimulated with PPD (an antigen that usually favors the development of Th1-like cells) in the presence of exogenous IL-4.[121] IL-4 added in bulk culture before cloning inhibited not only the differentiation of PPD-specific T cells into Th1-like clones, but also the development of their cytolytic potential. The depressive effect of IL-4 on the development of PPD-specific T cells with both Th1 profile and cytolytic potential was dependent on early addition of IL-4.[177] A preferential Th1-promoting effect by TGF-β on human CD4+ T cells has also been described.[190]

SOURCE OF IL-4 REQUIRED FOR THE INDUCTION OF TH2 DEVELOPMENT

The source of IL-4 which is required for priming naive T cells to develop into Th2 cells is still unclear. Five major candidates have been described. They include Fcε receptor 1-positive (FcεR1[+]) non-T cells, CD8[+] Tc2 cells, the LECAM-1[dull] Mel-14[low] subset of CD4[+] T cells, the CD4[+]NK1.1[+] subset and naive T cell themselves.

FcεR1[+] non-T cells

Several types of FcεR1[+] non-T cells are able to produce IL-4. First, murine mast cell lines capable of producing IL-4 have been described.[191] Then, non-T, non-B cells from mouse spleen and human bone marrow, probably belonging to the mast cell/basophil lineage, were found to be able to synthesize IL-4.[192,193] The IL-4-producing capacity of mouse non-T cells expands dramatically in *N. brasiliensis* infection and in association with anti-IgD injection,[194] suggesting that these cells play an important role in lymphokine production in helminthic infections and in other situations marked by striking elevations of serum IgE levels. These non-T/non-B cells represent the dominant source of IL-4 and IL-6 in the spleens of immunized animals. Exposing these cells to antigen-specific IgE or IgG in vivo (or in vitro) "armed" them to release both IL-4 and IL-6 upon subsequent antigenic challenge.[195] Accordingly, both human mast cells and basophils were found to produce IL-4 in response to several secretagogues.[196-199] More recently, it was found that activated human eosinophils can also release high IL-4 concentrations.[200-202] Thus, at least potentially, non-T cells may represent the "natural immunity" analog for the development of CD4[+] Th2 cells[178] and they might very well reflect a means through which Th2 cells can be strikingly amplified in vivo during allergic reactions and parasitic infestations. Cocultivation of naive T cells in the presence of anti-dinitrophenyl (DNP) IgE-loaded bone marrow-derived mast cells and bovine serum albumin-conjugated DNP led to the development of IL-4-producing Th2 cells, and this effect was inhibited by the addition of an anti-IL-4 antibody. In contrast, IL-12 addition did not inhibit the development of IL-4-producing cells, but favored the development of cells producing high amounts of both IL-4 and IFN-γ.[203] These data suggest that IgE-activated mast cells, basophils or eosinophils can bias an emerging T cell dependent immune response towards a Th2-dominated reaction by the initial production of IL-4. However, it is unlikely that parasites or allergens would be able to crosslink their receptors prior to a specific immune response that had produced parasite-specific IgG and IgE antibodies. On the other hand, mast cell-deficient mice develop normal Th2 responses.[204] Finally, in IL-4-deficient mice only those mice which are reconstituted with IL-4-producing T (but not with IL-4-producing non-T) cells produce antigen-specific IgE.[205] Thus, IL-4 production by mast cells/basophils or eosinophils triggered by antigen-IgE antibody immune complexes may play a role in amplifying secondary responses to parasites, but cannot account for the Th2 development in primary immune responses. A way out of this dilemma may be a pathway of IL-4 secretion independent from FcεR crosslinking. It has been suggested that both helminth products and some allergens may induce FcεRI+ cells to release IL-4 because of their proteolytic activity.[206] Some compounds, such as mercuric chloride ($HgCL_2$), can indeed induce the release of IL-4 by rat mast cells.[207] Likewise, the bee venom component phospholipase A_2 is also able to induce IL-4 release in rodent mast cells because of its catalytic activity.[208] Finally, IL-3/C5a-mediated IL-4 expression was found in human basophils.[209] Intriguingly, *Selistosonia mansoni* (*S. mansoni*) eggs were also found to be able to trigger IL-4 release by basophils from healthy subjects previously unexposed to *S. mansoni*, via an IgE-dependent mechanism.[210] However, obvious mechanisms of FcεR-independent IL-4 production for the great majority of allergens or helminth components have not been identified yet.

CD8+ Tc2 cells

The recent demonstration that under certain experimental conditions both murine and human CD8+ T cells can develop into Tc2 cells,[22,60-63] raises the possibility that IL-4 produced by CD8+ Tc2 cells may influence the development of Th cells. However, even if it is possible that IL-4-producing CD8+ T cells can have some effect in some pathological conditions (severe atopy, lepromatous leprosy, AIDS?), it is highly unlikely that they play a physiologic regulatory role on the development of Th2 cells.

CD4+ memory T cells

The L-selectin marker (detected by the Mel-14 antibody) has been used to separate naive and memory/activated subsets of CD4+ T cells from immunized mice, with Mel-14[low] T cells containing the memory and Mel-14[high] the naive subset.[211] CD4+ memory T cells also have low expression of CD45RBO, but high expression of CD44 (Table 3.3). Only the Mel-14[low] subset which contains the majority of the memory/activated CD4+ T cells has been shown to secrete significant amounts of IL-4 upon primary stimulation in vitro.[212] These cells may be activated by a primary antigen challenge because of crossreactivity to previously encountered antigens (i.e., self antigens, normal intestinal flora and other environmental antigens), and thus induce the development of naive T cells into IL-4 secreting cells.

CD4+NK1+ T cells

These cells represent a specialized population of mouse CD4+ T cells that bear NK surface receptors, express high CD44 and low CD45RB and Mel 14 (Table 3.3), and have T cell and NK-like functions. Their

Table 3.3. Surface markers and TCR repertoire of murine conventional (naive and memory) CD4⁺ T cells and CD4⁺NK1⁺ cells

Marker	Naive T	Memory T	NK1⁺ T
CD4	+	+	+ or −
NK1.1	−	−	+
CD44 (Pgp-1)	Low	High	High
CD45RB	High	Low	Low
CD62L (Mel 14)	High	Low	Low
CD24 (HSA)	Low	Low	Low
TCRVβ	All	All	2, 7, 8.2
TCRVα	All	All	14

TCR repertoire is very restricted, using a single invariant TCR α chain, Vα14-Jα281, paired with Vβ8⁺, Vβ7⁺ or Vβ2⁺ TCR chains.[213] In addition to CD4⁺NK1.1⁺ T cells, CD4⁻CD8⁻, but not CD8⁺, NK1⁺ T cells exist. NK1⁺ T cells are detectable in both thymus (where they account for up to 20% of the adult mature thymocyte compartment) and periphery.[213] NK1⁺ T cells were recently shown to be specific for the nonpolymorphic, β₂-microglobulin (β₂m)-associated MHC class-I-like CD1 molecules encoded outside the MHC region.[214] Since the most striking property of NK1⁺ T cells is the ability to secrete large amounts of IL-4 upon primary stimulation in vivo,[215,216] it was suggested that the CD1/NK1⁺ T cell pathway may direct the Th2 differentiation of some immune responses and that induction of CD1 during immune responses may recruit and activate NK1⁺ T cells.[217,218] Interestingly, indeed, β₂m-deficient mice (which are also deficient in CD1 expression) do neither produce IL-4 nor IgE, after injection of anti-IgD antibody;[219] moreover, SJL mice that are unable to produce IgE neither possess CD4⁺NK1⁺ T cells nor express mIL-4 following in vivo injection of anti-CD3 antibody.[220] The observation that CD4⁺NK1⁺ cells are downregulated in the liver of mice infected with *L. monocytogenes*,[221] which consistently promotes IL-12 production and Th1-dominated immune responses (see below), also provides indirect support for a role of these cells in promoting the Th2 cell development. Therefore, it is possible that immunogens, having associated superantigens that could interact with a sufficiently large fraction of these cells, may promote a pulse of IL-4 being available at the time when naive CD4⁺ T cells were responding to antigen for the first time. It is unlikely, however, that all antigens able to promote the differentiation of naive Th cells into the Th2 pathway should necessarily activate CD4⁺NK1⁺, CD1-restricted, T cells. This does indeed not seem to be the case of *L. major* antigens. In susceptible mice (see below), *L. major* induces very rapid IL-4 production by CD4⁺ T cells, which are NK1⁻,[222] suggesting that at least in this model NK1⁺ cells are not responsible for early IL-4 production leading to Th2 cell development. On the other side, at least in humans, a major class of microbial antigens presented to T cells by CD1 molecules are mycobacterial lipoglycans and such cells produce IFN-γ and are cytolytic. Moreover, CD1 proteins are highly expressed in the lesions of patients with the self-healing (Th1-dominated) form of leprosy,[223] suggesting that CD1-restricted antigens do not selectively evoke Th2 responses.

Class I-selected CD4⁻CD8⁻TCR⁺ T cells

In addition to CD4⁺NK1⁺ cells, a thymic population of cells showing TCRαβ but neither CD4 nor CD8 expression, preferential responsiveness to IL-7, and MHC class I restriction has been shown to produce high amounts of IL-4 in vitro in response to CD3 or TCR crosslinking.[224] A similar effect has also been shown in vivo. Following injection of anti-CD3 antibody, mRNA for IL-4 is expressed in CD4⁻CD8⁻TCR⁺ splenic T cells from both wild and MHC class II- but not MHC class I-deficient mice, suggesting their restriction by MHC class I or class I-like CD1 molecules.[225]

CD4⁺ naive T cells

Another possibility is that the source of IL-4 in the primary response is the naive CD4⁺ T cells themselves. These cells have low expression of CD44 but high expression of both CD45RB and Mel-14 (Table 3.2). The possibility that CD4⁺ naive T cells can provide IL-4 which is required for their development into Th2 cells has recently been supported by several findings. First, low intensity signaling of TCR, such as that mediated by low peptide doses or by mutant peptides, led to secretion of low levels of IL-4 by murine naive T cells.[143] Naive T cells, recently activated in the presence of costimulatory molecules-expressing fibroblasts (in the absence of outside influences from other cells), required two or more stimulation events to produce IL-4 and IL-5 and this induction of Th2-type cytokine secretion was blocked by inhibiting IL-4 action, suggesting that it was due to endogenous IL-4 produced by the naive T cells themselves.[226] Likewise, human CD45RA⁺ (naive) adult peripheral blood T cells, as well as human neonatal T cells, were found to develop into IL-4-producing cells in the absence of any preexisting source of IL-4 and despite the presence of anti-IL-4 antibodies.[227-229] Finally, high proportions of T cell clones showing a clear-cut Th2 profile of cytokine production could be generated from single CD4⁺ T cells isolated from thymus of small children.[161] A significant fraction of uncommitted T cells may be primed for a Th2 phenotype independent of antigen and IL-4 if they are exposed to IL-2 and simultaneously interact with accessory cells bearing the natural CD28 ligands B7-1 and B7-2. When stimulated by specific antigen, such primed Th2 precursor cells may provide a source of IL-4 to promote Th2 immunity.[104] Thus, evidence is accumulating suggesting that the maturation of naive T cells into the Th2 pathway mainly depends on the levels and the kinetics of autocrine IL-4 production at priming. This can be induced without exposure to IL-4 by accessory cells and may likely be determined by: (1) the genetic background of the individual; (2) the nature and the intensity of TCR signaling by the peptide ligand. Obviously, when CD1-restricted antigens are expressed on APC, CD4+NK1+ T cells which rapidly release high IL-4 amounts may also contribute to the development of the Th2 pathway. Likewise, cytokines from other cells (e.g., mast cell IL-4, macrophage IL-12), hormones, and other possible microenvironmental factors may also influence such an autocrine pathway.

ROLE OF OTHER CYTOKINES IN FAVORING THE TH2 DEVELOPMENT

An addition of IL-10 during primary stimulation of TCR-transgenic T cells did neither upregulate IL-4 or IL-5 nor inhibit IL-2 production. However, IL-10 decreased IFN-γ production slightly but reproducibly, compared to control cultures, during primary stimulation when either splenocytes or dendritic cells were used as APCs.[79,163] Neutralization of endogenous IL-10 with an anti-IL-10 antibody led to increased IFN-γ production and reduced IL-4 and IL-5 production, but only when irradiated BALB/c or SCID splenocytes were used as APCs in the priming cultures. Although only the addition of IL-4, but not IL-10, increased IL-4 and IL-5 production, the emergence of Th1 phenotype caused by neutralization of IL-4 could be partially reversed by IL-10 when irradiated splenocytes were used as APCs.[79] These findings suggest that there is a distinguishing mechanism of action between IL-4 and IL-10 for Th-cell phenotype development. IL-10 inhibits the development of a Th1 phenotype by inhibiting the production of IL-12 by macrophages,[230] but only IL-4 will directly skew toward the Th2 phenotype.

Studies with established cloned murine CD4+ lines have demonstrated that a competitive antagonist of IL-1 (IL-1RA) can block the proliferative response of some Th2 clones, suggesting that IL-1 is a costimulator of Th2, but no Th1, cells.[231,232] Indeed, murine Th2, but no Th1, cells have been found to be able to produce IL-1α in its active form in the absence of APCs, and this cytokine acted as an autocrine growth factor for Th2 cells.[233] On the other hand, it was found that macrophage-derived IL-1 is required for the development of Th1 cells stimulated with SEB,[234] and that IL-1 and TNF-α were required for induction of maximal levels of IFN-γ upon restimulation of Th1 cells.[163]

In the human system, we have found that IL-1 was neither apparently required for the proliferative response of already established Th1 and Th2 clones, nor for the in vitro development of PPD-specific T lymphocytes into Th1-like cells. However, IL-1 neutralization in bulk culture favored the development of Der p 1-specific T cell lines and clones producing high concentrations of IFN-γ and no, or low concentrations of, IL-4 in comparison to T cell lines and clones generated in the absence of IL-1 blockers or competitive antagonists, which usually exhibited a Th2-like profile.[235] In conclusion, IL-10 appears to act as a Th2-promoting factor, whereas the role of IL-1 is controversial. However, both IL-1 and IL-10 certainly play a minor effect in Th cell development in comparison to IL-4 and IL-12.

HORMONES

The role of hormones in promoting the differentiation of Th cells or in favoring the shifting of already differentiated Th cells from one to another cytokine profile has also been suggested.

GLUCOCORTICOIDS

It has been reported that in mice physiologic doses of glucocorticoids (GCS) enhance the production of IL-4, whereas "supraphysiologic" doses are required to inhibit production of IL-2, suggesting that some of the antiinflammatory effects of GCS are actually being mediated indirectly through a biologic effect of secreted IL-4.[236] A similar promoting effect by GCS on Th2 cytokine responses was also observed in rats.[237] However, a more complex pathway in the regulatory activity of GCS on the human Th cell response has been described. At high doses, GCS inhibited the production of both IFN-γ and IL-4, but at the lowest doses tested both hydrocortisone and hydrocortisone 17-butyrate had a stimulatory effect on IL-4 production.[238] Low GCS concentrations also favored the development of effector cells from both naive and memory Th cells, which upon restimulation produced large amounts of IL-10, but low amounts of IL-4, IL-5 or IFN-γ. Interestingly, GCS displayed different effects if they were added only during the restimulation of effector cells. In the effector T cells generated from the naive subset, GCS induced production of IL-4 and IL-10, but blocked production of IL-5 and IFN-γ. In effector T cells generated from the memory subset, GCS blocked production of IL-4, IL-5 and IL-10, but even at very high concentrations inhibited production of IFN-γ by only 50%.[239] These results indicate that GCS have the potential to increase or suppress IL-4 and IL-10 production depending on the stage of T cell activation.

ANDROGEN STEROIDS

An additional class of steroid hormones having important immunomodulatory function in vivo are androgens. Mice treated with metyrapone showed enhancement of IL-2 and IFN-γ production upon activation.[240] Metyrapone is a glucococorticoid inhibitor which causes an increase in the production of dihydroxyepiandrosterone (DHEA) (one of several steroids that circulate as inactive prohormones, becoming activated in target organs). Accordingly, DHEA when tested on normal cells stimulated with anti-CD3 antibody enhanced the secretion of IL-2 but not IL-4.[240] Testosterone, a DHEA metabolite, is a prohormone in many tissues and needs to be enzymatically converted to hydrotestorone (DHT). DHT is capable of depressing, but not abrogating, the quantity of IL-4, IL-5 and IFN-γ produced by activated T cells without affecting their capacity to produce IL-2.[241] It is of note that DHEA falls to extremely low levels in old age, and DHEA supplements can correct many of the immunological defects seen in old mice.[242,243] These results suggest that changes in the concentrations of steroid hormones may profoundly affect the patterns of lymphokines produced in a subsequent immune response. Hormonal control over T cells was found to exist in specific anatomic compartments. T cells isolated from nonmucosal tissue sites produced IL-2 as their predominant lymphokine upon activation. By contrast, T cells isolated from lymphoid organs draining mucosal sites, such as Peyer's patches, produced IL-4 as their major cytokine. Systemic treatment of mice with DHEA resulted in increased production of IL-2 by T cells from all lymphoid organs.[244]

CALCITRIOL

Another major prohormone, 25-hydroxy cholecalciferol (25 (OH) vitamin D3) may have a reverse effect on the Th1/Th2 balance. There is intense conversion of 25 (OH) vitamin D3 to 1,25 (OH)2 vitamin D3 (calcitriol) that is able to decrease output of IL-2 and IFN-γ and, when administered peripherally with antigen, evokes a Th2 pattern of response localized to mucosal surfaces.[245,246] More importantly, calcitriol analogs can rival cyclosporin A in their ability to prolong survival of skin grafts by inhibiting Th1 activity.[247] There is intense conversion of 25 (OH) vitamin D3 to calcitriol in the lesions of chronic T cell-dependent inflammatory disorders, such as tuberculosis or sarcoidosis,[248] as well in Hodgkin's disease.[249] The enzyme responsible, 1-α–hydroxylase, is upregulated in macrophages exposed to IFN-γ or to bacterial components, such as lipopolysaccharide (LPS). In the lymphoid compartments, calcitriol is an important regulator of T cell function. It decreases output of IL-2 and IFN-γ[250] and, when administered peripherally with antigen, it evokes a Th2 pattern of response that tends to localize to mucosal surfaces.[245] The Th2-promoting activity of calcitriol is probably due to its inhibitory effect on the production of IL-12 by both monocytes and B cells which leads to the activation and differentiation of Th1 cells. In addition, calcitriol directly inhibits IFN-γ secretion by Th1 clones, whereas it has little effect on IL-4 secretion by Th2 clones.[250]

PROGESTERONE AND RELAXIN

Recently, we found that progesterone (PG) favors the in vitro development of human Th cells producing Th2-type cytokines and promotes both IL-4 production and membrane CD30 expression in established human Th1 clones.[251] This may represent one of the mechanisms involved in the Th1/Th2 switch which has been hypothesized to occur at the maternal-fetal interface in order to improve fetal survival and promote successful pregnancy[252](see below). In more recent experiments, relaxin (RLX), another corpus luteum-derived hormone, was found to favor the development of IFN-γ and TNF-β producing cells, without having any influence on IL-4 and IL-5 production, thus showing an opposite effect compared to progesterone.[253] Therefore, increasing evidence is accumulating to suggest that hormones and peripherally activated prohormones may regulate the Th1/Th2 balance.

TCR REPERTOIRE

The observation that certain types of antigens preferentially induce Th1 or Th2-type responses raised the possibility that the TCR repertoires of IL-4 and IFN-γ producers were different. As mentioned above, the analysis of TCR expressed by mouse T cell clones specific for leishmanial antigens revealed that the same TCR was utilized by clones that made IFN-γ as well as by clones that made IL-4.[137] These experiments demonstrate that there can be no exclusivity in the use of one or another set of germline V or Ja segments in the expressed repertoires. However, more subtle differences in repertoire cannot be excluded. When TCR Vβ8+ and Vβ8-activated T cell blasts were cocultured with a mitogenic anti-Vβ8 antibody, restimulation of separated Vβ8+ and Vβ8-T cells revealed that IL-4 production was induced and IL-2 release was downregulated in Vβ8+ cells only.[254,255]

OTHER INFLUENCES

Several other substances capable of exerting some influence in the development of Th1 and Th2 cells have been described. PGE_2 and forskolin differentially modulate cytokine secretion profiles of adult human Th lymphocytes by inducing a higher elevation of intracellular cAMP levels in Th0 and Th1 than in Th2 clones.[256] However, in cord blood naive T cells PGE_2 inhibits acquisition of ability to produce IFN-γ and IL-2 but not IL-4 and IL-5, thus showing a clear promoting effect towards the Th2-cell development.[257] Nitric oxide (NO), which is produced by Th1, but no Th2, cells selectively inhibits the proliferation and the production of IL-2 and IFN-γ by Th1 cells, whereas it has no effect on IL-4 production by Th2 cells.[258,259] However, such a selective effect on Th1 cells has not been confirmed in another study.[260] Ultraviolet radiation (UVR) also suppresses Th1 responses, while leaving Th2 responses intact, by stimulating IL-10 production by both keratinocytes[261] and Th2 cells themselves.[262] IL-10 is indeed constitutively produced by keratinocytes and UVR upregulates both mRNA IL-10 expression and IL-10 protein production.[263] Interestingly, IL-12 neutralized the activity of UVR-induced suppression.[264] $HgCL_2$, a chemical responsible for autoimmune manifestations in Brown Norway rats, induces early and high expression of IL-4 mRNA in T cells from these animals.[265] Likewise, gold salts promote autoimmune manifestations and the development of Th0/Th2 cells in the same animals.[266] Thalidomide also enhances the production of IL-4 and IL-5, while inhibiting at the same dose IFN-γ production.[267] In contrast, thiols decrease production of Th2-derived cytokines without affecting production of IL-2 and IFN-γ.[268] Naturally occurring flavonoid compounds, such as rutin (a polyphenol-containing glycoprotein from tobacco), preferentially activate Th2 cells.[269] Vitamin A deficiency results in a strong regulatory T cell imbalance with excessive Th1 response and insufficient Th2 cell development and function. At least three vitamin A activities that balance Th1 and Th2 functions were identified, downregulating Th1 cell IFN-γ secretion directly, decreasing activated APC function, and promoting Th2 cell growth and/or differentiation.[270] The inhibition of IFN-γ synthesis by retinoic acid is probably due to blocking some step in the CD28 pathway.[271] Interestingly, dietary retinoic acid supplementation downregulates the level of constitutive IL-12 and IFN-γ transcription.[272] Finally, CKS-17, a synthetic retroviral peptide, modulated the Th1/Th2 balance in favor of Th2 cells by inhibiting IL-12 production and stimulating production of IL-10.[273]

ROLE OF GENETIC BACKGROUND IN THE TH OUTCOME

From the above mentioned findings, it appears clearly that, although the type of antigen and of antigen presentation plays an important role in the Th cell differentiation (intracellular pathogens usually promote Th1-dominated responses, whereas extracellular pathogens, soluble antigens and oral immunization preferentially promote Th2-dominated responses), there are striking differences in Th outcome depending on the genetic background of the host. The first example was provided by the demonstration that MHC controls the cytokine phenotype of CD4+ T cells responding to collagen IV,[274] as well as to allo-4-hydroxyphenylpyruvate dioxygenase.[275] The clearest example of genetic control of the Th1/Th2 responses, however, is provided by murine *L. major* infection. Transgenic T cells from both the B10.D2 and BALB/c backgrounds showed development toward either the Th1 or Th2 phenotype under the strong directing influence of IL-12 and IL-4, respectively. However, when T cells were activated in vitro under neutral conditions in which exogenous cytokines were not added, B10.D2-derived T cells acquired a significantly stronger Th1 phenotype than T cells from the BALB/c background, correspondent with in vivo Th responses to *L. major* in these strains.[276] Another interesting example is provided by the different effect exerted by HgCl2. In Brown Norway rats HgCl2 induces early and strong IL-4 expression and autoimmunity, whereas it does not affect IL-4 expression in Lewis rats who do not develop autoimmunity.[265] Other well-characterized examples of genetic differences in Th cell development include murine candidiasis[277] and malaria,[278] autoimmune diabetes,[279] intestinal helminth infections,[280] Lyme disease[281] and atopic disorders[282] (see also below). At least in the *L. major* model, the effects of genetic background on Th phenotype development seem to reside within the T cell, and not the APC compartment.[276] Common cytokine receptor usage and related transcription factors pathways are areas where minor polymorphism could regulate major differences in Th cell development.

Recently, it has been found that T cells from B10.D2 mice (a murine strain easily inducible to Th1 responses) have an intrinsically greater capacity to maintain IL-12 responsiveness under neutral conditions in vitro compared to T cells from BALB/c mice (a strain inducible to Th2 responses), allowing for prolonged capacity to undergo IL-12-induced Th1 development.[283] The locus controlling this genetic effect was localized in a region of chromosome 11, containing a cluster of genes important for T cell differentiation, including IL-4, IL-5, IL-3 and interferon regulatory factor-1 (IRF-1),[284] which is syntenic with the homologous gene cluster on human chromosome 5 linked to several phenotypic markers of atopy (see below).

=========== CHAPTER 4 ===========

Th1/Th2 Cells and Intracellular Signaling

Although much is known about the functions of Th1 and Th2 cells as regulators of specific immune responses, relatively little is known about the biochemical basis for the differential production of cytokines by these cell types. Likewise, the intracellular signalings involved in the development of one or the other phenotype are still poorly understood.

INTRACELLULAR SIGNALING IN ESTABLISHED TH1 AND TH2 CELLS

Several studies have shown that there may be differences in TCR-mediated signaling mechanisms between Th1 and Th2 cell clones. Th2 cells make significantly more cAMP in response to TCR signals than do Th1 cells.[285] Importantly, cAMP has been shown to inhibit IL-2 production, in part by blocking NF-κB activation.[286] Other studies suggest that increases in cytoplasmic calcium upon TCR stimulation occur in Th1 cells but not in Th2 cells.[287,288] Transcriptionally active levels of the critical IL-2 transcription factor, nuclear factor of activated T cells, (NF-AT) occurred only in Th2 cells overexpressing the eukaryotic initiation factor 4E (eIF-4E), but not in normal Th2 cells, thus indicating that the inability of Th2 cells to express IL-2 was associated with inadequate levels of at least one transcription factor, NF-AT.[289] A failure to induce IL-2 gene promoter activity in a TCR-stimulated Th2 cell clone, and an associated lack of NF-κB binding factors in Th2 cell clones, has also been reported.[290] Taken together, these results suggest that TCR signaling differences in Th1 and Th2 cells may be responsible for the failure to induce the full set of *trans*-acting factors required for IL-2 gene transcription.[291,292] The IL-2 gene enhancer contains a number of *cis*-acting regulatory elements, including an OCT-1 binding site called NFIL-2A, proximal and distal NF-AT and AP-1 sites and a single NF-κB site. All these enhancer elements play a coordinated role in regulating IL-2 gene transcription. Direct comparison of nuclear factors specific for these IL-2 enhancer elements showed that there were no detectable differences in NFIL-2A, NF-AT and AP-1 binding factors in TCR-stimulated Th1 and Th2 clones, but there was a clear difference in nuclear NF-κB factors. In particular, TCR stimulation of IL-2-producing Th1 and Th0 cell clones led to a reversal in the nuclear ratio of p50 homodimers to p65(RelA)p50 heterodimers, while it did not occur in Th2 clones.[290] This was due to the nuclear influx of p65(RelA) in Th1 but not in Th2 cells, suggesting that this factor is sequestered in the cytoplasm of Th2 cells, probably because of the activity of NF-κB inhibitors, such as the members of the IκBα family.[293]

INTRACELLULAR SIGNALINGS INVOLVED IN TH1/TH2 CELL DEVELOPMENT

The appreciation that cytokines present in the microenvironment at the time of antigen presentation (IL-12/IFN and IL-4) play a critical role in favoring the differentiation of Th cells towards the Th1 or the Th2 profile has opened the question of the intracellular signaling involved in the Th1/Th2 development. Cytokines exert their effects on cells by interacting with specific receptors expressed at the cell surface. This results in receptor homo- or hetero-dimerization and triggering of intracellular signals. One of the earliest signaling events is the activation of protein tyrosine kinases (PTKs), which are physically associated with the receptor.[294] After activation, receptor-associated PTKs phosphorylate several substrates critical for signal transduction, including specific tyrosine residues in the cytoplasmic domains of the receptors. One important component of cytokine signaling is the specific transcriptional activation of target genes, which is very rapid and does not require the synthesis of new proteins. PTKs utilized by cytokine/cytokine receptor complexes for the signal transduction comprise two families of essential elements, which are known as the JAK-STAT pathway.[295-297]

THE JAK-STAT PATHWAY

The Janus family of kinases (JAK) contains the members JAK1, JAK2, JAK3 and TYK2. These kinases preferentially and constitutively associate with the intracellular domains of cytokine receptors and become activated following ligand-induced assembly of receptor subunits at the cell surface (Table 4.1). The second family comprises of src homology 2 (SH2) domain-containing, latent cytosolic transcription factors, known as signal transducers and activators of transcription (STATs). To date, six members of the STAT family, STAT1 through STAT6, have been identified and characterized (Table 4.1). STATs are widely expressed in different cell types and tissues, except for STAT4, which is expressed predominantly in testis and in cells of hematopoietic origin. Typically, stimulation by a particular cytokine results in the activation of a distinct pair of two of the four known JAK ki-

Table 4.1. JAK kinases, STATs and their extracellular ligands

Receptor	Activated JAKs	Activated STATs
IFN-α	JAK1, TYK2	STAT1, STAT2, STAT3
IFN-γ	JAK1, JAK2	STAT1
IL-2	JAK1, JAK3	STAT3, STAT5
IL-12	JAK2, TYK2	STAT3, STAT4
IL-4	JAK1, JAK3	STAT6
IL-10	Unknown	STAT1, STAT3
IL-13	Unknown	STAT6

nases. JAK kinases are required for tyrosine phosphorylation and activation of STATs, although it is not yet clear whether JAKs phosphorylate STATs directly. After tyrosine phosphorylation and subsequent activation, STATs translocate to the nucleus and bind specific, but related, DNA sequences to promote transcription of unique, but overlapping, patterns of cytokine-responsive genes (Fig. 4.1).

The rapid elucidation of the JAK-STAT pathway has been made possible in part through the detailed investigation of IFN signaling. Both JAK1 and JAK2 are required for IFN-γ signaling, while JAK1 and TYK2 are involved in IFN-α signaling.[298] STAT1, STAT2 and STAT3 are activated by IFN-α,[299] while only STAT1 is activated by IFN-γ.[300] The analysis of the IFN signaling has then shown that ligation of IFN-γ receptor leads to rapid phosphorylation of a particular tyrosine-containing sequence near the carboxyl terminus of the receptor α chain, thereby forming a specific docking site on the receptor for STAT1.[301] After docking with the receptor, STATs become thyrosine-phosphorylated, dissociate from the receptor and form dimers in a process that may be guided by the relative affinity of STAT SH2 domains for various phosphotyrosine-containing sequences[302] (Fig. 4.1). Binding of STAT1 to the ligand-induced receptor docking site is specific, of moderately high affinity, mediated by the STAT1 SH2 domain, and required for subsequent STAT1 activation. These observations have formed the basis of the hypothesis that the unique pattern of STAT proteins activated by each cytokine is determined by the ability of each STAT protein to bind through its SH2 domain to specific docking sites generated in the intracellular domains of the different cytokine receptors following activation. Further fine-tuning of specificity may occur through interaction of STATs with other receptor-associated molecules, including previously recruited STATs or the JAK kinases. However, the lack of correlation between activation of specific JAKs with related STATs suggests that the JAK kinases may be relatively nonspecific.

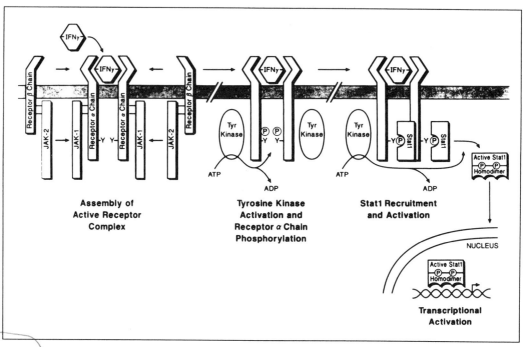

Fig. 4.1. Model of human IFN-γ signal transduction. In an unstimulated cell, the human IFN-γ receptor α and β polypeptides carry distinct JAK kinases in inactive form, but are not preassociated with one another. JAK-1 constitutively associates with the receptor α chain intracellular domain. JAK-2 constitutively associates with the receptor β chain. Signal transduction through the IFN-γ receptor is initiated following binding of a IFN-γ homodimer to two IFN-γ receptor α chains, thereby inducing α chain dimerization. The receptor β chain then associates with the ligand-receptor α chain complex, thereby bringing the intracellular domains of the receptor polypeptides and the kinases that are associated with them into close juxtaposition. This event forms on the dimerized receptor polypeptides two moderately high affinity, specific, and juxtaposed docking sites for latent STAT1. STAT1 molecules then bind directly to each phosphorylated receptor α chain via the STAT1 SH2 domains and are thereby brought into close proximity with the activated receptor-associated tyrosine kinases. STAT1 is subsequently activated by phosphorylation of a specific tyrosine residue. The rapid dissociation of the STAT1-receptor complexes, which are in close proximity with one another, favors the in situ formation of STAT1 homodimers, which are stabilized by reciprocal SH2 domain binding. This event thereby releases STAT1 from its receptor tether allowing the activated complex to translocate to the nucleus and induce gene transcription. Reprinted with permission from Greenlund AC et al, Immunity 1995; 2:677-687.[301]

INTERACTIONS OF STATS WITH DNA SEQUENCES

STAT binding sequences in DNA can vary considerably from a consensus palindromic sequence $TTCN_{(2-4)}GAA$, and can be divided into two groups: sequences that bind several different STAT complexes, and sequences that preferentially bind a particular STAT. Conversely, a particular STAT complex can bind to several different sequences, although the apparent affinity of binding is variable. Spacing between the palindromic half-sites is important in determining which STATs are able to bind, although the spacer and flanking nucleotides also play a role.[297] This pattern of binding specificities suggests a framework for explaining overlapping patterns of gene that are induced by different cytokines. Furthermore, it is likely that the opposing actions of some cytokines may be achieved through activation of distinct sets of effector genes. STAT-binding activity typically disappears within several hours of stimulation, presumably through the action of protein-tyrosine phosphatases (PTPs), thus providing an important mechanism of negative regulation for STAT-induced activation.

IL-12 INDUCES ACTIVATION OF STAT4

It has clearly been shown that IL-12 directly influences T cells for the induction of Th1 differentiation.[147,153] Therefore, signals delivered by IL-12 at the T cell surface would be an important step in inducing Th1 development from naive T cells. Treatment of murine TCR-transgenic T cells with IL-12 produced an electromobility shift assay (EMSA) complex containing STAT3 and STAT4, whose mobility was distinct from that of complexes induced by IL-2 and IL-4, which contain STAT5 and STAT6, respectively.[303] Interestingly, activation of EMSA complexes containing STAT3 and STAT4, as well as STAT4 phosphorylation, are evident in early Th1 cells. Th2 cells did not respond to IL-12, although they maintained the capacity to respond to several other cytokines, including IL-2, IL-4, IFN-γ (involving activity of JAK1 and JAK2) and IFN-α (involving activity of JAK1 and TYK2). The lack of STAT4 phosphorylation in Th2 cells was not due to a lack of STAT4 protein, since Th2 cells expressed similar levels of STAT3 and STAT4 compared to Th1 cells, but to the failure to phosphorylate JAK2, STAT3 and STAT4.[304] This implies that the defect in Th2 cells for IL-12 responses is upstream of the STATs and the kinases, and may involve an unidentified component of the IL-12 receptor itself[13] (Fig. 4.2).

In human T cells, IL-12 induces thyrosine phosphorylation of JAK2 and TYK2, whereas JAK1 and JAK3, which are phosphorylated in response to IL-2, are not phosphorylated after IL-12 treatment.[305] More importantly, IL-12 induces tyrosine phosphorylation and activation of STAT4-, but not of STAT1- or STAT2-containing complexes, which bind to the GRR DNA sequence.[306]

ROLE OF STAT6 IN IL-4 SIGNALING AND REGULATION OF THE IL-4 GENE EXPRESSION

The recognition that IL-4 expression during immune responses is critical for determining the development of Th2 cells has intensified interest in the molecular basis of its regulation. It is now clear that following the interaction between IL-4 and its receptor on a given cell the IL-4-induced STAT protein, initially designated IL-4 STAT[307] and hereafter termed STAT6, is activated. STAT6 is related in primary amino acid sequence to STAT1, yet encoded by a different gene.[297] The

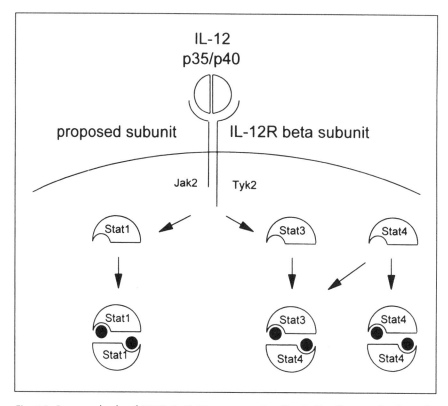

Fig. 4.2. Proposed role of STATs in IL-12 receptor signaling in T cells. In early Th1 cells, interaction of IL-12 with its receptor activates JAK-2 and TYK-2 which promote STAT4 phosphorylation and production of specific electromobility shift assay (EMSA) complexes containing STAT3 and STAT4. Since Th2 cells express similar levels of STAT3 and STAT4 compared to Th1 cells, this implies that the inability of Th2 cells to respond to IL-12 is upstream of the STATs and the kinases and involves a receptor component itself. Reprinted with permission from O'Garra A et al, Chem Immunol 1996; 63:1-13.[13]

essential role of STAT6 in IL-4 signaling has clearly been demonstrated in STAT6-deficient mice. In these animals, T cells are indeed unable to develop into Th2 cells and production of IgE and IgG$_1$ is virtually abolished.[308,309]

The mechanisms governing the IL-4 gene expression in T cells, however, are very complex and still unclear. Analyses of the human and mouse IL-4 genes have identified multiple *cis*-elements that regulate the proper tissue-specific and developmental expression of the genes.[310-314] In the mouse, several positive regulatory elements (PRE) have been identified. An 11-base pair DNA motif (P sequence, -78GAAAATTTCCA-68) in the 5' flanking region of the human IL-4 gene was initially identified as an enhancer element sharing a sequence (CLEO-like) with other cytokine gene promoters, such as GM-CSF, IL-2 and IL-5.[310] One of the binding factors, the NF(P) factor, appears closely related to the cytoplasmic component of NF-AT, the nuclear factor of activated T cells essential for IL-2 gene induction. Another binding factor possessed biochemical and immunological features identical to the transcription factor AP-1. NF-AT- and AP-1-related factors can cooperatively activate the transcription of reporter genes driven by composite OAP_{40}/P sequence repeats. The AP-1 component binding to the IL-4 NF-AT/AP1 composite site may contain Fra-1, Fra-2, JunB and JunD.[314] Although the AP-1 family members utilized by this composite site differ from those reported to be present in the IL-2 NF-AT/ AP-1 site, the two composite sites appear functionally interchangeable and do not, by themselves, determine Th1/Th2-specific promoter activity.[314] An essential region of the IL-4 promoter is located immediately upstream of the TATA element. Included in the region are overlapping binding sites for the cyclosporin A-sensitive factor NF-ATp and a novel constitutively expressed factor designated PCC.[315] Of note is that mice with a null mutation in the NF-ATp gene have splenomegaly with hyperproliferation of both T and B cells and a striking defect in early IL-4 production after ligation of the TCR complex by anti-CD3 treatment in vivo, suggesting that NF-ATp may be involved in cell growth and play a role in the balanced transcription of the IL-4 gene during the course of an immune response.[316]

Four promoter elements have been implicated in the transcriptional regulation of the human IL-4 gene: the positive (P) sequence, the positive regulatory element (PRE) and two negative regulatory elements (NRE)s,

Table 4.2. Regulation elements of murine and human IL-4 gene promoter and relative nuclear factors

Promoter Element	Nuclear Factors (NF)
Murine	
P elements (P1, P2, P3, P4)	Nuclear factors (P) (NF-Y + NF-ATp)
CLE-0	NF-CLE-Oa, NF-CLE-0b Related to NF(P), NF-ATc, AP-1
Consensus sequences (CS1, CS2)	Not identified
Y box	NF-Y
OAP sites	OAP-40
Human	
Positive (P) element	Nuclear factors (P) (NF-Y + NF-ATp)
Positive regulatory elements (PRE)	POS-1, POS-2
Negative regulatory elements (NRE)	Neg-1, Neg-2

NRE-I and NRE-II (Table 4.2). PRE-I is a strong enhancer element essential for the expression of human IL-4 gene.[317] NRE-I is a 9-bp element for the T cell-specific factor Neg-1, whereas NRE-II is a 13-bp element for the ubiquitous factor Neg-2. Functional suppression of IL-4 transcription was only achieved when the binding sites for both Neg-1 and Neg-2 were intact.[311]

It recently has been shown that the human IL-4 proximal promoter exists in multiple allelic forms and that one of the cloned alleles has a markedly enhanced promoter strength relative to the others.[318] In view of the central role the P sequence plays in the transcriptional activity of the human IL-4 promoter and the documented importance of AP-1 family members interacting with the OAP_{40} site in stabilizing NF-AT interaction with the P sequence, an enhanced affinity for AP-1-related factors in a particularly potent allele of the IL-4 promoter, or a decreased affinity for repressor proteins, may result in overexpression of the gene in Th cells, biasing Th cell development down the Th2 pathway.

CHAPTER 5

CROSSREGULATORY ACTIVITY

It is well-established that some lymphokines produced by Th1 and Th2 cells can exert mutual regulatory interactions (Fig. 5.1). In particular, IL-4 and IFN-γ, the principal products of Th2 and Th1 cells, respectively, often oppose one another's actions. IL-10 which is mainly produced by Th2 cells but also by macrophages and B cells exerts negative regulatory effects on some Th1 cell functions. By contrast, the Th1-derived cytokine IFN-γ, as well as IL-12 and IFN-α, which are not a product of Th1 cells but act as Th1 inducing cytokines, downregulate the function of Th2 cells.

CROSSREGULATION BY TYPE 2 CYTOKINES

IL-4

There is considerable evidence that IL-4 prevents priming of naive Th cells to become IFN-γ producers. In fact, IL-4 is able to strikingly inhibit IL-2 production by naive T cells in response to anti-CD3 antibody and APCs or, when transgenic T cells are used, to antigen and APCs.[319] In contrast, IL-4 has little effect on IL-2 or IFN-γ production by established T cell lines or by T cells that have been already primed in vitro. The suppressive effects of IL-4 on priming for IFN-γ production are markedly diminished in the presence of IL-12. Thus IL-12 not only enhances the priming of naive Th cells to become IFN-γ producers, it also diminishes their sensitivity to inhibition by IL-4 from >90% to about 50%.[320] However, IL-4 inhibits the IFN-γ-mediated positive feedback stimulation of IL-12 production by macrophages.[321]

IL-10

IL-10, another cytokine selectively produced by murine Th2 cells,[28] but common to all types of human Th cells,[25] inhibits lymphokine production by Th1, but not by Th2 clones.[322] This inhibition is somewhat selective in that secretion of IFN-γ and IL-3, lymphokines secreted mainly at later times after stimulation, is substantially inhibited

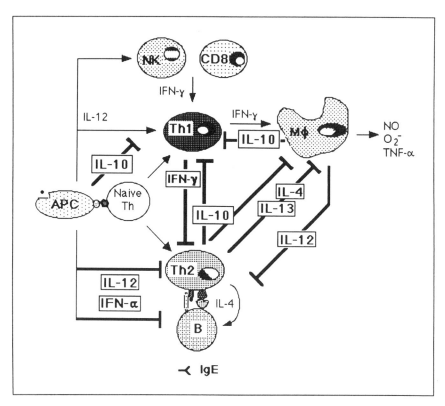

Fig. 5.1. Crossregulatory effects of Th1- or Th2-inducing and Th1- or Th2-derived cytokines. IL-12 and IFN-α produced by APC inhibit both the development of Th2 cells and their B cell helper activity for IgE synthesis, whereas IL-10 produced by the same cells and by Th2 cells inhibits both the development and function of Th1 cells, as well as several macrophage functions. IFN-γ produced by Th1 cells (as well as by NK cells and CD8+ T cells) inhibits the development and the proliferation of Th2 cells. IL-4 and IL-13, produced by Th2 cells, inhibit several functions of macrophages activated by Th1 cells (——⊣ = inhibitory effect).

while secretion of GM-CSF and TNF-β, lymphokines secreted mainly at early times, is inhibited slightly if at all; the effect on IL-2 production often is less than the effect on IFN-γ production.[322] IL-10 also inhibits the IFN-γ-mediated positive feedback stimulation of IL-12 production by macrophages[321,323] and by suppressing costimulatory molecules such as TNF-α and IL-1 inhibits the stimulatory effects of IL-12 on T and NK cells. This results in downregulation of Th1 cell differentiation.[324] IL-10 also inhibits the synthesis of IFN-γ by CD8+ CTL clones, although the extent of inhibition is somewhat lower that observed with Th1 clones.[325] Because IL-10 inhibits secretion of IL-2 by Th1 cells while IL-2 causes proliferation of CD8+ T cells through a paracrine pathway, Th2 cells and other cells that secrete IL-10 regulate clonal expansion of those subsets that produce IFN-γ.

IL-13

As mentioned above, production of IL-13 is a property of murine Th2 cells, whereas it is less restricted in human Th cells. In any case, IL-13 cannot exhibit direct crossregulatory activity on Th1 cells because both murine and human Th cells appear to be insensitive to the activity of IL-13.[326] However, IL-13 modulates several macrophage functions: (1) it enhances the expression of integrin super gene family, CD23 and MHC class II antigens; (2) it downregulates the production of NO and (3) it downregulates the production of cytokines, such as IL-1, IL-6, TNF-α, IL-12 and IFN-α, and of chemokines, such as IL-8 and MIP-1α.[327] Thus, since IL-12 and IFN-α are important in the differentiation of Th1 cells, the inhibitory activity of IL-13 on their production may represent another important mechanism of indirect crossregulation for Th1 cells.

CROSSREGULATION BY TYPE 1 CYTOKINES

IFN-γ

The addition of IFN-γ to cultures containing optimal amounts of IL-4 failed to inhibit the priming of CD4+ T cells from TCR transgenic mice to develop into IL-4-producing T cells. However, when suboptimal concentrations of IL-4 were used for priming, IFN-γ caused a significant decrease in the amount of IL-4 produced after restimulation.[60] This result is consistent with the observation that few IL-4-producing T cell clones emerge from a culture containing IFN-γ.[325] Indeed, IFN-γ, at relatively low concentrations, inhibits proliferation of murine Th2 clones stimulated with antigen, mitogens or anti-TCR antibodies; however, secretion of lymphokines including IL-4 in response to these stimuli is not affected.[325] IFN-γ also inhibits proliferation of murine Th2 clones exposed to IL-2 or IL-4.[328,329] IFN-γ does not affect proliferation or lymphokine production by Th1 cells or other CD4+ or CD8+ clones that secrete IFN-γ. Although not absolute, the inhibitory effect of IFN-γ on proliferation of murine Th2 cells is significant and seems to be sufficient to limit the clonal expansion of such cells. While IFN-γ does not inhibit lymphokine secretion by stimulated Th2 cells, IFN-γ does inhibit many of the agonist effects of those secreted cytokines. For example, IFN-γ inhibits proliferation of murine bone marrow cells stimulated with IL-3, IL-4 or GM-CSF.[330] In addition IFN-γ can inhibit IL-4-dependent B cell differentiation.[331] The proliferation of human Th2 clones is also inhibited by IFN-γ.[25]

IFN-α

As IFN-γ, IFN-α plays a negative regulatory role in the development of Th2 cells. In particular, in the mouse, IFN-α was found to be able to suppress increases in the level of splenic IL-4 mRNA induced by either treatment with anti-IgD antibody or infection with

N. brasiliensis, whereas in both conditions the levels of IFN-γ mRNA were increased.[332,333] In the absence of IFN-γ, IFN-α augments IL-12 effects on inhibition of subsequent IL-4 production rather than enhancing IL-12 priming for subsequent IFN-γ production.[171] The regulatory activity of IFN-α has also been demonstrated in the human system. IFN-α inhibited the development of allergen-specific T cells into Th2-like cells.[177,179,180] This effect is probably related to a selective antiproliferative activity on T cells planned to the production of Th2 cytokines, inasmuch as addition of IFN-α in bulk culture before cloning resulted in the development of allergen-specific T cell clones showing not only a different cytokine profile (Th1 or Th0 versus Th2), but also different TCR repertoire and peptide reactivity.[179]

IL-12

In addition to its well-known ability in priming Th cells to produce IFN-γ, and therefore to develop into Th1 cells,[147,150] IL-12 also inhibits the differentiation of T cells into IL-4-secreting cells, i.e., into Th2 cells.[150,153] This inhibitory effect is in part a direct effect,[165] in part it is mediated by its activity on APCs,[158] and in part by its stimulation of IFN-γ synthesis.[150,153,334] IL-12 also inhibits the production of at least one cytokine, IL-3, that is not generally regarded to be strictly Th1- or Th2-associated,[335] as well as it inhibits switching to IgE secretion to a greater extent than switching to other Ig isotypes.[335,336] IL-12 is not capable, however, of suppressing a Th2 cell recall response.[337] Interestingly, IL-12 may also limit its own effects by inducing the production of a cytokine, such as IL-10, that downregulates both IL-12 production and IL-12-induced IFN-γ production.[321,324,335,338] When IL-12 and IL-4 are present together, paradoxically IL-4 suppresses the IL-12-induced priming for IL-10 production, but only minimally decreases the priming for high IFN-γ production.[324] The in vivo effects of IL-12, however, appear to be, to a large extent, IFN-γ-dependent.[334,335]

CHAPTER 6

TOLERANCE AND APOPTOSIS IN TH1 AND TH2 CELLS

During development in the thymus, T cells expressing self-reactive TCR are deleted or rendered functionally anergic (central tolerance). However, clonal anergy acts as an important mechanism of tolerance even for mature T cells reactive with self-antigens that are not expressed in the thymus, as well as for T cells that escape intrathymic clonal deletion (peripheral tolerance). Two main mechanisms seem to account for the induction of peripheral tolerance: (1) apoptotic cell death and (2) anergy of the effector cell or its suppression by a regulatory T cell.

APOPTOTIC CELL DEATH IN TH1/TH2 CELLS

When a naive T cell is subjected to inadequate stimulation, apoptosis or programmed cell death (PCD) occurs. PCD is prevented by IL-2, which promotes both proliferation and differentiation. Repeated antigenic stimulation of the activated T cell can also result in apoptosis or activation-induced cell death (AICD), which is increased by IL-2.[336] AICD occurs with superantigens, activated T cells and high doses of anti-TCR or anti-CD3 antibody; it requires the presence of APC and is mediated by Fas/Fas ligand (FasL) interaction. Fas and FasL are members of the TNF/nerve growth factor receptor family and of the TNF family, respectively.[337] Although Fas/FasL interaction probably provides a costimulatory signal in resting T cells, its critical involvement in AICD is generally accepted. Several data demonstrate that chronically activated T cells express high amounts of Fas and are susceptible to Fas-mediated killing.[338-340] FasL was originally identified on a CD8+ T cell hybridoma and, although it is not the primary cytotoxic molecule associated with the induction of target cell lysis, it can act as a second, perforin-independent mechanism by which CD8+ T cells induce target cell cytolysis.[341] The ability of CD4+ T cells to act as cytolytic effector cells in the absence of perforin-containing granules suggests that CD4+ T cells also use the Fas pathway.

The expression of Fas and FasL has recently been evaluated in Th-cell subsets, focusing on expression of these molecules by Th1 and Th2 cells. Fas is expressed by both subsets, whereas FasL is expressed predominantly, but not exclusively, by Th1 and Th0 cells.[343,344] Interestingly, the differential expression of FasL by Th1 and Th2 cells correlates with the ability of these cells to undergo AICD. Whereas Th1 clones are highly sensitive to AICD, Th2 clones are relatively resistant. However, the Th2 clones do express Fas because these cells are sensitive to the apoptotic effects of FasL expressed by Th1 cells.[345] The preferential expression of FasL by Th1 cells also accounts for the deletion of activated macrophages in the course of Th1-dominated responses. When macrophages were pulsed with antigen and then incubated with either Th1 or Th2 cell lines or clones, Th1, but not Th2, T cells induced lysis of 60-80% normal macrophages, whereas macrophages obtained from mice with mutations in the Fas were totally resistant to Th1-mediated cytotoxicity.[346] These results may account for previous findings showing that human Th1, but not Th2, cells induce cytolysis in B cells acting as APC in the presence of the specific antigen.[29] Thus, it is likely that FasL expression in human Th cells is also predominantly expressed by, or operating in, the Th1 subset. The fact that Th1 cells possess both FasL and Fas, whereas Th2 cells express Fas, but low FasL, suggests that Th2 cells are susceptible to AICD in the presence of Th1 cells, whereas Th1 cells can be killed by interacting among themselves rather than with Th2 cells (Fig. 6.1). This 'competitive disadvantage' of Th1 cells has been envisaged to lead to the preferential loss of Th1 cells and to the proposed skewing of the immune system in favor of Th2 responses in HIV infection (see below).

RESPONSE OF TH1 AND TH2 CELLS TO TOLEROGENIC SIGNALS

Several data indicate that at least in vitro both Th1 and Th2 cells can be tolerized,[347] even if Th1 cells are more susceptible to tolerogenic signals than Th2 cells.[348-350] In the Th1 subset, indeed, TCR engagement without costimulation does not provide adequate signaling to induce proliferation.[348-351] Disruption of a putative tyrosine kinase network seems to account for Th1 cell anergy during restimulation,[352] which probably consists of early cell sequestration in the G_{1a} phase of cell cycle.[353] Stimulation of Th1 clones with altered peptide ligands and live APC, a combination that partially activates the T cells but does not induce proliferation, also results in unresponsiveness to future stimulation with the immunogenic peptide.[347] Interestingly, treatment of cloned Th0 cells with anergizing stimuli resulted in the selective loss of Th1 characteristics and retention of a Th2 phenotype.[354]

The higher susceptibility of Th1 cells to tolerogenic signals is strongly supported by experiments performed in vivo. Injection of high doses

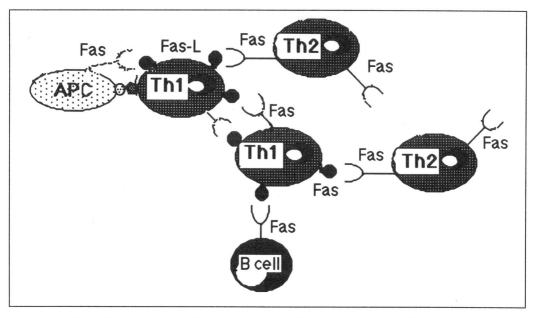

Fig. 6.1. Th1/Th2 cells and apoptosis. Th1 cells express both Fas and Fas-L, whereas Th2 cells express high Fas but low Fas-L. Therefore, Th1 cells can kill and be killed, whereas Th2 cells can only be killed via Fas-mediated apoptotic mechanisms. Macrophages and B cells can also be killed by Th1 cells.

of aqueous antigens induces in vivo tolerance selectively or prevalently in Th1 cells.[355-357] This is probably because high doses of aqueous antigen administered parenterally are picked up and presented by APC that do not express costimulatory molecules. Thus defective expression of costimulators and/or defective production of IL-2 resulting from injection of high doses of aqueous antigens may account for the selective anergy inducible in Th1 cells. However, this does not represent the unique mechanism of Th1 tolerance. It has been suggested that neonatal tolerization may induce a vigorous unipolar Th2 response rather than tolerance in the immunological sense[131] (see above). The function of residual Th1 cells can indeed be rapidly suppressed by IL-10, which is produced by the newly developed Th2 cells and by TGF-β (Fig. 6.2). This possibility has also been clearly demonstrated by experiments showing induction of anergy or active suppression following oral antigen administration.[10,358] At high doses, oral antigen may induce deletion of antigen-specific T cells, which is mediated by apoptosis. Conditions for generating Th2 cell tolerance were different from those required to generate tolerance in Th1 cells: these included extended continuous exposure to high dosages of antigen, rather than a single or intermittent feeding regimen which was sufficient to induce tolerance in Th1 cells.[359] At lower doses, however, T cell deletion was not observed; instead, there was induction of antigen-specific cells that produced TGF-β, IL-4 and IL-10.[87,358] However, the role of Th2 cytokines in oral tolerance has been questioned.[360]

Fig. 6.2. Th1/Th2 cells and peripheral tolerance. Immunization with high doses of aqueous antigens induces anergy of Th1 cells, and therefore favors the expansion of Th2 cells. Cytokines produced by Th2 cells (mainly IL-10 and IL-4) suppress both the development and the activity of Th1 cells, thus further promoting the outcome of a Th2-dominated response.

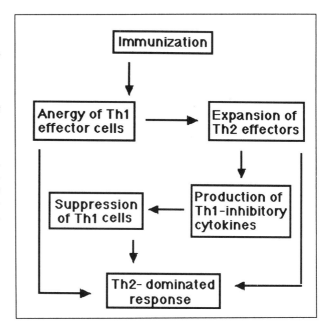

CHAPTER 7

ROLE OF TH1/TH2 CELLS IN PROTECTION AGAINST INFECTIOUS AGENTS

PROTOZOAN INFECTIONS

The outcome of a microbial infection is a dynamic process that depends on factors derived from both the microorganism and the host. In chronic human infections, the specific immune response to the pathogen may be of vital importance to host defense. However, an inappropriate response may not only result in lack of protection, it may even contribute to the induction of immunopathology. Thus, although at least some intracellular protozoan parasites are relatively harmless when they are met by an appropriate immune response, an inappropriate T cell response against them can cause severe diseases (Table 7.1).

LEISHMANIA MAJOR

Experimental infection with *L. major* is considered to be the simplest in vivo example for the existence of the Th1/Th2 paradigm. The first observation was that nonhealing BALB/c mice infected with *L. major* contained transcripts for IL-4 in their draining lymph node cells, in marked contrast to C57BL/6 mice that expressed transcripts for IFN-γ but not IL-4.[361] This finding was confirmed by studies demonstrating differences in cytokine production from parasite-specific T cell lines that were capable or incapable of transferring resistance.[362] The capacity of *L. major*-specific CD4+ T cells to passively transfer resistance or exacerbation of disease to immunodeficient or sublethally irradiated naive hosts correlated with their production of Th1 or Th2 cytokines, emphasizing the ability of only committed CD4+ T cells to confer the entire phenotype of the murine disease.[363] Although certain studies have suggested that some antigens with Th1- or Th2-type tendencies may account for such a difference,[138,159,364-367] the bulk of experimental data suggests both that most naive T cells have the potential to mature into

Table 7.1. Potential role of T-cell subsets in protozoan diseases

Protozoan	T-Cell Subset	Suggested Function
L. major	Th1	Protection
	Th2	Exacerbation
L. donovani	Th1	Protection ?
L. brasiliensis	Th1	Protection ?
T. gondi	Tc1, Th1	Protection
T. cruzi	Tc1, Th1	Protection
P. chabaudi		
erythrocyte	Th1 and Th2	Protection
cerebral	Th1	Immunopathology

either a subset of effector cells and that critical cytokines supplied at the time of T cell priming mediate this differentiation (Fig. 7.1). During the first few days after infection with *L. major* of both resistant and susceptible mice, a strong mixed response in the CD4[+] population consisting of IL-2, IL-4 and IL-13 (that peaks on day 4) can be observed. Importantly, however, healer strains rapidly downregulate IL-4 transcription, whereas BALB/c mice continue to express IL-4 levels consistent with Th2 cells.[366] Recently, however, the unique role for IL-4 in determining the susceptibility of BALB/c mice to infection with *L. major* has been questioned. Indeed, IL-4 gene knockout BALB/c mice, despite the absence of IL-4, remain susceptible to *L. major* infection.[368] Moreover, IL-4 gene disruption in 129 Sv x C57BL6 mice inhibited disease progression during *L. mexicana* infection but did not increase control of *L. donovani* infection.[369] On the other hand, IL-12 produced by infected macrophages, together with IFN-γ produced by NK cells, was found to be responsible for the development of the protective Th1 response in healer mice.[370-373] However, addition of IFN-γ to the parasite inoculum, although substantially reduced the IL-4 produced in BALB/c mice,[370] did not reverse the ultimate progressive course of disease.[186,370] By contrast, injection with anti-IL-4 antibody or IL-12 administered with infection could change the phenotype of susceptible BALB/c mice, provided that they were given within the first week of infection.[25,186,374] The injection of anti-IL-12 antibody abrogated healing in resistant C57BL/6 mice,[372] suggesting that endogenous IL-12 is required for effective control of infection. The IL-4 suppressive activity of IL-12 in susceptible mice was independent of IFN-γ, as demonstrated by using IFN-γ knockout mice or injection of anti-IFN-γ antibody,[165,170] and it was lost once naive CD4[+] T cells had differentiated to effector Th2 cells.[373] However, when BALB/c mice with established

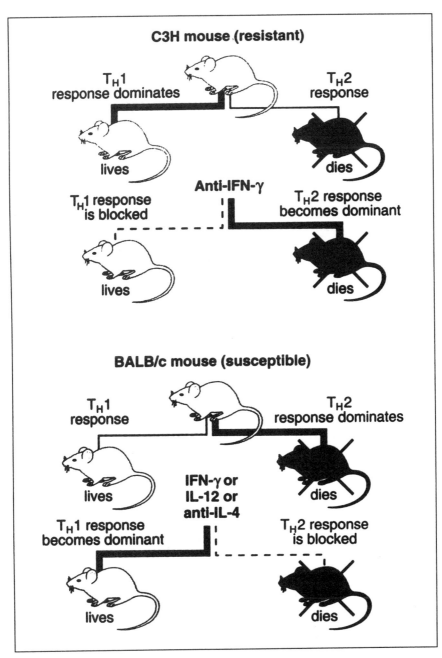

Fig. 7.1. The L. major *model of Th1/Th2 response. C3H strain mice infected with* L. major *develop a Th1-dominated response and are resistant to the disease. However, if C3H mice are injected with anti-IFN-γ antibody at the time of* L. major *infection they develop a Th2-dominated response and die. By contrast, BALB/c mice infected with* L. major *develop a Th2-dominated response and die; however, they mount a prevalent Th1 response and become resistant to* L. major *infection if injected with IFN-γ, IL-12 or anti-IL-4 antibody at the time of infection. Reprinted with permission from Romagnani S, Science & Medicine 1994; 1:68-77.[1]*

infection were treated with both IL-12 and Pentostam (a leishmanicidal drug), they were able to completely heal their lesions and became resistant to rechallenge infection.[375] The genetic ability of T cells from B10.D2 mice to maintain responsiveness to IL-12 has been found to play a major role in the resistance of this mouse strain in comparison with the BALB/c susceptible mice, whose T cells rapidly lose IL-12 responsiveness.[376] A possible explanation for the different behavior of susceptible and resistant mice may lie in the CD4⁺NK1⁺ T cell subset.[216] However, CD4⁺ T cells that provide early IL-4 in susceptible mice appear to be NK1⁻, suggesting that at least in this infection CD4⁺NK1⁺ cells do not contribute to the early IL-4 response.[225] Genetic analysis suggests indeed that both T cell and non-T cell compartments can independently determine resistance to *L. major*.[377] Interestingly, it has recently been shown that susceptibility of BALB/c mice to infection with *L. major* may also derive from the loss of ability to generate IL-12-induced Th1 responses rather than from an IL-4-induced Th2 response.[283] A single locus on chromosome 11 seems to regulate the differential maintenance of IL-12 responsiveness.[284] Other data suggest that the susceptible BALB/c mice carry a defect expressed in CD4⁺ T cells such that IL-4 production becomes overabundant during priming, perhaps due to a failure to suppress transcription or to unusual message stability.[366] Taken together, these findings underline the role of both genetic and environmental factors in determining the type of Th cell development and therefore the outcome of leishmanial infection. However, in spite of its apparent simplicity compared with other infections, there remain many unanswered questions about Th1 and Th2 cell subsets in this disease.

Attempts have been made to identify a role for Th1/Th2 dichotomy in the response of human CD4⁺ T cells to *Leishmania* parasites and to relate cytokine patterns to disease severity. Patients suffering from visceral leishmaniasis have elevated circulating levels of IL-4.[378] Furthermore, PBMC from patients with visceral leishmaniasis do not produce IFN-γ in response to stimulation with *Leishmania* antigens, due to the large production of IL-10.[379,380] In the early stages of infection with *L. donovani*, lack of IFN-γ production by PBMC predicts progression of the infection into fulminant visceral leishmaniasis, whereas individuals whose cells produce large amounts of IFN-γ usually remain asymptomatic.[381] More recently, it was found that individuals with a history of *L. major* infection, either as uncomplicated cutaneous leishmaniasis or as a subclinical infection, have strong Th1 responses to *Leishmania* antigens. By contrast, individuals cured from visceral leishmaniasis recognize Leishmania antigens both with Th1 and Th2 cells.[382] Analyses of mRNA for various cytokines have shown that Th1-type lymphokines are prevalent in the skin of patients with localized and mucocutaneous leishmaniasis, whereas in the skin of patients with diffuse, chronic or destructive forms of cutaneous leishmaniasis and in bone marrow of those with active visceral leishmaniasis increased mRNA expression of Th2-type lymphokines was found.[383-387] High concentrations of both IFN-γ and IL-10 were found in the serum of Sicilian patients with active visceral leishmaniasis that returned to the normal level following successful chemotherapy.[388] It is also noteworthy that IFN-γ in combination with pentavalent antimony was effective in treating patients with severe or refractory cases of visceral leishmaniasis.[389] Thus, there is now strong evidence for a correlation between differential activation of T cell subsets and severity of disease in human leishmaniasis. Thus, although the polarization of human T cell response into Th1 and Th2 is not as clear-cut as in the experimental animal system, probably due to both variations in the virulence and inoculum size of parasite strains and heterogeneity of the genetic background of the hosts, strategies based on the use of one or more immunodominant antigens,[159,390] in combination with IL-12 or an adjuvant capable of inducing endogenous IL-12, may be used in order to create successful vaccine candidates. Moreover, combination of IL-12 with suboptimal chemotherapeutic regimens may also be envisaged to redirect towards a more protective phenotype established effector response.

TOXOPLASMA GONDII

The intracellular protozoan *Toxoplasma gondii* (*T. gondii*) is a ubiquitous parasite of man and animals, which after infection remains indefinitely quiescent in the central nervous system (CNS) and other host tissues. The quiescent nature of chronic toxoplasmosis is attributed to the induction of strong CMI against *T. gondii*, which is crucially underscored in clinical situations of immunodeficiency. In particular, toxoplasmosis has emerged as a major opportunistic infection in patients with acquired immunodeficiency syndrome (AIDS).[391] Evidence has been accumulated in animal models of *T. gondii* infection to suggest that Th1 cells play a crucial role in establishing this protective immune response.[392]

In mice chronically infected with *T. gondii* stimulation of spleen cells with infected macrophages of soluble tachyzoite antigen results in high levels of IFN-γ production, whereas neither IL-4 nor IL-5 are evident. This apparent Th1 response has been shown to be the product of both CD4+ and CD8+ T cells.[393] In addition to CD8+ lymphocytes, NK cells have also been implicated as effector cells of IFN-γ dependent resistance to *T. gondii* in a model employing β2-microglobulin (β2m)knockout mice. These animals, despite their deficiency in CD8+ cells, display nearly the same level of resistance to *T. gondii* challenge as control littermates, due to the development of a population of NK1+ cells which replaced CD8+ T lymphocytes as the major effectors of IFN-γ dependent immunity.[394] Indeed, the production of IFN-γ was ablated by depletion of NK cells in vivo or in vitro, thereby revealing NK cells as the source of IFN-γ.[395,396] The selective Th1 induction in

T. gondii-infected animals depends on two main mechanisms. First, *T. gondii* infection induces the production of IL-12, TNF-α and IL-1β by macrophages.[393,395,396] Together IL-12 and TNF-α activate NK cells to produce IFN-γ. IL-1β also plays an important role in the IL-12-mediated stimulation of NK cell production of IFN-γ.[397] IFN-γ in turn activates macrophages to inhibit/kill parasite replication and to mediate nonspecific resistance to infection (Fig. 7.2). Thus, the activation of NK cells to synthesize IFN-γ early after infection appears to be the primary mechanism of IL-12-dependent resistance in *T. gondii*-infected SCID mice. In conventional mice the effects of early IL-12 are likely to be pleiotropic, including NK cells, as well as CD4+, CD8+ and γδ T cell populations. In particular, the early presence of IL-12 and IFN-γ influences the development of T cells toward a Th1 type response, which is also associated with protective immunity to intracellular parasites.[392] In contrast to other intracellular parasites, however, production of monokines in response to *T. gondii* occurs independently of IFN-γ, but is clearly augmented when IFN-γ is present.[398] Indeed, early IL-12 production was also detected in *T. gondii*-infected IFN-γ knockout mice confirming the IFN-γ independence of IL-12 induction by this pathogen.[399] The importance of both IL-12 and IFN-γ in determining the protective Th1 pattern seen in *T. gondii* infection was also supported by the demonstration that neutralization of either cytokine during acute infection resulted in the appearance of IL-4 production together with uncontrolled parasite growth leading to death of the animals.[398] Thus, in contrast to infection with *L. major*, early IL-4 production appears to be universally suppressed in the case of *T. gondii* and cannot exert a genetically regulated effect on CD4+ differentiation.[392] The second mechanism involved in the Th1 induction is related to the presence in the pathogen of a superantigen capable of expanding Vβ5+ T cells. Interestingly, the Vβ5+ population expanded in vitro is predominantly CD8+ and produces high levels of IFN-γ,[392] which may provide an additional source of early IFN-γ important in driving T cell differentiation toward the Th1 phenotype. While the mechanisms responsible for the initiation of innate and adaptive immunity to *T. gondii* are sufficiently clear, those involved in maintaining IFN-γ-dependent immunity during chronic infection have not yet been clarified. Thus, while neutralization of IFN-γ at 4 weeks of infection results in rapid reactivation of latent infection, anti-IL-12 treatment at the same stage fails to increase parasite mortality and in vitro neutralization of IL-12 in spleen cell cultures from chronically infected mice does not substantially affect the levels of Th1 and Th2 cytokines produced in these cultures.[398]

IL-12 production and function is also tightly regulated during *T. gondii* infection. A role for TGF-β in limiting the action of IL-12 is suggested by the demonstration that a TGF-β-specific neutralizing

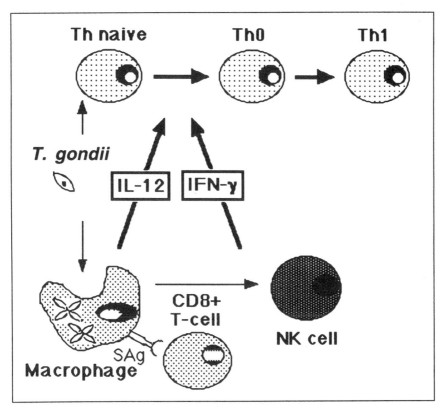

Fig. 7.2. The T. gondii *model of Th1 response. The selection of Th1 responses by* T. gondii *is dependent on the interaction of the parasite with macrophages, NK cells and CD8+ T cells, which produce the Th1-differentiating cytokines IL-12 and IFN-γ. Reprinted with permission from Jankovic D et al, Chem Immunol 1996; 63:51-65.*[392]

antibody increased IFN-γ synthesis by *T. gondii*-exposed SCID spleen cell cultures.[400] More importantly, the therapeutic effects of recombinant IL-12 in *T. gondii*-infected SCID mice were abolished by simultaneous treatment with anti-TGF-β, suggesting that endogenous TGF-β may antagonize IL-12 function via its ability to inhibit NK cell-derived IFN-γ synthesis during *T. gondii* infection.[399] Another major regulator of IL-12 production and function during *T. gondii* infection is IL-10. IL-10-knockout mice succumb to acute infection, not because of rapid tachyzoite growth, but rather with the overproduction of inflammatory cytokines (IL-12, TNF-α, IFN-γ) during the first week of infection. Indeed, treatment of these animals with anti-IFN-γ antibody at day 5 significantly prolongs their survival. Based on these findings, it has been postulated that both IL-10 and TFG-β are stimulated by the parasite to prevent the host-detrimental effects of excessive Th1 cytokine and monokine production.[399,401]

PLASMODIUM

Multiple immune mechanisms are involved in controlling malaria infection and these vary depending upon the stage of parasite development. Humoral immunity can protect in blocking merozoite invasion of erythrocytes and attack their differentiated forms that infect mosquitoes (gametocytes). CMI is directed primarily against the infected hepatocyte, but can also act against blood stages. The mechanism of CMI is not clear at present, but it could occur as a result of direct contact between the T cell and the hepatocyte, with resultant lysis or apoptotic death of the hepatocyte, or through the release of cytokines, which induce the hepatocyte to produce substances toxic for the parasite. At least in the models of experimental infection, both Th1 and Th2 cells may be involved in the cytokine response. By adoptive transfer of cloned T cell lines, direct evidence was provided that both Th1 and Th2 subsets of CD4+ T cells can protect mice against *Plasmodium chabaudi* (*P. chabaudi*) infection.[402,403] Th2 clones derived after further exposure to parasite appear to be as protective as Th1 clones derived at a relatively early stage of infection, suggesting that immunity to *P. chabaudi* is a biphasic process.[404] In the host resistance to blood-stage *P. chabaudi*, the early Th1 activation mediates NO-dependent mechanisms which are toxic to the parasite[405] and resolve the acute parasitaemia, while the later Th2 cell activation mediates B cell activation and strong malaria-specific IgG_1 production to clear and sterilize the infection by antibody dependent mechanims.[406] The presence of B cells is critical for switching the balance between CD4+ T cells from Th1 to Th2 and eliminating the infection.[407] As in the *L. major* model, high levels of IFN-γ were detected during the early phase of the infection in (resistant) C57BL/6 mice, while higher levels of IL-4 transcripts were detected in the spleens of (susceptible) A/J mice.[403] Moreover, administration of low doses of recombinant IL-12 to susceptible A/J mice during the first week of infection promoted an increase in resistance. Conversely, treatment of resistant C57BL/6 mice with anti-IL-12 antibody resulted in higher parasitaemia. Injection of IL-12 also protected BALB/c mice against a nonlethal strain of *P. yoelii*, a highly infectious agent of malaria in rodents.[408] The IL-12-induced protection against blood-stage *P. chabaudi* AS requires both IFN-γ and TNF-α.[409] Likewise, protection against *P. yoelii* was eliminated in all mice by administration of an anti-IFN-γ antibody and in 50% of mice by a competitive inhibitor of inducible NO synthase.[410] Of note is that cerebral complications of malaria also are probably due to the activity of IFN-γ and TNF-α and therefore associate with the protective Th1 response.[411] Thus, the T cell subset involved in pathology is the same as that implicated in protection.

In human malaria, epidemiological data suggest that individuals at risk of major complications, including severe anemia and cerebral malaria, are those who contract the disease for the first time, or who have been only slightly exposed to the parasite and develop important CMI responses. In the early phase of *P. falciparum* sporozoite-induced human infection, a predominant Th1 response appears, as revealed by a brisk increase in IFN-γ in the sera of infected volunteers before fever or an increase in C-reactive protein,[412,413] as well as by the high levels of IFN-γ in the serum of children living in endemic areas.[414] The Th1 response in naive people probably represents the main mechanism responsible for protection. Indeed, IFN-γ levels decrease drastically after the age of eight, the age of acquisition of premunition, whereas IL-4 becomes detectable.[414] In some individuals, however, the massive activation of Th1 cells leads to the overproduction of IFN-γ and especially of TNF-α, the key cytokine involved in cerebral malaria.[411] Both IFN-γ and TNF-α contribute to the upregulation of adhesion molecules on brain microvascular endothelial cells, which in turn allow for the sequestration of either parasitized erythrocytes or activated leukocytes and increase platelet adherence and fusion to endothelial cells.[415] Conditions and intensity of stimulation, quality of parasite antigens, duration of activation, as well as site of inappropriate activation of these cells may be among the crucial parameters that will determine the balance between protection and pathology.[416]

CRYPTOSPORIDIUM

Cryptosporidium parvum (C. parvum) is a parasitic protozoan that invades intestinal epithelial cells of human and numerous domesticated and wild animals. Suckling mice are considerably more susceptible to *C. parvum* infection than adults, and both CD4⁺ T cells and IFN-γ have roles in protecting mice against infection.[417] In BALB/c mice there was a correlation between the development of immunity to *C. muris* infection and the production of cytokines. IFN-γ and IL-2 were detected on day 14 after infection and their concentrations increased between day 21 and 26, whereas IL-4 was not detected until day 21.[418] Recently, it has been shown that treatment of immunodeficient neonatal or immunocompetent mice with a single dose of IL-12 prevented the establishment of *C. parvum* infection through a IFN-γ-dependent mechanism, whereas treatment of *C. parvum*-infected animals with exogenous IL-12 did not terminate, and only measurably ameliorated, *C. pervum* infection.[419]

BACTERIAL INFECTIONS

Bacteria represent a heterogenous family of pathogens that in a very simplified scheme can be grouped as follows: (1) toxin-producing bacteria; (2) extracellular bacteria; and (3) intracellular bacteria. Each group of bacteria causes the host a different problem of protection. In the case of toxin-producing bacteria (e.g., *Clostridium botulinum, Corynebacterium diphteriae*) the most important problem is not the elimination of the pathogen, but rather toxin neutralization, which may be introduced into the body even independently of infection. Therefore, toxin neutralization by specific antibodies is of central importance for protection against toxin-producing bacteria. Extracellular bacteria (e.g., gram-negative and gram-positive cocci and many enterobacteriaceae) cause an acute-type disease soon after host invasion due to various harmful factors which promote their colonization and invasion. Once specific antibodies have been produced against these structures, bacteria are opsonized, phagocytozed and rapidly killed by professional phagocytes, resulting in a purulent reaction in the site of destruction; therefore, the production of opsonizing and complement-fixing antibodies is central to protection against extracellular bacteria. Intracellular bacteria (e.g., *L. monocytogenes, Mycobacteria, Salmonellae*) are capable of surviving within mononuclear phagocytes or other host cells, a lifestyle which makes these pathogens insensitive to antibody attacks and enables T lymphocytes to be central to protection via the activation of antibacterial capacities in the infected macrophages. An optimum host response against such diverse microbial strategies demands for highly specialized reactions which are primarily controlled by CD4 Th-cell subsets (Table 7.2).

LEISTERIA MONOCYTOGENES

L. monocytogenes is a gram-positive bacillus, which belongs to the group of facultative intracellular bacteria. All the main T cell subsets, CD4$\alpha\beta^+$, CD8$\alpha\beta^+$ and $\gamma\delta^+$ cells, as well as NK cells, contribute to optimal protection against *L. monocytogenes*. According to their cytokine profile, *L. monocytogenes*-reactive CD4$^+$ cells almost exclusively belong to the Th1 subset.[420] The predominance of Th1 cells in leisteriosis can be attributed to innate immune responses at the

Table 7.2. Potential role of T-cell subsets in bacterial diseases

Bacterium	T-Cell Subset	Suggested Function
L. monocytogenes	Tc1, Th1	Protection
M. tuberculosis	Tc1, Th1	Protection
M. bovis (B.C.G.)	Tc1, Th1	Protection
M. leprae		
TT	Tc1, Th1	Protection
LL	Tc2, Th2	Susceptibility
B. Burgdorferi	Th2	Protection
	Th1	Immunopathology
B. pertussis	Th1	Protection
Chlamydia	Th1	Protection

onset of infection. *L. monocytogenes*-infected macrophages produce IL-12 which effectively activates NK cells to secrete IFN-γ,[421] and depletion of IL-12 renders mice more susceptible to listeriosis.[147,421] IL-1β seems to be important in favoring the IL-12-mediated stimulation of NK cell production of IFN-γ,[367] and IFN-γ itself exerts a potent amplification loop for IL-12 production.[422] TNF-α also plays a protective role in the innate immunity against *L. monocytogenes*, inasmuch as its neutralization results in increased susceptibility to *L. monocytogenes* infection.[423] By contrast, IL-10, which is produced by *L. monocytogenes*-infected macrophages especially in the presence of immune complexes or PGE$_2$,[423,424] inhibits the production of IFN-γ by NK cells by altering their ability to respond to either IL-12 or TNF-α.[425] Neutrophils, which are also capable of producing IL-12, participate in the protection provided by the innate immunity mainly by favoring the lysis of infected hepatocytes in early infection.[426] Experiments performed in TCRδ knockout mice suggest that γδ⁺ cells also provide help for IFN-γ production.[278]

The sterilizing immunity against *L. monocytogenes*, however, requires the activation of the adaptive cellular immunity with the generation of antigen-specific CD4⁺ lymphocytes showing a Th1 cytokine profile,[427] and the macrophage-derived IL-12 is the main inducer for the development of *L. monocytogenes*-specific naive Th cells into the Th1 phenotype.[147] IL-12 levels in IFN-γ receptor-knockout mice were even higher than in wild mice, suggesting that compensatory mechanisms had evolved in the absence of IFN-γ receptivity. Indeed, IFN-γ (and in its absence IFN-α) is also involved in the process of Th1 differentiation, probably by augmenting production of IL-12 and TNF-α by macrophages.[171] In contrast to primary response, however, secondary response to *L. monocytogenes* infection still requires IFN-γ, but is partially independent of IL-12.[425] Although the mouse model suggests that resistant mice are protected because of strong Th1 responses,[428] genetic differences in natural resistance of mouse strains seem to correlate with the level of IL-4 produced.[429] IL-4 is produced early in listeriosis, and probably plays an inhibitory role in the initial cellular immune response. In fact, administration of anti-IL-4 antibody enhances the resistance of mice to *L. monocytogenes* infection.[428] However, IL-4 is produced in low concentrations and by cells other than Th2 cells.[430,431] A possible source of early IL-4 production in leisteriosis may be CD4⁺ NK1.1⁺ cells. These cells indeed disappear soon after infection with *L. monocytogenes* and this effect can be partially reversed by neutralization of IL-12 with specific antibody and mimicked by administration of recombinant IL-12.[221] It, therefore, appears that IL-4-producing cells are not simply ignored in leisteriosis, but rather actively impaired. In addition to IL-4, IL-10 appears to be involved in the regulation of early immune responses to *L. monocytogenes*. In fact, macrophages from *L. monocytogenes*-infected mice produce IL-10 and IL-10 neutralization renders mice more resistant to *L. monocytogenes* during the early phase, whereas at later stages this treatment impairs bacterial clearance.[432] In conclusion, experimental leisteriosis is characterized by an almost exclusive Th1 response and even interferes with Th2 stimulation.

MYCOBACTERIA

Mycobacteria are a group of ubiquitous intracellular bacteria that include a few pathogenic species, such as *M. tuberculosis*, *M. bovis*, *M. leprae* and *M. avium*. These bacteria are readily taken up by macrophages and during the first weeks their numbers are mainly controlled by nonspecific resistance, but 2-3 weeks later protective immunity develops.[433] However, mycobacteria employ various strategies to evade the bactericidal mechanisms of their host cells and they are usually not completely eradicated, resulting in a balanced state between host immunity and persistent pathogens. Thus, when immune surveillance is insufficient or depressed, *M. tuberculosis* organisms multiply and severe disseminated infection develops.[434] Leprosy appears as spectral disease with several clinical forms ranging between two extreme poles. Tuberculoid leprosy (TT) is characterized by few *M. leprae* organisms in skin lesions and development of effective CMI, while an enormous load of *M. leprae* organisms in the skin, and suppressed immunity, is typical for lepromatous leprosy (LL).[435] Likewise, tuberculosis can manifest as reactive or unreactive disease.

Although all three T cell subsets, CD4$\alpha\beta^+$, CD8$\alpha\beta^+$ and $\gamma\delta^+$ cells, participate in optimal protection against mycobacteria,[436,437] activation of macrophages and blood monocytes, which is the central step in the elimination of mycobacteria, crucially depends on both the Th1-type cytokine IFN-γ and TNF-α.[438-441] Unequivocal proof for a vital role of IFN-γ was provided by use of IFN-γ or IFN-γ-receptor gene disruption mutant mice, which are highly susceptible to *M. tuberculosis* and *M. Bovis* BCG infections and develop disseminated disease.[440,442] TNF-α production is also required for protection.[441] Although protection against mycobacterial infections are predominantly controlled by Th1 cells, Th2-type cytokines have been detected during infection with *M. tuberculosis* or *M. Bovis*. It has been suggested that Th1 and Th2 responses in the mouse do not occur simultaneously. Rather it appears that Th1-type cytokines dominate the first (protective) phase of *M. tuberculosis* infection, whereas Th2-type cytokines lead to detrimental effects in the late phase of infection.[443] Interestingly, activation of IL-4-producing cells was seen after infection with *M. bovis* or vaccination with killed, but not live, BCG.[446]

The role of IFN-γ in controlling human mycobacterial infections is stressed by the observations that: (1) treatment of patients suffering from disseminated *M. avium* infections with recombinant IFN-γ in addition to chemotherapy caused clinical improvement and (2) local administration of IFN-γ induces marked bacterial clearance in LL lesions.[445]

The protective role of Th1 cells in human mycobacterial infections is also indirectly supported by the demonstration that PPD-specific CD4$^+$ T cells from healthy individuals usually develop into Th1 clones.[18,20] Accordingly, there is preferential mRNA expression of Th1-type cells (IFN-γ^+, IL-2$^+$) in classic DTH reactions in human skin.[447] The kinetics and frequencies of cytokine-producing cells were also studied by immunofluorescent visualization of intracellular cytokines in healthy individuals vaccinated with BCG. Early, at days 4 and 5, there was a marked production of Th1 cytokines, IL-2, IFN-γ and TNF-β, but late in the reaction, at days 10-12, a Th2 response with IL-4, IL-5 and IL-10 was detected, whereas the synthesis of Th1 cytokines and monokines declined.[448] Finally, bioactive IL-12 was detectable in supernatants of pleural fluid cells stimulated with *M. tuberculosis*.[449] However, *Mycobacterium*-reactive T cell clones from health donors, as well as PPD-specific T cell clones generated from cells present in the pleural fluid of patients with *M. tuberculosis* infection can exhibit a Th0-like profile (ref. 450 and De Carli et al, unpublished). Moreover, Th2-type cytokines have been detected during infection with *M. tuberculosis* or *M. bovis*, although at low levels.[433,443] These data clearly demonstrate that IFN-γ is the major cytokine induced by mycobacteria in healthy individuals, but also suggest that Th2 cytokines participate in the response. Both protective and detrimental functions have been associated with Th2-type cytokines. IL-4 and IL-6 may contribute to protective immunity, as shown by inhibition of mycobacterial growth in murine bone marrow macrophages, which had been treated with IL-4 or IL-6 after infection with *M. bovis*.[451] Yet, Th2-type cytokines also indicate progression of infection, since PBMC from tuberculosis patients with active disease produce elevated levels of IL-4.[452,453] Moreover, IL-10 neutralization augments mouse resistance to systemic *M. avium* infection.[454] Recently, we have looked at the presence of sCD30 in the serum of a number of tuberculosis patients as possible indicator of predominant and persistent Th2-cell activation. Significantly higher levels of sCD30 were found in the sera of patients with stage III-IV (unreactive) in comparison with patients with stage I-II (reactive) tuberculosis (unpublished data), suggesting that the Th2-dominated responses against *M. tuberculosis* result in more severe and long-lasting disease. Other findings, however, do not support this hypothesis. Although *M. tuberculosis*-induction of Th1 cytokines IFN-γ and IL-2 is depressed in tuberculous patients, compared to healthy tuberculin reactors,[453,455] tuberculosis patients had no enhanced mRNA expression or production of the Th2 cytokines IL-4, IL-10 and IL-13, suggesting that the reduced Th1 response is not mediated by a strong Th2 response.[455] The Th1 response in tuberculosis may be depressed through mechanisms independent of Th2 cells, such as disregulation of costimulatory molecules, anergized Th1 cells and enhanced production of immunosuppressive monokines, including TGF-β.[456]

PBMC from healthy leprosy household contacts usually produce IFN-γ when restimulated with PPD in vitro, whereas those from persons who subsequently developed active disease fail to do so.[457] Activated CD4+ *M. leprae*-reactive T cell clones derived from TT patients exhibit a clear-cut Th1 profile.[20] Expression of IL-2 and IFN-γ mRNA, but not IL-4, IL-5 and IL-10, mRNA is detected in skin lesions of patients with TT, whereas in skin lesions of LL patients, mRNA for IL-4, IL-5 and IL-10 is readily detectable, suggesting a prevalence of Th1 reactions in TT and a prevalence of Th2 reactions in LL.[22,458] Accordingly, high expression of CD26, which has been considered an operational Th1 marker, was found in TT in contrast to no or very little expression in LL.[44] However, no difference in the accumulation of CD30-positive cells between the tuberculoid and lepromatous form of leprosy was found.[51] Moreover, while these patterns are observed in skin lesions, the situation in the peripheral blood of leprosy patients is different, and Th1 responses are found across the whole leprosy spectrum. Based on all these data, the following possibility may be suggested: as long as Th1 reactions predominate in the response to mycobacteria, the bacterial number can be controlled and the host appears asymptomatic or suffers from a milder form of disease. However, if the balance shifts toward the Th2 cells, severe and chronic forms of disease develop. So far it is not known which parameters determine whether infection with mycobacteria results in protective (Th1-mediated) immunity or severe (Th2-dominated) infection. Genetic predisposition and/or early immune responses may be involved. The fact that 10-fold IL-12 is produced by TT patients than compared to LL patients suggests a critical role for IL-12 in this scenario.[459,460] IL-12, indeed, increases resistance of BALB/c mice to *M. avium* [461] and to *M. tuberculosis* infection, but this occurs only in the presence of IFN-γ since its activity is abolished in mice in which the IFN-γ gene has been disrupted.[462] Some mycobacteria, such as *M. bovis* BCG, almost exclusively stimulate Th1 responses, suggesting some role for the pathogen in the early induction of IL-12 production, even though after the initial Th1 response a switch to the production of Th2 cytokines seems to occur.[448] In contrast, *M. tuberculosis* and especially *M. leprae* can concomitantly activate both Th1 and Th2 reactions and, at least with regard to the *M. leprae*, the developed Th phenotype is stable and uninfluenced by related antigens of the microbe.[458] Thus, in these infections, host genetic differences in the early innate immune system may act as a decisive control point of the ensuing specific immune response (Fig. 7.3).

Borrelia Burgdorferi

Borrelia burgdorferi (*B. burgdorferi*) is a gram-negative spirochete that can cause Lyme disease (also called Lyme borreliosis) in humans.

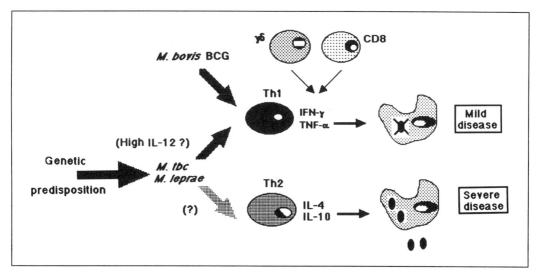

Fig. 7.3. Schematic representation of the mechanisms governing cellular immune response against Mycobacteria. Infection with M. bovis BCG generally results in a Th1 response, whereas infection with M. tuberculosis (tbc) or M. leprae may result either in a prevalent Th1 or Th2 response, probably according to different genetic predisposition. In subjects showing a Th1 response, protection is provided through the activation of bactericidal macrophages by both IFN-γ and TNF-α and results in mild or no disease. CD8⁺ T cells and γδ⁺ T cells also participate in the protective response. In subjects showing Th2-dominated responses, severe and chronic disease develops.

Since *B. burgdorferi* is an extracellular bacterium, antibodies play an important role in protective immunity. However, *B. burgdorferi*-reactive Th1-type CD4⁺ T cells seem to be involved in the pathogenesis of Lyme disease. CD4⁺ T cell clones generated from the sinovial fluid of patients with Lyme arthritis produce IFN-γ, but not IL-4 or IL-5.[21] Second, in experimentally induced Lyme arthritis, lymph nodes from C3H susceptible mice that develop a severe disease produce IFN-γ, whereas lymph nodes from BALB/c susceptible mice that develop only mild symptoms produce IL-4.[463,464] Administration of recombinant IL-4 to susceptible CH3 mice augments resistance to *B. burgdorferi* infection.[464] Finally, neutralization of IL-4 in resistant BALB/c mice resulted in more severe arthritis whereas neutralization of IFN-γ in susceptible C3H mice attenuated the severity of disease.[465] Thus, the same Th1 cells seem to be responsible for both protection (via the production of opsonizing and complement-activating antibodies) and immunopathology.

Yersinia Enterocolitica

Yersinia enterocolitica (*Y. enterocolitica*) is a gram-negative enterobacterium which causes enteritis, lymphadenitis or sepsis, and reactive arthritis in genetically selected (HLA-B27) individuals. Mouse strains

are naturally resistant or susceptible to *Y. enterocolitica* and early production of IFN-γ is associated with resistance to infection, whereas
lower concentrations of IFN-γ are found in susceptible strains.[466,467]
Yet, administration of anti-IL-4 antibody before or during infection
increases resistance to *Y. enterocolitica* in susceptible strains.[466] Treatment of *Y. enterocolitica*-infected cells with IFN-γ or IL-4 in vitro inhibits or promotes bacterial growth, respectively.[468] IL-12 is essential
for resistance against *Y. enterocolitica* by triggering IFN-γ production
in NK cells and CD4⁺ T cells.[469]

The situation in humans is slightly different. Reactive arthritis
develops after *Y. enterocolitica* infection has cleared, i.e., in resistant
individuals, and *Y. enterocolitica*-reactive T cell clones from the inflamed
joints of patients with reactive arthritis produce IFN-γ but no IL-4,
i.e., they are of the Th1 type.[468,470] Thus, *Y. enterocolitica*-reactive Th1
cells seem to be at the same time protective against the pathogen and
responsible for the immunopathological reaction at articular level.

CHLAMIDIA TRACHOMATIS

The intracellular obligate bacterium *C. trachomatis* is the etiologic
agent of trachoma and genito-urinary infection. *C. trachomatis* microorganisms are taken up as infectious extracellular elementary bodies
by host cells, and then multiply and differentiate into intracellular re-
ticulate bodies. Anti-*C. trachomatis* antibodies are detected in the sera
of infected individuals, but protective immunity is mainly mediated
by both CD4⁺ and CD8⁺ T lymphocytes.[471,472] The majority of human
C. trachomatis-reactive CD4⁺ and CD8⁺ T cell clones produce IFN-γ,
but about one-third of them also produce IL-4,[472,473] suggesting that
immunity to *C. trachomatis* is dominated by Th1 cells with some
contribution of Th0 cells.

BORDETELLA PERTUSSIS

Bordetella pertussis (*B. pertussis*), another gram-negative bacterium,
is the etiologic agent of whooping cough. Resistance to *B. pertussis*
seems to correlate with specific antibodies, but complete bacterial clearance depends on CMI. Vaccination of mice with the whole cell vaccine induces a high degree of protection, and stimulated T cells produce IFN-γ and IL-2, but no IL-4.[474,475] Likewise, pertussis toxin
(PT)-specific CD4⁺ T cell clones generated from normal individuals
(who had suffered from natural immunization) show a clear-cut Th1
profile.[476] In contrast, antigen-specific T cells derived from mice immunized with the acellular vaccine were almost exclusively of the Th2
cell type.[477,478] Moreover, soluble PT represents a good adjuvant for
Th2 cells causing especially IgE antibody production.[479,480] Yet, it also
induces IFN-γ and IL-4 production in immunized mice.[481] These data
suggest that despite the Th2-inducing property of PT, the whole
microrganism is able to activate the Th1-inducing potential of the invaded

macrophage. Thus, both Th1 and Th2 cells may be involved in order to achieve optimum mucosal protection against *B. pertussis*, even if their respective role is not yet clearly defined.

BRUCELLA ABORTUS

The gram-negative bacterium *Brucella abortus* (*B. abortus*) is a facultative intracellular parasite responsible for a chronic granulomatous infection of cattle that can be transmitted to man through direct contact with contaminated meat, dairy products or still-borne fetuses. If *B. abortus* microrganisms are not confined in draining lymph nodes, severe lesions systemically develop in infected tissues.[482] Both CD4+ and CD8+ T cells contribute to protection against *B. abortus* and IFN-γ certainly plays a crucial role in the resolution of *B. abortus* infection. First, IFN-γ is able to activate antibacterial functions of *B. abortus*-infected macrophages.[483] Second, administration of IFN-γ prior to infection increases resistance to *B. abortus* in mice, whereas IFN-γ neutralization enhances mouse susceptibility to infection.[484,485] *B. abortus* has indeed been found to preferentially stimulate Th1 cells in vivo,[486] whereas IL-10 downmodulates CMI to *B. abortus*, as shown by elevated IFN-γ levels in anti-IL-10-treated spleen cells, and decreased bacterial loads in anti-IL-10-treated *B. abortus*-infected mice.[487] A preventive role of anti-IgG2a antibody directed against a major surface antigen of *B. abortus* has also been demonstrated, whereas IgG1 antibodies only diminish infection.[488,489] Inasmuch as production of the IgG2a isotype is induced by Th1 cells, it is obvious that protective immunity to *B. abortus* strongly depends on Th1 cells both at the cellular and the humoral levels.

SALMONELLA SPECIES

The gram-negative enterobacteriaceae *Salmonella typhy* (*S. typhy*), *S. paratyphy* and *S. thyphimurium* are facultative intracellular pathogens responsible for human or murine typhoid, respectively. Innate resistance in the early phase of infection as well as adaptive immunity in the later phase contribute to the protection against *Salmonella* infections. Nude mice are indeed initially resistant to *S. typhimurium*, but fail to control disease in the late phase of infection.[490] Both CD4+ and CD8+ T cells can adoptively transfer resistance to *S. typhimurium*, whereas depletion of both CD4+ and CD8+ T cells does not affect resistance during the first 2 weeks, but in both cases infection is exacerbated at later stages.[490] Production of IFN-γ, IFN-α and TNF-α seems to play a major role in immunity to these pathogens.[491-494] Mice infected orally with the attenuated *S. dublin* strain exhibit early expression of IL-12 mRNA in the Peyer's patches and in the mesenteric lymph nodes.[495] In vivo neutralization of IL-12 reduced host resistance to virulent oral challenge with *S. typhimurium*.[496] Finally, recombinant *S. typhimurium* expressing a leishmanial surface protein, or tetanus toxoid, induces protective Th1 responses.[497,498] Taken together, these findings suggest a preferential stimulation of Th1 cells in immunity to *Salmonella*.

LEGIONELLA PNEUMOPHILA

The facultative intracellular bacterium *Legionella pneumophila* (*L. pneumophila*) is amoebae's parasite when living in water, but its airborne-transmitted infection especially in older or immunocompromised individuals results in severe pneumonia, known as 'Legionaires disease.' Since in the infected individuals *L. pneumophila* lives and replicates within macrophages, protective responses against *L. pneumophila* are mainly based on NK cells and specific T cells able to produce IFN-γ, which can activate bactericidal mechanisms of *L. pneumophila*-infected macrophages.[499,500] Interestingly, immunity to *L. pneumophila* is suppressed by delta-9-tetrahy-drocannabinol (THC), the psychoactive component of marijuana, which is also able to induce IL-4 secretion by spleen cells in vitro.[501,502] Thus, there is evidence, although indirect, to suggest that the protective immunity against *L. pneumophila* is mainly mediated by Th1 cells.

FRANCISELLA TULARENSIS

The gram-negative bacterium *Francisella tularnesis* (*F. tularensis*) is the etiologic agent of human tularemia, which is transmitted by direct contact with infected wild mammals, especially rabbits, or by insect bites. Tularemia usually starts as a local skin ulcer, but after bacteria have reached draining lymph nodes hematogenic dissemination leads to severe systemic infection. Protective immunity against *F. tularensis* is probably based on different mechanisms, including innate resistance, humoral immunity and CMI. Both CD4+ and CD8+ T cells contribute to immunity, but even in the absence of both subsets, mice are able to control (but not to resolve) the infection, thus suggesting a major role for innate resistance. Accordingly, an attenuated live *F. tularensis* vaccine available in humans, which stimulates T cells and the production of IFN-γ, IL-2 and TNF-α, does not ensure absolute protection.[503,504] Transfer of immune serum to naive mice does not protect by itself, but increases resistance to challenge with this vaccine suggesting an ancillary role for humoral immunity.[505] However, the main role in protection is played by Th1 cytokines. Treatment of mice with anti-IFN-γ or anti-TNF-α antibodies prior to infection exacerbates disease, whereas administration of anti-IL-4 antibody does not significantly alter resistance.[506] Analysis of cytokine mRNAs in the liver of infected mice revealed expression of IFN-γ, TNF-α, IL-10 and IL-12, but no IL-4.[507] Taken together, these findings suggest a major role for Th1 cells in protective immunity to *F. tularensis*.

RICKETTSIA SPECIES

All members of the genus *Rickettsia* (*R.*) are obligate intracellular parasites transmitted to men or animals by bites of infected insects. Although the diagnosis of rickettsial diseases is based on the detection of specific antibodies in the serum, the protective immunity mainly depends on CMI responses sustained by Th1 cells. In the murine model of infection with *R. tsutsugamushi*, IFN-γ production appears to be necessary for the activation of bactericidal mechanisms of macrophages in vitro and also plays a critical protective role in vivo.[508,509] Moreover, protective immunity could be transferred by a CD4+ T cell line showing a Th1-like phenotype,[509] and an epitope of the 47 kD membrane antigen of *R. tsutsugamushi* stimulates the proliferation of Th1 cells.[510]

TREPONEMA PALLIDUM

Infection with the spirochete *Treponema pallidum* (*T. pallidum*) evokes a Th1-type response. Both primary and secondary syphilis lesions contain indeed mRNA for IL-12, IFN-γ, but not for IL-4, IL-5 and IL-13.[511] The protective Th1 response, however, may be downregulated because of the potent activity of *T. pallidum* in inducing macrophage production of PGE_2. This may result in selection for Th2 predominance accounting for effective stimulation of B cell responses to a variety of treponemal epitopes. Th2 lymphokines, such as IL-4 and IL-10, could further dampen Th1 capabilities. The few remaining treponemes that escaped the activated macrophages must multiply slowly, possibly held in check by the high levels of antibody. This pathway would explain the early resolution of the acute infection and the establishment of lifelong chronic infection.[512]

In conclusion, a growing body of evidence suggests that the human immune response to bacterial infections is mediated by T cell subpopulations secreting specific cytokine patterns. In general, the proper opponent of bacterial toxins is the Th2 cell, which produces cytokines that favor B cell maturation and production of appropriate antibody isotypes. In contrast, Th1 cells produce cytokines which activate macrophage and cytolytic T cells for protection against intracellular bacteria. Combat of extracellular bacteria involves antibodies which first neutralize invasion and adhesion factors and second opsonize bacteria for phagocytosis. Probably, these bacteria are best counteracted by a combination of Th2 and Th1-type cytokines, e.g., by Th0 cells. The predominance of the Th1 or Th2 phenotype is probably modulated by both the pathogen and the genetic background of the host, and the decisive control point is the response of the innate immunity. Bacteria possess indeed several components that trigger IL-12 production by macrophages at the very outset of infection, thus favoring the Th1 development. These 'Th1 inducers' include the lipoarabinomannan of mycobacteria, teichoic acids of gram-positive bacteria and LPS of gram-negative bacteria. In this regard, it is of interest that lipoteichoic acid preparations of gram-positive bacteria have recently been found to be able to induce IL-12 production by macrophages through a CD14-dependent pathway.[513] Bacterial components which preferentially stimulate Th2 cell development are chemically less well-defined. The role of genetic differences in the production of IL-12 and other 'natural' cytokines, the expression and function of their receptors, as well as of other costimulatory molecules that contribute to determine the ensuing specific immune response also remains to be clarified. It also appears that strong and/or persistent Th1 responses against bacteria may often result in genetically predisposed individuals in immunopathological reactions.

FUNGAL INFECTIONS

CANDIDA ALBICANS

Infection by *Candida albicans* (*C. albicans*) has certainly been the best-studied fungal infection with respect to the Th1/Th2 paradigm. Th1-biased underlying immunity and Th1 cytokines (IL-2 and IFN-γ) characterize mice with mucosal yeast colonization,[514,515] a condition that simulates the saprophytic yeast carriage of healthy human subjects. Interfacial and hence continuously critical in the mucosal association between the yeast and its host, the role of Th1 cells becomes operative in deep-seated systemic infections when recruitment of antigen-specific lymphocytes and locally high cytokine concentrations are needed for full expression of the anti-candidal potential of nonspecific effectors. Indeed, any alteration leading to suppressed Th1 function may result in impaired ability to control infectivity of the yeast, focus an infection, or clear the yeast from infected tissues.[277] This has been shown in mixed Th1/Th2 responses, such as those occurring in mice with systemic yeast infections, in which Th1 cells are subjected to deactivation by IL-4 and IL-10. Th2 cytokines clearly outweight Th1 responses, masking any protective role of Th1 cells.[516] In contrast, selective blockade of Th2 cell development results in Th1-associated curative responses.[517,518] At least three cytokines (IL-12, IFN-γ and TGF-β) were found to be required for optimal in vivo development of Th1 cells leading to long-lived anticandidal resistance.[519] Although neutralizing antibodies to these cytokines may each block Th1 development, neither IFN-γ[518] nor TGF-β[519] is a correlative of Th1 development as is IL-12.[518] Surprisingly, however, injection of IL-12 not only did not exert beneficial action in systemically infected nonhealer mice, but could also have an exacerbating effect in the mucosal infection model, where the spontaneous development of Th1-associated resistance was somewhat impaired to the benefit of an emerging Th2-biased reactivity. To explain these findings, the IL-12-mediated induction of an IL-10 crossregulatory response, which may blunt the Th1-inducing potential of IL-12 itself, has been suggested.[520,521]

It is highly likely that Th1-type CD4[+] T cells are also critical in resistance to mucocutaneous infections in humans. The possible involvement of Th2 cytokines in modifying the host response so as to contribute to the parasite persistence has indeed been suggested in conditions, such as chronic mucocutaneous candidiasis, recurrent vaginal candidiasis, atopy and AIDS. However, direct evidence for such an involvement is still lacking.

ASPERGILLUS FUMIGATUS

In a murine model of allergic aspergillosis, exposure to particulate, but not soluble, *Aspergillus fumigatus* (*A. fumigatus*) antigens elicits a strong Th2 response, characterized by elevated levels of circulating IgE, increased production of IL-4 and IL-5, and eosinophilia.[522] In allergic bronchopulmonary aspergillosis, both specific and total serum IgE levels, peripheral and lung eosinophilia, and the frequency of CD4[+] Th2 cells specific for *Aspergillus* antigen were found to be elevated.[523] Likewise, patients with allergic bronchopulmonary aspergillosis demonstrated significantly increased levels of IL-4 and IL-5 in BAL fluid, with low but significantly elevated concentrations of IL-2 and IFN-γ.[524]

VIRAL INFECTIONS

As different cells (NK cells and CD8[+] CTL) are major players in protection against viral infections as compared with protozoan, fungal, bacterial or parasitic infections, it might be predicted that cytokine responses to viral infections will not directly parallel responses to these other antigens. IFN-α/β production and NK cell responses to acute primary viral infections are indeed induced early, whereas T cell responses are induced late. Moreover, stimulation of T cell responses may occur first in the context of class I MHC antigen presentation pathways and later, when viral particles may be taken up from outside host cells, in the context of class II antigen presentation pathways. Although both pathways can be in place, conditions in many viral infections are such that there is an acute preferential expansion of CD8[+] over CD4[+] T cells. Thus, the overall conditions and requirements for cytokine support of protective immune responses to viral infections are different from the type 1 or type 2 responses associated with most protozoan, fungal, bacterial, or helminthic infections.[525]

In general, the activation of Th1 cells leads to several effector functions causing cytotoxicity and so progression of an immune response towards a Th1 pathway would probably be most appropriate for dealing with intracellular organisms such as viruses. Moreover, CD8[+] CTL synthesize a pattern of lymphokines very similar to that of Th1 cells[59] and, therefore, activation of CTL may influence activation of Th cells in favor of Th1 cells. On the other hand, activation of Th1 cells leads to the production of IFN-γ, which has been shown to have anti-viral activity, and cytolytic activity in synergy with Th1-cell derived lympho-toxin would presumably promote the eradication of the virus.[526,527] Further support for a protective role of Th1-type response in viral infections is provided by the demonstration that infection with a large panel of RNA and DNA viruses resulted in a preponderance of comple-ment-fixing, cytotoxic IgG2a antibodies, some with nonviral specifici-ties, in contrast to IgG1 in anti-protein and IgG3 in anticarbohydrate responses.[528] Finally, in a recent study, it has been shown that the synthetic double-stranded (ds) RNA poly I-poly-C is able to shift the development of allergen-specific T cells from the Th0/Th2 to the Th1 profile.[180] This effect was prevented by addition of a mixture of anti-IL-12 and anti-IFN-α antibodies, but not by anti-IL-12 or anti-IFN-α antibody alone. Since many pathogenic viruses, such as influenza vi-ruses, rhinoviruses, and Coxsackie viruses, replicate through dsRNA intermediates, it is possible that they promote predominant Th1 re-sponses by stimulating the production of both IFN-α and IL-12 by macrophages. The ability of dsRNA to induce IL-12 production by macrophages has recently been confirmed in mice, as well.[529] More-over, it has been shown that IL-12 also plays a protective role in vivo in the CNS infection induced by ssRNA vescicular stomatitis virus,[530] as well as in acute infections sustained by murine cytomegalovirus or lymphocytic choriomeningitis virus (LMCV).[531] Studies devoted to char-acterize the functional profile of virus-specific human Th cells begin to become available (Table 7.3).

Table 7.3. Potential role of T-cell subsets in viral infections

Virus	T-Cell Subset	Suggested Effect
LMCV	CD8+, CD4+ Th1	Virus clearance
HSV	CD4+ Th1	Protection; induction
HSK	CD4+Th2	of HSK remission
Influenza	CD8+, CD4+ Th1	Virus clearance
Measles	Th0/Th2	Suppression of DTH
HBV	Th0	High viral load
HCV	Th1	Low viral load
MAIDS	Early Th1	Disease
	Late Th2	Not required for progression
HIV	Early Th1	Transient protection
	Late Th2	Progression

SINDBIS VIRUS

Sindbis virus causes an acute encephalomyelitis in mice. After intracerebral inoculation with Sindbis virus, T cell dependent mRNA expression of IL-4 and IL-10, as well as IL-2 and IFN-γ mRNA, is apparent in the brain. As IL-4 and IL-10 mRNAs are more persistent and more easily detectable than IL-2 and IFN-γ mRNA, it is likely that the response to Sindbis virus is mainly of the Th2 type.[532] However, as the magnitude of relative IFN-γ induction is similar to that of IL-4 and IL-10, the profiles of mRNA expression do not fit those of other Th2 responses.[525]

LYMPHOCYTIC CHORIOMENINGITIS VIRUS

The protection against lymphoctyic choriomeningitis virus (LMCV) is mainly mediated by in vivo activated LMCV-specific CD8+ CTL, but CD4+ T cells are required for clearance of this virus.[533] Although the infection induces systemic IFNα/β production, T cell-derived IFN-γ also plays a role in the defense against LMCV.[534] Interestingly, the administration of IL-12 at low concentrations induced enhancement of CD8+ T cell expansion and increased the resistance to virus infection in LMCV-infected C57BL/6 mice. However, administration of anti-IL-12 antibody failed to inhibit any of the endogenous T cell responses to LCMV, suggesting that these responses can even proceed through IL-12-independent mechanisms. Moreover, at doses known to enhance resistance to parasites or tumors, IL-12 induced dramatic immunotoxicity in LCMV-infected mice[535] (Fig. 7.4). The IL-12 immunotoxicity was mainly related to the release of high amounts of TNF-α and appeared to be dependent upon endogenous immune response and genetic sensitivity to the factor.[536] Thus, although the studies in several viral models support the importance of IL-12 for promoting defense against disease (see below), these findings remind us that it can also synergize with other factors to induce systemic and immunologic toxicities[537] (Fig. 7.4).

HERPES SYMPLEX

Herpes simplex type 1 virus (HSV) causes skin and/or mucous membrane lesions at various anatomic sites in a portion of the human population worldwide. Ocular disease resulting from HSV infection is a common cause of blindness, which results from a tissue-destructive inflammation in the corneal stroma. The mouse has provided to be a useful model for studying herpetic stromal keratitis (HSK). There is general agreement that CD4+ are the principal mediators of tissue damage, whereas the pathogenic role of CD8+ T cells is minimal.[538,539] Initially, only T cells with the characteristic Th1 profile could be demonstrated in cell populations derived from the eyes of HSV-infected mice and cultured for various time periods with or without antigen or nonspecific stimulants.[540] Interestingly, these HSV-induced Th1 cells, which

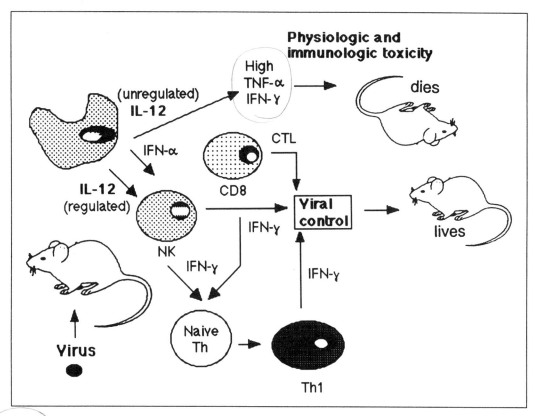

Fig. 7.4. Immune protection in viral infections. CD8+ CTL and NK cells play a central protective role against viruses, but CD4+ Th1 cells are also involved in protection. Both IL-12 and IFNs produced by macrophages, CD8+ T cells, and NK cells contribute to the Th1 response. Low doses of endogenously synthesized and/or administered IL-12 have beneficial effects by promoting protective NK responses and Th1-cell development. However, high concentrations of IL-12 during viral infection may result in toxicity and promote the death of virus-infected animals. Modified and reprinted with permission from Biron AC et al, Res Immunol 1995; 146:590-597.[537]

appear to play an essential role in the induction of HSK, also protect against dissemination of the virus in the skin surrounding the eye.[541] These data have been challenged on the basis of adoptive transfer experiments with a HSV-specific clone, showing that cells with a Th2-like profile could rather contribute to lesions.[542] More recently, reassessment of HSK with a more sensitive technique (RT-PCR) showed that the profile of cytokine expression may change during the course of infection. Initially, Th1 cytokines, particularly IFN-γ, are predominant,[543] and HSV-induced IL-12 production in the eye acts as the triggering event that biases HSV-specific immunity to the Th1 response.[544] As the disease regresses, Th2 cytokines become prominent and can be associated with lesion remission.[543] Thus, the HSV infection seems to represent another model in which the Th1 response is protective against the virus spread but can result in tissue damage, whereas the shifting to a Th2-dominated response associates with resolution of immunopathology.

Although limited, studies in human HSV infection suggest that a Th1-like cytokine response may be associated with resistance to naturally occurring episodes of *herpes labialis*.[545]

INFLUENZA VIRUS

The patterns of cytokine mRNA expression in mice with primary or secondary influenza pneumonia have been assessed in cells from both the mediastinal lymph nodes and the virus-infected lung. The initial response occurred in regional lymph node tissue, with the effector T cell later moving to the lung. CD8+ T cells are normally the key mediators of virus clearance, though CD4+ effectors may also function with varying success depending on the virulence of the challenge virus.[546] Mice lacking CD8+ T cells as a consequence of β2m gene disruption, as well as mice treated with anti-CD4 or anti-CD8 antibody clear influenza virus infection, whereas an elimination of both T cell subsets leads to a failure to clear virus and eventual death.[547,548] The γδ+ T cells are also an active component of influenza pneumonia, but they express mRNA for all cytokines tested, with IL-2, IL-4 and IFN-γ predominating among those recovered from the inflammatory exudate.[549] Among CD4+ αβ+ T cell subsets, transcripts for IFN-γ and TNF-β were most commonly found in the CD8+ population and in the early CD4+ T cell response, whereas mRNA for IL-4 and IL-10 was much more prevalent in later CD4+ T cell response.[549] Neutralization of IFN-γ prolongs viral persistence in CD8+ T cell-knockout mice, but there was no defect in the capacity of IFN-γ-knockout mice to deal with influenza virus, suggesting that this cytokine is not operating effectively to limit viral replication before the onset of the virus-specific T cell response.[550,551] However, influenza virus-specific Th1 clones are protective against lethal challenge with virus in vivo, whereas Th2 clones are noncytolytic and not protective.[552] Moreover, influenza virus clearance is accelerated by Th1 cells in the nasal site of mice immunized intranasally with adjuvant-combined recombinant nucleoprotein, indicating that the latter cells are important in protection.[553]

SYNCTYTIAL VIRUS

Respiratory synctytial virus (RSV) is a paramyxovirus responsible for the majority of serious viral respiratory illnesses in children and adults. The need for an effective vaccine against RSV has been apparent for many years, but none is yet available. Not only have vaccines failed to protect, but administration of formalin-inactivated RSV causes

Table 7.4. Effect of different treatments on the type of immunity and
pathology in RSV-infected mice

Treatment	T-Cell Subset	Pathology
Vaccination with:		
Live RSV	Th1	Mild illness
Formalin- inactivated RSV	Th2	Severe illness

Formalin-
    inactivated RSV +
    anti-IL-4 antibody
	Th1	Mild illness

Transfer of RSV protein:		
22K	CD8+	Rapid virus clearance 'Lung shock'
F	CD8+, CD4+ Th1	Mild illness
G	CD4+ Th2	Severe illness with lung eosinophilia

enhanced lung disease during subsequent natural infection.[554] Interestingly, upon RSV challenge, mice previously immunized intramuscu-
larly with inactivated whole virus express a Th2 pattern of cytokine
mRNA, while mice immunized with live virus either intranasally or
by parenteral routes express a prevalent Th1 pattern.[555] This is probably due to the fact that mice sensitized to individual RSV proteins
exhibit distinct patterns of immunity and pulmonary pathology when
challenged with live virus (Table 7.4). In mice primed with recombinant vaccinia, viruses expressing the major glycoprotein (G) T cells
were mostly CD4+, whereas priming with the second matrix (22k) protein
prevalently induced specific CD8+ CTL and priming with the fusion
protein (F) induced both CD4+ and CD8+ T cells. F-specific T cell
lines released an excess of IL-2, but little IL-4 or IL-5 (Th1-like pattern), whereas G-specific T cell lines produced IL-4 and IL-5, but little
IL-2 (Th2-like pattern). This observation suggests that, if activation
of both CD4+ and CD8+ T cells occurs simultaneously (as in F- and
22k-specific priming), Th1 rather than Th2 cells predominate. In contrast,
predominance of CD4+ T cell activation (as in G-specific priming) leads
to preferential expansion of the Th2-like cells.[556] Mice infected intranasally with RSV showed mild illness and recovered fully but developed respiratory distress after intravenous injection of T cells. Dose-
for-dose infected mice receiving F-specific T cells (consisting of both
CD8+ and Th1-like CD4+ T cells) developed minimal enhancement of
pathology, whereas 22k-specific T cells (mainly CD8+ T cells) caused

rapid RSV clearance from the lungs, but also a sometimes fatal disease reminiscent of shock lung, and G-specific T cells (Th2-like CD4+ T cells) induced a severe disease with a quite distinct pattern characterized by intense pulmonary eosinophilia, which resembles human asthma.[557] Treatment with anti-IL-4 at the time of immunization with inactivated RSV reduces clinical illness after live virus challenge and this is associated with an augmented CD8+ CTL response, increased expression of IFN-γ mRNA relative to IL-4 mRNA and a higher titer of RSV-specific IgG2a antibody.[558] Moreover, a formalin-inactivated RSV vaccine primes production of IL-4 and IL-10 after RSV infection which yields enhanced pulmonary histopathology.[559] RSV also potently enhanced IL-10 production in human cells, which functioned biologically to inhibit the expression of critical immunoregulatory cytokines.[560] Taken together, these findings provide another interesting model of how the degree of both protection and immunopathology can be determined by the pattern of Th1/Th2 cytokines. In the case of RSV infection, such a pathway appears to be strongly influenced by the type of individual RSV protein.

MEASLES VIRUS

Measles virus infection in the murine model of experimental measles virus-induced encephalitis is successfully controlled by virus-specific Th lymphocytes. T cells from BALB/c mice that are resistant to measles virus encephalitis have a Th1 profile, whereas Th cells from measles virus-infected susceptible C3H mice produce little IFN-γ. Moreover, neutralization of IFN-γ in vivo reverts the phenotype of measles virus-specific Th cells from BALB/c mice from Th1 to Th2 type, results in measles virus encephalitis and impairment of viral clearance from the CNS.[561] These data suggest that IFN-γ plays a significant role in the control of measles virus infection of the CNS.

Natural measles virus infection in humans is well recognized for causing prolonged abnormalities in immune responses, the best known being suppression of DTH skin test responses.[562,563] After vaccination with the attenuated live measles virus became available, similar abnormalities were observed, including suppression of DTH, and depression of antigen- and mitogen-induced lymphoproliferation.[564-566] Changes are dependent on use of live measles virus vaccine since they do not occur after immunization with killed measles virus vaccine.[567] During natural infection, the immune response to measles virus is characterized by the appearance of measles-specific cytotoxic CD8+ T cells, which clear the virus from tissues[568] and by the production of high levels of antibodies, including IgE,[569,570] whereas there is no induction of skin test reactivity[571] and proliferation of lymphocytes to measles virus antigens is low to undetectable.[572] Taken together, these findings suggest a preferential activation of Th2 cells. Indeed, plasma IL-4 levels were found to be elevated after resolution of the rash and remained elevated in some patients through a 7-week study period.[573] Accordingly, large amounts of sCD30 were found in the sera of all measles-infected subjects, which remained at high levels for several weeks.[574] Finally, an analysis for cytokines showed spontaneous production of high levels of IL-4 accompanied by low levels of IFN-γ by PBMC from children after vaccination with measles virus.[575] Very recently, it has been shown that infection with measles virus inhibits the production of IL-12 by macrophages.[576] This finding may explain the occurrence of a prevalent Th2-like response following natural measles infection or vaccination with attenuated live measles virus. The resulting IL-4- and/or IL-10-mediated downregulation of Th1 responses may also account for the well-documented consequences of measles virus infection and vaccination, such as suppressed DTH responses and lymphocyte proliferation.

HEPATITIS B AND C VIRUSES

Hepatitis B virus (HBV) and hepatitis C virus (HCV) are two hepatotropic viruses showing totally different biological features. HBV is a DNA virus apparently unable to cause a direct cytopathic effect. Chronic infection is generally characterized by high antigen concentrations in the serum and a wide spread of the virus within the liver.[577] HCV is a RNA virus that probably induces hepatocellular damage by both cytopathic and immune-mediated mechanisms, but generally it does not cause high viremia.[578]

In experimental models of HBV infection it has been shown that both the genetic background and the nature of HBV peptide antigens play a role in determining the cytokine profile of the immune response and the outcome of HBV infection. Examination of HBeAg-specific T cell cytokine production in B10.S Tg e/e and B10 Tg e/e mice provided indeed evidence of differential T cell response and T cell tolerance in these two strains. The T cell response in B10.S mice is highly focused on residues 120-131 and is predominantly Th1-like, whereas in B10 mice it appears exclusively focused on residues 129-140 and is predominantly Th2-like.[579] Moreover, a preferential ability of Th2-like cells to escape from tolerance induction was shown. These data suggest that Th cell recognition of HbeAg/HbcAg may result in Th1 cells which are able to clear the virus but are easily tolerized, thus skewing towards the Th2 subset in chronically HBV-infected individuals.[580] A low of dose IL-12 administered to vivo in HbeAg-expressing transgenic mice, which is dependent on self-reactive Th2 cells, was indeed able to inhibit autoantibody production by shifting the Th2-mediated response toward Th1 predominance.[581]

The possibility that a preponderance of HbeAg-specific Th2 cells occurs in chronic HBV patients is suggested by serological studies.[582,583] More importantly, CD4+ CD56+ T cell clones specific for HBV envelope antigen isolated from the liver of patients with HBV-induced chronic hepatitis were found to possess cytolytic potential and to express a clear-cut Th1 profile.[584] By contrast, when CD4+ T cell clones were derived by stimulation of single T cells with PHA from the liver of patients with HBV-induced hepatitis, they exhibited the ability to produce high amounts of Th2 cytokines and low levels of IFN-γ.[585] This picture was different when T cell clones were generated under the same experimental conditions from the liver of patients with HCV-induced hepatitis. Virtually all CD4+ T cell clones expressed both cytolytic activity and production of high concentrations of IFN-γ.[585] Based on these data, it is reasonable to suggest that HCV-specific Th1-like responses, although insufficient to cause complete viral clearance, could well contribute to keep the viral load at low levels. On the other hand, the prevalence of Th0-like cells may account for the high antigen load observed in HVB-induced hepatitis.

Mouse Retrovirus-Induced Immunodeficiency

Mouse retrovirus-induced immunodeficiency (MAIDS) is a syndrome of progressive lymphoproliferation and increasingly severe immunodeficiency that develops in mice following adult infection with retrovirus mixtures containing an etiologic replication-defective murine leukemia virus (MuLV) designated BM5def or Du5H.[586] Studies of MAIDS have evaluated both acute immune responses to infection and immune responsiveness in the chronic phase of infection. While at 1 week of postinfection there is a heterogenous cytokine pattern, at later times of postinfection a shift to predominant production of IL-4 and IL-10 occurs.[587,588] Thus, mixed Th1- and Th2-type responses are elicited during acute retroviral infection, but chronic infections result in immune cell populations that have lost the ability to produce Th1-type cytokines and/or preferentially produce Th2-type cytokines in response to new stimuli. However, Th2-type cytokines, IL-4, IL-6 and IL-10, are not required for induction or progression of MAIDS, since mice homozygous for knockouts of each of these genes, or doubly homozygous for knockouts of IL-4 and IL-10, develop MAIDS with a time course indistinguishable from that of wildtype mice.[589,590] Studies employing two independent systems have shown that, at least in B6 mice, IFN-γ is an important mediator of disease. First, mice homozygous for a knockout of the IFN-γ gene developed MAIDS with a substantially prolonged course.[591] Second, mice chronically treated with neutralizing anti-IFN-γ antibody exhibited delayed development and progression of lymphoadenopathy, immunodeficiency and elevations of serum Ig levels.[588] It has been postulated that production of IL-12 by MuLV-activated macrophages may stimulate production of IFN-γ by both NK cells and T cells, but also induce a translational block in anergic populations of T cells. IFN-γ at low levels is stimulatory to B cells, inducing activation, proliferation and differentiation to Ig secretion.[591] However, while the administration of recombinant IL-12 to MuLV-infected B6 mice at suboptimal doses resulted in an acceleration of lymphoproliferation, optimal IL-2 doses induced dramatic normalization of T cell functions and reduction in the severity of the disease.[592] Thus, IL-12 and IFN-γ may have opposite effects in MAIDS.

FRIEND IMMUNOSUPPRESSIVE VIRUS-2

Friend immunosuppressive virus type 2 (FIS-2) is a low oncogenic murine leukemia virus (MuLV) that induces lymphoadenopathy and immunosuppression in NMRI mice. In cultures from FIS-2-infected mice, the antibody response was reduced, compared to cultures from uninfected mice, and the production of the Th2 cytokines IL-4 and IL-6 was elevated, whereas the Th1 cytokines IL-2, IFN-γ and TNF-α were reduced. The suppressed antibody response in cultures from mice infected with FIS-2 seemed to be caused by an insufficient production of IL-2, since addition of recombinant IL-2 stimulated the antibody response. A switch to a Th2-cell response and suppression of IL-2 production was suggested to play a central role in the immune cell dysfunction induced by FIS-2.[593]

HUMAN IMMUNODEFICIENCY VIRUS

Progressive depletion of CD4⁺ T cells is one of the most dramatic effects of HIV infection. However, in a number of asymptomatic human immunodeficiency virus (HIV)-infected individuals, in spite of adequate CD4⁺ T cell counts, an early impairment of immune responses, particularly at the CD4⁺ T cell level, can also occur.[594] The observations that in certain murine and human diseases the Th1 response is usually associated with resistance to infection, whereas the Th2 pattern is more often related to disease susceptibility, raised the hypothesis that a switch from the Th1 to the Th2 cytokine pattern may occur and become relevant to the progression of HIV infection.[595]

The "Th1/Th2 switch" hypothesis in HIV infection

Two distinct observations were provided to substantiate the hypothesis of a Th1/Th2 switch in HIV infection. First, in HIV-seronegative individuals, who tested negative for HIV-specific antibodies in spite of exposure to the virus, evidence was found of HIV-specific CMI, as assessed by IL-2 production in cultures of PBMC stimulated with HIV envelope peptides.[596] In addition, the decrease of IL-2 responses to soluble antigens or HIV peptides was often associated with an increase of IL-4 and IL-10 production in response to mitogens.[597] In more recent experiments, it was found that both defective T cell proliferation and IL-2 production to influenza virus and HIV envelope peptides could be restored by addition in culture of IL-12.[598] Finally, increased expression of mRNA for, and production of, IL-10 upon mitogen stimulation was found in virtually all HIV-infected individuals, with a direct relationship between IL-10 levels and the severity of immunodeficiency. Neutralization of IL-10 by specific antibodies apparently restored the proliferative response to HIV peptides.[599] Recently, the possibility that HIV-related *nef* gene expression may be responsible for the downregulation of Th1 cytokines IL-2 and IFN-γ, without affecting the production of Th2 cytokines (IL-4, IL-9, IL-13), has been suggested.[600]

Several attempts have been made to prove or disprove the Th1/Th2 switch hypothesis in HIV infection. The most direct approach to the issue was to search for the persistent expression of mRNAs for IL-2, IL-4, IL-10 and IFN-γ in freshly isolated MNC and sorted CD4+ and CD8+ T cells from PB and lymph nodes of HIV-infected individuals. No evidence for IL-4 mRNA expression was found in any cell subset from PB or nodes, whereas IFN-γ and IL-10 mRNA expression could be observed, but only in CD4− T cells.[601] In another study based on the same experimental approach, abundant IFN-γ and low IL-2 gene transcription were reported, but no significant change in IL-4 mRNA expression was found in comparison with controls.[602] Finally, constitutive IL-10 mRNA expression was observed in a minority of HIV-infected individuals, but it was found to reflect the activity of non-T cells rather than T cells.[603] Thus, the analysis of constitutive cytokine expression in lymphoid tissues of HIV-infected individuals argues against a persistent HIV-induced expression of IL-4 mRNA as a proof for a Th2 switch occurring in vivo.

The search for changes in the cytokine profile of cells stimulated in vitro has also been partially disappointing. By using the same model of short-term PBMC cultures stimulated for 3 days with polyclonal activators, such as PHA or PMA plus anti-CD3 monoclonal antibody (mAb), production of IFN-γ was decreased or not significantly affected; however, production of both IL-4 and IL-10 was not increased (but rather decreased) in comparison with IL-4 and IL-10 production by matched HIV-sero-negative donors.[604-607] More importantly, PBMC from HIV-infected patients with reduced CD4+ T cell counts produced lower amounts of IL-4, IL-5 and IL-10 in comparison with HIV-infected patients showing quite normal or only slightly decreased CD4+ T cells.[605] In contrast, higher levels of PHA-induced IL-4 and IL-5, and lower levels of IL-2 and IFN-γ, were found in children with perinatal infection showing depressed response to alloantigens and soluble antigens than in those who responded to antigenic stimulation.[608]

Cytokine production in long-term cultures of CD4+ T cells such as T cell clones generated by stimulation with PHA from the PB of HIV-infected patients was also assessed. The proportions of CD4+ T cell clones inducible to IFN-γ production were comparable in HIV-sero-positive and HIV-sero-negative subjects, whereas the proportions of clones inducible to IL-4 and IL-5 production were significantly lower in HIV-infected individuals due to their selective reduction in patients with low CD4+ T cell counts.[605] However, when the cytokine secretion profile of antigen-specific T cell clones was assessed, a different pathway was found. About 40% of CD4⁺ T cell clones specific for *T. gondii* generated from HIV-sero-negative subjects showed a Th1 profile (production of IFN-γ and TNF-β, but not IL-4 or IL-5), whereas the remaining 60% exhibited a Th0 phenotype. In contrast, virtually all CD4⁺ *T. gondi* -specific T cell clones generated from HIV-sero-positive donors produced not only IFN-γ and TNF-β, but also IL-4, IL-5 and IL-10. Likewise, the great majority (80%) of PPD-specific T cell clones derived from controls were Th1, the other were Th0; in contrast, the majority of PPD-specific clones (71%) derived from HIV-sero-positive donors exhibited a Th0 phenotype and only a minority (29%) were Th1, suggesting a general shift at the level of memory CD4⁺ T cells towards the Th0 profile.[605] Similar results were reported by Meyaard et al[609] who found increased proportions of Th0-like clones in the clonal progenies of PHA-stimulated PB T cell suspensions of HIV-infected individuals enriched for CD45RO⁺ (memory) T cells.

The next approach was to assess the cytokine secretion profile of T cell clones derived from skin biopsy specimens obtained from HIV-infected patients. As controls, skin biopsy specimens derived from healthy volunteers or patients with atopic dermatitis were used. Skin fragments were cultured with IL-2 in order to expand in vivo activated T cells already expressing IL-2 receptor. The great majority of clones generated from both healthy subjects and patients with atopic dermatitis were CD4⁺ (86% and 73%, respectively), whereas the great majority of skin-derived clones (89%) in HIV-infected patients were CD8⁺ and only 11% were CD4⁺. The proportions of IL-4-producing CD4⁺ T cell clones were significantly higher in both HIV-infected patients and patients with atopic dermatitis in comparison with healthy individuals.[605] Taken together, these data suggest that in vitro activated CD4⁺ memory T cells from HIV-infected individuals develop into T cell clones that retain the ability to produce Th1 type cytokines, like their counterparts from anHIV-sero-negative subject, but acquire a greater ability to produce Th2 type cytokines. These findings do not fully support the "Th1/Th2 switch" hypothesis; at most, they indicate that a shift in a proportion of CD4⁺ memory T cells from the Th1 to the Th0 pattern can occur in some HIV-infected asymptomatic individuals.[610-612]

Enhanced proportions of CD8⁺ Tc2 cells in HIV-infected subjects

As mentioned above, the proportions of IL-4-producing CD8⁺ T cell clones generated from the skin of HIV-infected individuals were significantly higher in comparison with both healthy subjects and patients with atopic dermatitis, and an unusual number of CD8⁺ clones showing a Tc2 profile was found. The existence of unusual CD8⁺ T cells with Tc2 profile in HIV infection was subsequently confirmed by experiments performed in HIV-infected individuals suffering from adult-onset Job's-like-syndrome and/or showing high serum IgE levels and hypereosinophilia.[66,67] Most CD3+ T cell clones derived from both PB and the skin of HIV-infected patients with Job's-like syndrome were CD4−CD8+ or CD4−CD8−. However, all produced large amounts of IL-4 and IL-5 but no IFN-γ, exhibited reduced cytolytic activity, and provided helper function for IgE synthesis. These cells resemble the CD4−CD8− cells resulting from murine CD8+ cells incubated in vitro with IL-4,[61] suggesting they might result from an in vivo switching of CD8+ T cells, originally cytolytic and Th1-like, into poorly cytolytic Th2-like cells possibly conditioned by IL-4 present in their microenvironment. Interestingly, virtually all CD8+ Tc2 clones generated from HIV-infected patients consistently expressed surface CD30+ (a molecule preferentially associated with the production of Th2-type cytokines—see above) and produced high levels of sCD30 in their supernatants.[73] The mechanisms responsible for the possible shift of CD8+ T cell clones from HIV-infected patients from the Tc1 to the Tc0 or Tc2 profile have also been investigated. When CD8+ T cell clones from HIV-sero-positive individuals were generated by using irradiated cells from HIV-infected patients as feeder cells the shift toward the Tc2 profile was even more marked, but it could be completely prevented by the addition of IL-12 and an anti-IL-4 antibody in bulk culture before cloning. Accordingly, when CD8+ T cells from healthy HIV-sero-negative individuals were cloned by using cells from HIV-sero-positive individuals as feeder cells, a clear shift toward the development of Tc0/Tc2 clones was observed in comparison to the pathway obtained by using feeder cells from HIV-sero-negative individuals. These data suggest that the defective production of Th1-inducing cytokines by APCs, or the early IL-4 production by some still unknown cell type, may favor the shift of CD8+ T cells of HIV-infected individuals from the Tc1 to the Tc0/Tc2.

Defective production of IL-12 and IFN-α (both Th1-inducers) in HIV-infected subjects

The possibility that a defective production of Th1-inducing cytokines is involved in the shift of CD8+ T cells and possibly also of CD4+ T cells, towards the production of Th2-type cytokines is substantiated by several experimental data. First, despite the fact that both macrophages from HIV-infected individuals and normal macrophages infected in vitro with HIV usually produce normal or increased amounts of IL-1β, TNF-α, IL-6, GM-CSF and IL-10,[613] production of a powerful Th1-inducing cytokine, such as IL-12, in response to pathogenic bacteria and parasites is strongly defective.[614] Moreover, IL-12 was found to induce an irreversible priming for high IFN-γ production in both CD4+ and CD8+ T cell clones derived from HIV-infected patients,[615] which probably represents the most important mechanism by which IL-12 induces Th1 differentiation.[153,154] Finally, HIV-infected monocytes produced little or no IFN-α before or after treatment with poly(I)-

poly(C), Newcastle disease virus, or HSV, which induce high levels of IFN-α in noninfected monocytes.[616] Of note is that IFN-α has been shown to play an ancillary role in the IL-12-mediated in vivo development of murine Th1 cells[171] and a major role in the in vitro development of human Th1 cells.[177,179]

Th2-dominated responses favor HIV replication and disease progression

The studies mentioned above suggest that HIV infection may result in enhanced Th2-type cytokine production in a proportion of patients at both CD4⁺ and CD8⁺ T cell level. However, they also indicate that a preferential depletion of Th2-type CD4⁺ T cells can occur in the advanced phases of HIV infection. Such a depletion was associated with markedly lower clonal efficiency in these patients, suggesting either in vivo selective destruction of these cells or their HIV-induced killing and/or apoptosis in vitro early upon PHA stimulation. Evidence in favor of this possibility was recently provided by both in vitro and in vivo studies. Two independent studies have analyzed the ability of already established Th1, Th0 and Th2 CD4⁺ T cell clones, infected in vitro with HIV, to support viral replication. In our study, CD4⁺ T cell clones specific for bacterial antigens or allergens derived from seronegative subjects were infected in vitro with HIV and 2-3 weeks later assessed for the presence of DNA provirus by PCR and for viral replication by measurement of p24 antigen (Ag) in the supernatant. In spite of the presence of DNA provirus, none of the Th1 clones produced p24 Ag in their supernatants, whereas all the Th2 and two-thirds of the Th0 clones showed both positive PCR and p24 Ag production.[605] Accordingly, in another study, in which T cell clones specific for HIV gag p24 were assessed, only Th2 clones showed HIV replication, whereas Th1 clones did not replicate the virus and even showed the ability to inhibit HIV replication in other HIV-infected cells.[617]

The possibility that Th2 cells, while allowing higher virus replication, favor at the same time their own killing and further spread of HIV, is supported by several in vivo observations. First, HIV-infected individuals with elevated IgE serum levels at the time of infection progress more rapidly to both CD4⁺ T cell depletion and full-blown disease than HIV-infected subjects exhibiting normal or low serum IgE.[610,618,619] Moreover, HIV-infected individuals infested by helminths progress more rapidly to AIDS.[620] Thus, one may suggest that disease progression in HIV-infected individuals is favored by active viral replication in CD4⁺ T cells, which are stimulated to produce Th2-type cytokines by environmental stimuli (e.g., common allergens, helminth infections or other), rather than by a Th1/Th2 switch which still remains to be proved. However, the mechanisms by which Th2-dominated responses favor HIV replication and a more rapid progression toward full-blown disease are still unclear.

Role of Th1 and Th2 cytokines in HIV expression

The ability of Th1- or Th2-type cytokines to regulate HIV replication is of great potential relevance, but data presently available on their actual role do not provide a convincing explanation. Some cytokines can upregulate HIV replication in a number of primary cell and cell line models. The best example of this class of cytokines is TNF-α[621] that is, however, produced by both Th1 and Th2 cells. In contrast, IL-13, which is also a product of both Th1 and Th2 cells, shows an exclusively suppressive effect on HIV replication.[622] The majority of both Th1- and Th2-type cytokines, such as IL-2,[623] IFN-γ,[624] IL-4[625,626] and IL-10,[627] can exert dichotomous effects on HIV replication depending on the experimental conditions. Both IL-4 and IL-10, however, were found to reduce the ability of CD8+ to suppress HIV replication, whereas IL-2 improved the ability of these cells to suppress HIV replication.[628] With regard to the Th1-inducing cytokines, IFN-α is a selective inhibitor of HIV replication, whereas both IL-12 and TGF-β exert inhibitory or dichotomous effects[613] (Table 7.5).

Role of CD30 in HIV expression

The demonstration that CD30, a member of the TNF receptor superfamily,[47] is preferentially expressed on, and its soluble form (sCD30) released by, both CD4+ and CD8+ T cell responses characterized by the production of Th2-type cytokines[48,73] prompted us and others to

Table 7.5. Differential effects of Th1- and Th2-related cytokine on HIV expression

Cytokine	Regulatory Effect on HIV Expression in:	
	T Cell	Macrophage
Th1-Inducing		
IFN-α	−	−
IL-12	+	
TGF-β	+ or −	+ or −
Th1-Derived		
IL-2	+	
TNF-α/β	+	+
IFN-γ	+ or −	+
Th2-Derived		
IL-4	+	+ or −
IL-10		+ or −
IL-13		−

investigate the possible role of CD30 in HIV expression. This is also because elevated levels of sCD30 have been detected in the serum of many HIV-infected patients, suggesting a high turnover of this molecule in HIV infection.[629] Biswas et al[630] have recently shown that crosslinking of CD30, which is constitutively expressed on the surface of the chronically HIV-infected human T cell line ACH-2, results in HIV expression. The induction of HIV expression is not due to increased proliferation or endogenous TNF-α production, but is mediated by NF-κB activation which leads to enhanced HIV transcription.[630] Accordingly, we have shown that CD30 ligation with an agonistic CD30-specific monoclonal antibody potentiated HIV replication induced by an insolubilized anti-CD3 antibody in T cell lines generated from HIV-infected individuals.[631] More importantly, paraformaldehyde-fixed CD8[+] T cell clones expressing the CD30 ligand (CD30L) enhanced HIV replication in anti-CD3-stimulated allogeneic or autologous CD4[+] T cell lines generated from HIV-infected individuals and such a potentiating effect was inhibited by an anti-CD30L antibody. The anti-CD30L antibody also exerted a suppressive effect on the spontaneous HIV replication occurring in lymph node cells freshly derived from an HIV-sero-positive patient showing CD30 expression in B cells and in a proportion of CD8[+] T lymphocytes.[631] Finally, CD30 ligation induced NF-kB activation in human T cell lines, as well as in human CD30-expressing Th0 and Th2 CD4[+] T cell clones.[53] More recently, infection in vitro with HIV of CD4[+] T cell clones was found to be able to enhance the expression of CD30, which often preceded, and is associated with, the death of clonal T cells.[1147] Thus, triggering of CD30, which is mainly and persistently expressed by activated Th0 and Th2 cells, may play an important role in both HIV replication and death of HIV-infected CD4[+] T cells.

Th1/Th2 cell-derived cytokines and apoptosis

Accumulating evidence points to the notion that accelerated lymphocyte apoptosis might be a major contributor to the depletion of CD4[+] T cells in HIV infection.[632,633] In addition, analysis of the phenotype of cells undergoing apoptosis has revealed that not only CD4[+] T cells, but also CD8[+] T cells undergo accelerated apoptosis in HIV infection.[634,635] Several mechanisms have been proposed for the observed accelerated T cell apoptosis, which can be categorized as: (1) HIV envelope protein-mediated clustering of CD4 molecules and subsequent aberrant signal to T cells; (2) involvement of APCs as an apoptosis inducer and as a result of defective antigen presentation; (3) possible superantigen activity encoded by HIV products or cofactors and (4) involvement of cytokine/cytokine receptors, including Fas/FasL system. There is now convincing evidence to suggest that enhanced apoptosis in HIV infection is mediated by Fas/Fas-L interaction.[636] However, the regulatory role of Th1/Th2 cytokines in the Fas/Fas-L system expression and apoptosis activation is still controversial. It has recently been shown that Th1 cells can express both Fas and Fas-L, whereas Th2 cells express Fas, but little Fas-L.[345,637] Therefore, Th2 cells may undergo apoptosis by activated CD4⁺ Th1 cells, but not by Th2 cells themselves.[637] However, the possibility that Th1 cells can undergo apoptosis by Th1 cells themselves has been suggested.[345] Moreover, the Th2 cytokines IL-4 and IL-10 exert a favoring effect on apoptosis,[607,638] whereas both IL-2 (a Th1-type cytokine) and IL-12 (a cytokine that upregulates Th1 functions) seem to play a protective role.[607,638,639] Finally, production of TNF-α and IFN-γ in the absence of IL-2, which occurs as a consequence of CD4 crosslinking, contributes to Fas upregulation and apoptosis induction.[639] It is of note that the production of protective cytokines (IL-2 and IL-12) is defective in HIV-infected patients, whereas the production of cytokines favoring apoptosis (IL-4, IL-10, TNF-α, IFN-γ) is not reduced or even increased.

In conclusion, because of the complex nature of cytokine crosstalk and because of the pleiotropic nature of cytokine function, the exact series of events occurring in Th cell responses during HIV infection are still enigmatic and need closer scrutiny. However, some important points can be hypothesized. Defective production of IL-12 and IFN-α by HIV-infected macrophages and dendritic cells probably favors the preferential development of Th0/Th2 responses even in response to pathogens that usually stimulate IL-12 and/or IFN-α production by APCs and, therefore, promote the development of Th1 cells. HIV infection of Th0/Th2 cells results in high HIV replication and HIV-induced cell death, due at least in part to CD30/CD30L interactions, which promote induction of NF-κB and activation of viral LTR. CD30 expression is indeed high and persistent in activated Th2 cells and seems to be enhanced by HIV infection, while CD30L is constitutively expressed by B cells, as well as by a proportion of activated macrophages and CD8⁺ T cells. Moreover, Th0 and Th2 cells express high levels of Fas and are therefore subjected to undergo apoptosis by both Fas-L positive Th1 cells and CD8⁺ T cells. Both HIV-induced death of Th2 cells at lymph node level (where cell-to-cell interactions can easily occur) and apoptosis may account for the lack of evidence of Th2 predominance in the majority of HIV-infected individuals. On the other side, Th1 cells that develop despite the defective production of IL-12 by the APC can receive inappropriate CD4 signaling by gp120/anti gp120 antibody which results in increased IFN-γ and TNF-α production in the absence of IL-2 production. This favors Fas upregulation that, in the absence of IL-12 (which is protective) and in the presence of even small amounts of IL-4 and IL-10 (which favor apoptosis), makes these cells susceptible to apoptosis induced by other Fas-L positive Th1 cells and/or CD8⁺ T cells (Fig. 7.5).

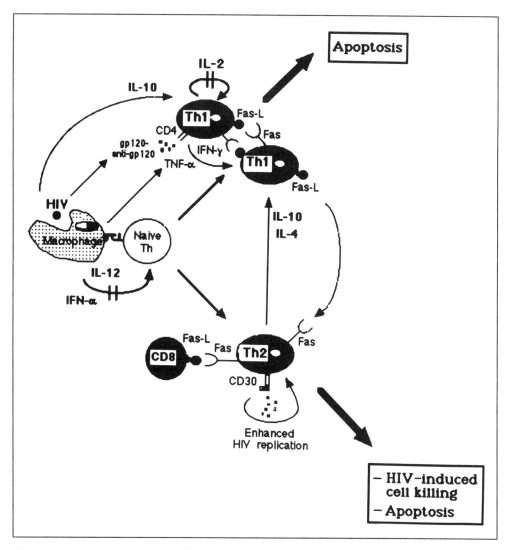

Fig. 7.5. Schematic view of the possible contribution of Th1 and Th2 cells to the immunopathogenesis of HIV infection. The defective production of IL-12 and IFN-α, together with the enhanced production of IL-10 by HIV-infected macrophages, may hamper the development of Th1 responses and favor the development of Th2-like cells. Th1 cells may die because of apoptosis promoted by either the binding of gp120/gp120 antibody complexes to CD4 in the presence of TNF-α and IFN-γ or the interaction between Fas and Fas-L under conditions of defective production of IL-2 and IL-12 (both of which prevent apoptosis), but enhanced production of IL-4 and IL-10 both of which favor apoptosis. Th2 cells may die because of either continuous HIV replication due to CD30L-CD30 interactions in lymphoid organs or apoptosis induced by interaction of their Fas with Fas-L expressed by both CD8+ and CD4+ Th1-like T cells.

HELMINTHIC INFECTIONS

Parasitic helminths are large multicellular organisms which, with few exceptions, exist extracellularly and are unable to replicate in the vertebrate host. The major immunologic hallmarks of helminth infections are eosinophilia, elevated IgE, and mastocytosis in the case of certain parasites that are stimulated by lymphokines or lymphokine combinations characteristic of Th2 cells.[640] Previous data have implicated eosinophils and IgE as major effector elements in the protective immunity against a number of different helminths.[641-643] A reevaluation of the question has recently led to a more complicated view of the role of these Th2-dependent responses in helminth immunity.[640,644] The possibility exists that Th2 responses are deliberately induced by worms to downregulate protective Th1 responses or by the host to avoid immunopathological reactions related to strong and persistent Th1 responses. An alternative hypothesis is that elevated IgE and eosinophilia play no protective role but are simply immunopathological manifestations of the dominant Th2 response induced by worms. Finally, recent data suggest that the helminth-induced Th2 response is indeed protective but involves cytokine-induced effector mechanisms that make the life environment unpleasant to the parasite without requiring IgE or eosinophils.[645] Some infections sustained by helminth parasites have been extensively investigated in both mice and humans (Table 7.6).

SCHISTOSOMA MANSONI

Schistosomiasis is a chronic and debilitating disease that affects over 200 million people worldwide. The pathology resulting from infection with *S. mansoni* is predominantly caused by the host's chronic granulomatous reaction to parasite eggs that are laid in the portal venous system and subsequently trapped in the liver and intestine. The associated fibrosis can lead to portal hypertension, which causes much of the morbidity and mortality associated with the disease. Granulomatous inflammation is a complex process involving multiple cell types and cytokines. In contrast to previous studies showing the capacity of rat

Table 7.6. Potential role of T-cell subsets in helminthic diseases

Helminth	T-Cell Subset	Suggested Function
	Th1	Protection/Immunopathology
S. mansoni (murine)	Th2	Immunopathology
H. polygirus	Th2	Protection
T. muris	Th2	Protection
N. brasiliensis	Th2	Protection
B. malayi	Th2	Protection
O. volvulus	Th2	Protection/Immunopathology
T. canis	Th2	Protection

or human eosinophils and IgE to participate in the in vitro killing of larval parasites in ADCC reactions,[642,643] the mouse model argued against a function of IgE and eosinophils and supported a role of Th1 cells in protection against schistosome.[646,647] More importantly, kinetic analyses of the cytokine response in infected mice revealed a downregulation of Th1 responses (revealed by early IFN-γ production) and a corresponding increase in Th2 cytokines at the time of egg laying, suggesting the involvement of Th2 rather than Th1 cytokines in lesion formation[648,649] (Fig. 7.6). Accordingly, it was shown that repeated injections of anti-IL-4 antibody given to acutely infected mice suppressed hepatic granuloma formation while increasing Th1-like cytokine production, whereas administration of recombinant IL-4 to chronically infected animals significantly enhanced the response.[650] Neutralization of IL-4 also suppressed pulmonary granuloma formation in sensitized hosts and, besides suppressing liver granuloma formation, significantly decreased hepatic collagen deposition.[651,652] Some studies, however, suggest that TNF-α production also contributes to the induction of the granulomatous response.[653,654] Moreover, other cytokines are involved in the regulation of schistosome egg granuloma formation. For example, the development of the Th2 response, in addition to being dependent on IL-4, is dependent on early IL-2 expression. In vivo treatment of infected mice with anti-IL-2 antibodies diminished the size of liver granulomas, IL-5 production, eosinophilia, and decreased hepatic fibrosis to half that in untreated animals.[655] Accordingly, administration of exogenous IL-2 to chronically infected mice increased the downregulated granulomatous response.[656] In contrast, IFN-γ plays a downregulatory role in schistosome granuloma formation. Neutralization of endogenous IFN-γ by anti-IFN-γ antibody significantly increased the lesion size and production of IL-4, IL-5 and IL-6.[657,658] Similar changes occurred when egg-injected mice were treated with neutralizing antibodies specific for IL-12 (a powerful IFN-γ inducer).[658] Moreover, sensitization with eggs plus IL-12 partly inhibits granuloma formation and dramatically reduces the tissue fibrosis induced by natural infection with *S. mansoni* worms.[659] Depletion of IFN-γ, but not IL-10, however, restored Th2 mRNA responses in IL-12-treated mice, arguing that the major suppressive effects of IL-12 on granuloma formation and Th2 cytokine expression were mediated through IFN-γ.[658] This finding was confirmed in egg-injected IFN-γ knockout mice treated with IL-12.[660] Surprisingly, no role for endogenous IL-10 in modulating schistosome granuloma formation has been detected.[657,658] Suppression of egg-induced primary Th2 responses by IL-12 suggested the possibility of protecting mice from granulomatous inflammation by sensitizing them to egg antigens plus exogenous IL-12.[660] This approach nearly completely inhibited granuloma formation after intravenous challenge with eggs while increasing Th1, and decreasing Th2, cytokine mRNA expression.[658] Endogenous IL-1 receptor antagonist (IL-1RA)

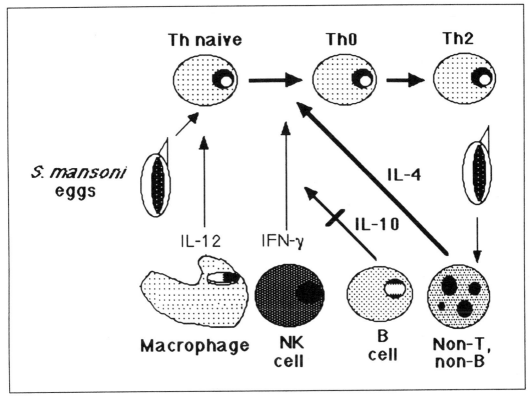

Fig. 7.6. The S. mansoni *model of Th2 response. The selection of Th2 responses by* S. mansoni *eggs appears to be the result both of the lack of a strong IL-12/IFN-γ stimulus combined with potent egg antigen driven T cell activation. In addition, the egg-induced Th2 response may be determined in part by the action of IL-4 derived from non-CD4+ cells and in part by the production of large amounts of IL-10 and PGE₂ (two molecules known to downregulate Th1 cells) by B cells stimulated by the egg antigen LNFP-III. Reprinted with permission from Jankovic D et al, Chem Immunol 1996; 63:51-65.[392]*

also downregulates the antigen-specific granulomatous response to schistosome eggs. In fact, in vivo depletion of IL-1RA by an anti-IL-1RA antibody augmented both the granuloma size and lymphokine (IL-2, IL-4, IL-10) production.[661] The factors and/or mechanisms that lead to the predominance of Th2-type responses in schistosome-infected mice have also been investigated. A non-T cell seems to be the major source of early IL-4 production, inasmuch as it is detectable after egg injection even in nude (T cell-depleted) mice.[662] One oligosaccharidic egg antigen, lacto-*N*-fucopentaose III (LNFP-III) induced production of large amounts of IL-10 and PGE₂ (two molecules known to downregulate Th1 cells) by splenic B cells of schistosome-infected and naive mice.[663] By contrast, a Ca⁺2 activated neutral proteinase of schistosome calpain seems to be one of the target antigens of the Th1-mediated protective response against invading schistosome larvae.[664]

The relation between human immune responses and protection against schistosome infection is more complex. In *S. haematobium* infected populations in the Gambia, IgE antibody responses increased progressively with age, and the high concentrations of IgE directed against adult worm antigens, and to a lesser extent egg antigens, were significantly associated with subsequent low intensities of reinfection. Individuals with the highest levels of IgE were ten times less likely to become reinfected after chemotherapy than those with the lowest levels, even after allowing for age and exposure.[665] Similar associations between high IgE responses and resistance to reinfection were described subsequently among Brasilians[666] and Kenyan[667] subjects exposed to *S. mansoni*. The cellular responses against *S. mansoni* have also been investigated. Antigen-induced stimulation of IL-5 production was particularly strong in many individuals, being inversely related to the production of IFN-γ and negatively correlated with intensities of reinfection.[668] Moreover, *S. mansoni*-specific T cell clones generated from subjects resistant to infection by *S. mansoni* are Th0/Th2, whereas clones of a sensitized adult from a nonendemic area are also Th0, but produce more IFN-γ than IL-4 (Th0/Th1).[669]

TRICHURIS MURIS

Trichuris muris (*T. muris*) or murine whipworm has an entirely enteric life cycle, maturing in the intestinal mucosa to the egg-laying adults that reside in the cecum and large bowel. There are, however, resistant (BALB/k) mice that expulse adult worms by 35 days and demonstrate immunity to rechallenge, and susceptible (AKR) mice that maintain persistent infection.[280] These disparate outcomes are correlated with Th2 or Th1 cytokine production by mesenteric lymph nodes in the resistant or susceptible strains, respectively. Neutralization of IFN-γ allowed susceptible strains to expulse worms, whereas blocking IL-4 using anti-IL-4 receptor antibody resulted in persistent infection in resistant mice. Further, administration of IL-4 (in the form of IL-4/anti-IL-4 complexes) conferred a resistant phenotype (worm expulsion) on the susceptible AKR strain.[280] Thus, only in this system was IL-4 demonstrated to be beneficial, and IFN-γ was demonstrated to be detrimental.

HELIGMOSOMOIDES POLYGYRUS

Heligmosoides polygyrus (*H. polygyrus*) also leads an enteric life, invading the mucosa to molt several times before emerging as egg-laying adults that reside in the upper small bowel where the worms reside for months. Infected mice are resistant to additional infestations if rechallenged, however, which is an example of concomitant immunity. The latter can be quantitated experimentally by drug-curing infected mice and demonstrating that rechallenge inocula are rapidly expulsed over 2-3 weeks. A highly specific and reproducible pattern of Th2 cytokine gene expression was detectable in the spleen, mesenteric lymph nodes and Peyer's patches in the first week after infection.[670] Such concomitant immunity was completely blocked by a single dose of either anti-IL-4 or anti-IL-4 receptor antibody, thus implicating IL-4 in mediating host defense.[671] Immunity was also absent when IL-4-knockout mice were infected, drug-cured, and secondarily challenged with *H. polygyrus*. Furthermore, recombinant IFN-γ and IFN-α exacerbate primary infections of mice with *H. polygyrus*.[206] In contrast, IL-4 treatment cured established infection in both immunocompetent and immunodeficient mice.[671] IL-4-mediated host protection acts on the adult parasite, is primarily antibody- and B cell-independent and is only partially dependent upon the presence of a specific immune response, since decreases in worm burden and egg production are seen in IL-4-treated SCID mice.[645] It rather reflects the ability of IL-4 to increase smooth muscle contractility, as well as to enhance intestinal chloride secretory response to mast-cell produced secretagogue PGE_2 with increased intestinal fluid content, decreased resistance to intestinal ion flow and decreased sodium adsorption in response to glucose. All these IL-4-induced changes in gut physiology interfere with parasite nutrition, thus making its life unpleasant within the host.[645]

NIPPOSTRONGYLUS BRASILIENSIS

N. brasiliensis is a rat parasite that has been adapted to the mouse through repeated passage. Larvae are inoculated subcutaneously, migrate to the vascular space, through the lungs, and up the trachea before being swallowed to gain access to the intestinal lumen. There, organisms begin laying eggs, although production is short-lived, and adults are expulsed by approximately 10 days. Secondary challenges are rebuffed more rapidly. Infection of both BALB/c mice and Brown Norway and Fischer-344 rats with *N. brasiliensis* generates intense Th2 responses[672,673] allowing interventions devoted to assess the components of normal immunity. As in the *T. muris* system, IFN-γ or IFN-α increased the duration of egg-laying and markedly delayed expulsion of the worms.[674] When administered during antigen priming, these cytokines shifted the response towards the Th1 phenotype. Moreover, IL-12 had similar but more profound effects, and these effects were correlated with the ability of IL-12 to enhance endogenous IFN-γ production while abrogating production of the Th2 cytokines IL-4, IL-5 and IL-9.[672] As predicted, such effects blocked intestinal mast cell hypertrophy, eosinophilia, and IgE synthesis. Coadministration of anti-IFN-γ antibody could abolish most of these effects, although eosinophilia remained curiously IFN-γ independent. Finally, administration during secondary rechallenge had little effect on worm persistence, egg-laying, or on the production of IL-4, IL-5 or IL-9 by mesenteric lymph node cells. Even in the primary infection, IL-12 had to be administered within the first 4-6 days in order to achieve maximum effects, suggesting that committed Th2 cells may not express IL-12 receptors like naive, Th0, or Th1 cells.[675] These studies raise some caution when considering the therapeutic role of IL-12 in boosting CMI, since immunity against these intestinal nematodes was clearly compromised because of the suppression of Th2 development. In contrast to the *H. polygyrus* infection, IL-4 was not required by BALB/c mice in order to expel *N. brasiliensis*, but can induce *N. brasiliensis* expulsion by SCID mice, or anti-CD4 antibody-treated BALB/c mice, which otherwise fail to expel this parasite.

One of the most fascinating aspects of these systems remain(s) the mechanism(s) by which worms are actually expulsed. IL-4 mediates expulsions by actions on the host, rather than directly on the worm. Observations that IL-4 is only partially effective at inducing anti-CD4 antibody-treated, mast cell-deficient mice (w/W^v mice or mice treated with anti-c-kit antibody), or 5-lipoxygenase-deficient (5LO-knockout) mice to expel *N. brasiliensis* suggest mast cell and leukotriene involvement in IL-4-induced worm expulsion. Increased nonpropulsive intestinal contractions are seen in IL-4-treated BALB/c mice and mice given a challenge infection with *H. polygyrus*, but not in IL-4-treated w/wv mice, 5LO-knockout mice or *H. polygyrus*-infected, anti-IL-4 receptor antibody-treated mice, and can be blocked in vitro by a specific inhibitor of the leukotriene D_4 receptor. In addition to induction of increased smooth muscle contractility, IL-4 treatment and *H. polygyrus* infection are associated with an increased intestinal chloride secretion response to mast cell-produced secretagogue PGE_2, which can be blocked in *H. polygyrus*-infected mice with anti-IL-4 receptor antibody, with increased intestinal fluid content, with decreased sodium adsorption in response to glucose.[645] In conclusion, several data indicate that IL-4 can protect hosts against gastrointestinal nematode infections and suggest that some of the protective effects of IL-4 are T and B cell-independent and are mediated by mast cell products that result in changes in gut physiology (increased intestinal contractions and net fluid content) that may interfere with parasite nutrition.

FILARIAE

The human lymphatic filariases, estimated to affect about 100 million people worldwide, are persistent infections that induce a breadth of host immune responses implicated in the pathogenesis of the different clinical manifestations of this infection. These responses in both brugian and bancroftian filariasis include: (1) intermittent lymphangitis and lymphoadenitis ("filarial fevers") that can lead to chronic lymphatic obstruction; (2) the syndrome of tropical pulmonary eosinophilia and (3) a condition in which individuals are asymptomatic, but have persistent microfilaremia. It has been postulated that these different clinical conditions reflect the nature of the host immune response to filarial infection.[676] BALB/c mice inoculated with live *Brugia malayi* (*B. malayi*) microfilariae, or immunized with a soluble *B. malayi* filarial extract developed a pronounced Th2 response over time.[677] Interestingly, establishment of a Th2 response by either inoculation of live micriofilariae or immunization with the soluble filarial extract before administration of a Th1-inducing antigen, such as PPD from *M. tuberculosis*, also skewed the PPD-specific response towards the Th2-like profile. This Th2 shift was prevented by in vivo neutralization of IL-4, suggesting that ongoing Th2 responses to microfilariae modulate the Th response to mycobacterial antigens by an IL-4-dependent mechanism.[677] The response to microfilariae was very different from that to adult worms. The most potent Th2 response was induced by the adult parasite females, whereas microfilariae induced a strong initial IFN-γ response. Moreover, the Th2 response induced by adult females could be modulated or downregulated by IFN-γ elicited by microfilariae.[678] Resistance to infection with the filarial nematodes does not seem, however, to be dependent on the Th2 response. Infection with *B. malayi* in IL-4-knockout mice results indeed in a dramatic change from a dominant Th2 to a Th1 response, but survival of infective larvae, adult worms or microfilariae in the peritoneal cavity was unaffected.[679] Prevalent Th2-type responses have also been demonstrated in human filariases, which seem to be mainly related to the action of parasitic antigens.[680]

ONCHOCERCA VOLVULUS

Onchocerca volvulus (*O. volvulus*) infects about 20 million people in Africa and Latin America and in a minority of subjects provokes severe pathologic consequences (blindness, skin disease) as a result of the immune response to parasite. Infection with *O. volvulus* is initiated by an infected blackfly feeding on a human, during which time infective third stage larvae are released into the skin. The larvae develop over many months into adult worms, which mate and release microfilariae into the skin. An association has been described between protection against *O. volvulus* infection and the presence of a Th2 response. Humans putatively immune to *O. volvulus* have been identified in *O. volvulus*-endemic regions. The principal immunologic difference between infected and immune individuals was that cells from immune individuals produced IL-2 and IL-5 after stimulation with antigen, whereas cells from infected individuals did not.[681] In mice immunized with *O. volvulus* IL-5, but no IFN-γ, were detected in the parasites' microenvironment. Depletion of either IL-4 or IL-5 caused a significant reduction in the level of protective immunity which developed after vaccination with irradiated larvae.[682] Thus, based on these results a role for both IL-4 and IL-5 in the protection against *O. Volvulus* infection was hypothesized. IL-5 may act by inducing the production and attraction of eosinophils, whereas IL-4 may participate in the protective immune response by inducing the production of parasite-specific IgG1 antibodies.[682]

TOXOCARA CANIS

Human infection with the nematode *T. canis* may result in two main clinical pictures: *visceral larva migrans* or ocular toxocariasis. Symptoms and signs are related to the number and location of parasite lesions, but in the majority of cases only asymptomatic eosinophilia and raised serum levels of IgE mark the presence of the parasite.[683] Human toxocariasis is quite rare but serum antibodies to various *T. canis* antigens have been found in 2-3% of the adult population and in 7-14% of school-aged children, probably reflecting simple exposure to *T. canis* antigens in the environment rather than current infection.[684] Interestingly, PBMC obtained from six out of eight randomly selected healthy donors, without history or serology suggestive for toxocariasis, showed strong proliferative responses to TES antigen(s). Moreover, TES-specific CD4$^+$ T cell clones with a characteristic Th2 lymphokine profile could be generated from these cultures, whereas PPD-specific T cell clones obtained from the same donors showed an opposite (Th1-like) profile.[18] Accordingly, patients affected by toxocariasis showed increased prevalence in their peripheral blood of IL-4- and IL-5-producing cells and increased production of IL-4 and/or IL-5 in response to mitogen stimulation.[685-687] The increased proportion of Th2-like cells in the PB of patients with toxocariasis normalized after appropriate treatment.[687] The ability of PB cells to produce IFN-γ was reduced in patients with toxocariasis or schistosomiasis, suggesting a worm-induced downregulation of Th1-type reactions.[687,688]

CHAPTER 8

ROLE OF TH1/TH2 CELLS IN PATHOPHYSIOLOGIC CONDITIONS

AGING

It has been widely observed that, with aging, substantial changes occur in both the functional and phenotypic profiles of T lymphocytes in experimental animal models and in humans.[689] These changes include a shift toward greater proportions of CD4+ T cells of memory (CD44hiCD45RO+) phenotype and fewer cells of naive (CD44loCD45RA+) phenotype.[690,691] Paralleling these phenotypic changes are functional changes that occur with aging, including alterations in the profiles of cytokines produced in response to T cell activation.[692-694] T lymphocytes from old mice tend to exhibit an enhanced capacity to release IL-3, IL-4, IL-5 and IFN-γ,[692-694] which is consistent with the shift toward higher proportions of memory versus naive T cells. Neonatal allograft-primed BALB/c mice contain higher ratios of Th2/Th1 CD4+ T cells compared with adult primed mice.[695] An enrichment for Th1 cells in the "naive" (Mel-14+) population of aged mice has been reported.[696] In other studies, however, the ability of T cells to produce IL-4 appears to be also increased[697] or unchanged[694] with aging. Thus, no clear evidence to suggest the occurrence of a Th1 or a Th2 shift with aging is available.

STRESS

Numerous studies have investigated the effects of environmental and psychologic stress on alterations in immune parameters, and in susceptibility to disease.[698,699] Stress mainly acts by activation of the hypothalamic-pituitary adrenal axis. As little as 5 minutes of restraint stress causes increased expression of mRNA for *c-fos* and corticotropin-releasing hormone (CRH) in the rat hypothalamus,[700] which leads to production of adrenocorticotropic hormone (ACTH) by the pituitary and consequently of GCS by the adrenal gland. An important effect of acute physiologic stress is a redistribution of immune cells between different body compartments and such a redistribution may have significant consequences for the immune response.[701] For example, this redistribution may ensure that appropriate leukocytes are present in the right place at the right time to response to an immune challenge that may be initiated by the stress-inducing agent (e.g., attack by a predator, invasion by a pathogen, etc.). The modulation of immune cell distribution by acute stress may be an adaptive response designed to enhance immune surveillance and to increase the capacity of the immune system to respond to challenge in immune compartments (such as the skin and epithelia of lung, gastrointestinal and urogenital tracts), which serve as major defense barriers for the body. Indeed, in animals sensitized with dinitrochloro benzene (DNCB) and subjected to acute stress, an increase of DTH response to the chemical was observed. However, when the stress is very intense and increased production of ACTH and GCS persists, the possibility that stress may drive the switch from a Th1 to a Th2 response cannot be excluded.[264] The possibility that immune responses and production of cytokines are at least partially under the control of the sympathetic nervous system has also been suggested. First, Th1 cells express a high-affinity β_2-adrenoreceptor, whereas Th2 cells do not.[702] Moreover, chemical sympathectomy increased antibody production in C57Bl6J mice, characterized by dominant CMI responses, but not in BALB/cJ mice, showing prevalent humoral responses.[703] Finally, the possibility that Th2 cells act as a peripheral target of melatonin has been suggested.[704]

Studies on the effects of stress on the function of human T cell subsets are still at anecdotical level. Students stressed about their exams show increased titers of antibody to Epstein-Barr virus (EBV), implying transient activation of the latent infection that is normally controlled by CTL. A study of the consequences of an intensely stressful training course to which the U.S. Rangers are exposed showed a loss of DTH responses with relative sparing of humoral immunity. Of note is that thyroid hormone levels also fell so dramatically that the subjects became clinically hypothyroid and testosterone fell to levels observed in castrated males.[705] Thus, the fall in the ratio between DHEA (Th1-inducer) and GCS (Th2-inducer) (see above) may account for a possible impairment of the Th1 pathway and subsequent shifting of the immune response towards a prevalent Th2 profile.[264] So far, however, the evidence suggesting a Th1/Th2 switch as a consequence of stress is not convincing.

PREGNANCY AND UNEXPLAINED RECURRENT ABORTIONS

Mammalian reproduction is initiated by the mating of individuals with distinct genotypes and, therefore, mammalian embryos express antigens belonging to both maternal and paternal MHC. Despite the fact that the embryo, because of the presence of paternal MHC antigens, is similar to an allograft and therefore represents a potential target for the maternal immune system, it is usually not rejected until the time of delivery. This means that maternal immunologic recognition of the developing fetal semi-allograft is a complex process that allows fetal survival and growth to occur (immunologic tolerance of the conceptus). Several studies have indeed shown that certain cases of habitual miscarriage are the result of inappropriate maternal immune reaction against the fetus. However, the mechanisms involved in the immunologic tolerance of the conceptus, as well as those responsible for its premature rejection, are still unclear. The human decidua which is in strict contact with the conceptus contains a relatively large number of T lymphocytes and macrophages.[706] These cell types are potentially able to promote the rejection of fetal semi-allograft, which is first mediated by the recognition of paternal MHC antigens and then by the activity of effector T cells via the release of various cytokines. Therefore, changes in the recognition mechanisms and/or in the pattern of cytokines produced by the activated T cells are involved in the immunologic tolerance of the conceptus during successful pregnancy, as well as in its premature rejection. There is now convincing evidence to suggest that maternal T lymphocytes play an important role in the development of placenta and in fetal survival. The injection of anti-T cell antibodies in MRL-lpr/lpr homologous mice, which exhibit excessive T cell proliferation and large placentas, reduced placental parameters to normal.[707] In normal mice, the same treatment decreased placental size and in some strain combinations caused fetal resorption.[708] Inasmuch as many T cell effects are mediated via the production of cytokines, it is likely that the maintenance of the feto-placental unit is mainly dependent upon the type of cytokines produced by infiltrating decidual T cells during pregnancy. Accordingly, the injection of TNF-α, IFN-γ and IL-2 can increase fetal resorption rates in abortion prone (CBA/J X DBA/2) and nonabortion prone (CBA/J X Balb/c, C3H X DBA/2) matings, whereas IL-3 and GM-CSF increase the chances of fetal survival when injected into abortion prone mice.[709,710] Moreover, in CBA X DBA/2 mice, which have placentae deficient in IL-4 and IL-10 and show elevated fetal loss (50-70%), intraperitoneal injection of IL-10 reduced fetal loss to normal levels (5%). On the other hand, the injection of either anti-IFN-γ antibody or pentoxifillin (an anti-TNF agent) partially reduced the rate of resorption. When given together, anti-IFN-γ antibody and pentoxifillin produced a synergistic remission of fetal loss. Finally, the local defect in IL-10 and IL-4 production in this abortion prone combination was corrected by in vivo injection of IFN-τ (ovine trophoblast protein).[710] Other studies have shown that Th1-type cytokines, especially IFN-γ and TNF-α, impair early embryo development, as well as trophoblast growth and function in vitro.[711-713] Recently, Lin et al[714] have reported that the Th2-type cytokines IL-4, IL-5 and IL-10 are detectable at the materno-fetal interface during all periods of gestation, whereas IFN-γ production is transient, being detectable only in the first period. Based on these findings, the existence of a bidirectional interaction between the maternal immune system and the reproductive system during pregnancy was hypothesized.[715] Since Th1-type cytokines promote allograft rejection and therefore may compromise pregnancy, the production at the level of materno-fetal interface of Th2 cytokines which inhibit Th1 responses may improve fetal survival.[715,716] Accordingly, non-gestating females have almost undetectable levels of IL-4-producing cells in the spleen, whereas in gestating females IL-4-producing cells formed clusters mainly at the periphery of the organ, a pathway that was altered by administration of IFN-γ.[717] More importantly, in pregnant mice, placental levels for IL-4 mRNA expression were found to be 5- to 10-fold higher than the blood mRNA expression.[718] In the first week, placental IFN-γ levels were below the levels detected in the blood, whereas in the last weeks of gestation the difference was reversed.[718] The possibility that at least in mice a successful pregnancy is a Th2-mediated phenomenon was then supported by studies designed to investigate the relationship between pregnancy and infection. Infection with *L. major* is eliminated in resistant mice by a strong Th1 response, but persists longer in pregnant mice. This was accompanied by reduced IFN-γ and TNF-α responses to *L. major* antigens.[719] In the reverse direction, *L. major* infection resulted in implantation failures and fetal resorptions.[720] Even in surviving placentas, the protective cytokine IL-10 was reduced, and the harmful cytokine IFN-γ was increased. This interaction may have considerable implication for vaccination and treatment of infections during pregnancy.[720]

Unexplained Recurrent Abortions

Evidence is accumulating to support the view that maternal immunity may also unfavorably affect human gestation. First, women with recurrent spontaneous abortion can deliver a normal child following immunization with paternal or pooled third party white blood cells.[721] Moreover, there is clinical evidence that pregnant women undergo immunological changes consistent with a weakening of Th1 responses and strengthening of Th2 responses. Approximately 70% of women with rheumatoid arthritis (RA), which is characterized by prevalent Th1 responses (see below), experience a temporary remission of their symptoms during gestation.[722] Systemic lupus eryhthematosus (SLE), in which the principal pathology is mediated by excessive autoantibody production, that probably means remarkable Th2 cell activation (see below), tends to flare up during pregnancy, especially in women with recently active disease before conception.[715] There are also a number of infectious diseases caused by intracellular pathogens (such as HIV infection, leprosy, tuberculosis, malaria, toxoplasmosis and coccidioidomycosis) which appear to be exacerbated by pregnancy,[723-727] although a good deal of controversy surrounds this subject because of the difficulty of designing proper control groups. We recently investigated decidual T cells of pregnant women during the first period of gestation (from 8-12 weeks) by comparing the cytokine profile of CD4[+] and CD8[+] T cell clones established from both decidua and blood of women with unexplained recurrent abortion (URA) or voluntary abortion (normal gestation), as well as from endometrium and blood of nonpregnant women. Interestingly, although the majority of T cell clones from the three groups studied showed a Th0-like profile, significantly higher numbers of Th1-like T cell clones were generated from the decidua of women suffering from URA. By contrast, no differences in the cytokine profile of T cell clones generated from the peripheral blood of the three groups were found (M-P. Piccinni et al). Furthermore, T cell clones generated from the decidua of women with URA produced significantly lower IL-4 and IL-10 concentrations than T cell clones generated from either the decidua of voluntary abortion or the endometrium of nonpregnant women, but there were no differences in both IL-4 amounts produced by blood-derived T cell clones from the three groups (M-P. Piccinni et al). These results suggest that local production of IL-4 may be important for the maintenance of pregnancy, whereas its reduced production can compromise pregnancy. We also observed production of high levels of IFN-γ by T cell clones generated from the endometrium of nonpregnant women, whereas such levels were significantly lower in T cell clones derived from the decidua of voluntary abortions, and still lower in those generated from the decidua of women suffering from URA. By contrast, the amounts of IFN-γ produced by blood-derived T cell clones were comparable in women with URA or voluntary abortion and significantly higher than those produced by blood-derived T cell clones of nonpregnant women (Piccinni et al, unpublished data). In order to explain these findings, one might speculate that some IFN-γ production at the materno-fetal interface is required for fetal maintenance. On the other side, the increased production of IFN-γ by peripheral blood T cells during pregnancy may reflect the necessity to potentiate at the systemic level the response against intracellular bacteria and viruses that could be dangerous if they reach the fetus. High production of embryotoxic factor activity (EFA), as well as IFN-γ, TNF-α and TNF-β, by trophoblast-activated PBMC from women with URA has also been reported.[728] By contrast, cells from parous women with a history of normal pregnancies failed to produce both EFA and Th1-type cytokines, but produced Th2-type cytokines (IL-4 and IL-10), in response to trophoblast antigens.[728] The high correlation between EFA and Th1 cytokines (particularly IFN-γ) implicates a Th1-type response to trophoblast antigens in women with URA. At present, however, the mechanism by which trophoblast antigen(s) induce PBMC from women with URA to produce Th1-type cytokines are unclear. One possibility is that these women have an inability to mount a Th2-type response to trophoblast or other fetal antigens that would serve to downregulate harmful Th1-type responses. Recently, we have shown that PG concentrations comparable to those present at the materno-fetal interface favor the development of human T cells producing Th2-type cytokines (i.e., IL-4 and IL-5).[251] Furthermore, we showed that PG promotes both IL-4 production and CD30 expression in established Th1-like clones. Interestingly, CD30 has also been found to be largely present in the human decidual tissue, thus supporting the view that the expression of this molecule may be regulated by PG.[729] In the course of the same study, the effect of human chorionic gonadotropin (hCG), another hormone present at high levels during pregnancy, was investigated. HCG apparently showed no significant effect on the differentiation of T cells into one or another pattern of cytokine production, as well as on the cytokine profile of established T cell clones.[251] However, hCG may have an indirect modulatory effect on the T cell cytokine pattern via the stimulation of other active hormone(s). It is of interest that PG is also able to inhibit production of both EFA and IFN-γ and TNF-α by PBMC from women with URA stimulated with trophoblast antigens (K. Polgar, personal communication). On the other hand, PG is well known because of its immunosuppressive properties.[730] PG-mediated immunosuppression is needed for the maintenance of normal gestation.[731] Postcoital administration of a mouse monoclonal antibody against PG prevents pregnancy in several species.[732] A factor secreted by splenocytes from pregnant mice upon PG induction can correct resorption rates in CBA X DBA/2 mating, as well as prevent the abortifacient effects of Poly I-Poly C.[733] Thus, it is reasonable to suggest that the high levels of PG present at the materno-fetal interface during gestation may contribute, at least in part, to the development of a prevalent Th2-type profile which allows successful pregnancy. More recently, we examined the effect of RLX in the same system used to assess the activity of PG (see above). RLX is a polypeptide hormone mainly produced by the corpus luteum of pregnancy, that is active on both the mammary gland and the female reproductive organs.[734] RLX regulates cervical softening, inhibits uterine contractility, stimulates uterine growth and exerts other functions which are needed for the maintenance of pregnancy and for normal delivery.[734] Preliminary results indicate that RLX, at the physiologic concentrations found during pregnancy, favors the development of human Th cells producing Th1-type cytokines. Indeed, antigen-specific human CD4+ T cell lines derived in the presence of RLX exhibited a significantly increased ability to produce TNF-β and IFN-γ in comparison to T cell lines derived in the absence of RLX. In addition, antigen-specific T cell lines generated in the presence of RLX developed into T cell clones producing high levels of TNF-β. Furthermore, stimulation of established CD4⁺ antigen-specific T cell clones produced higher levels of IFN-γ in the presence than in the absence of RLX (M-P Piccinni et al, unpublished data).

These findings raise the intriguing question of why the same tissue during gestation can secrete two hormones (PG and RLX) that, at least in vitro, apparently promote two opposite T cell cytokine profiles, since PG is a Th2-, whereas RLX seems to be rather a Th1-, promoting agent. A tempting, even if oversimplistic, speculation may be that the predominance of PG at the beginning of pregnancy is needed in order to orient the local immune response against the conceptus towards a Th2-like pattern. The Th2 cytokines downregulate the potentially dangerous Th1 response, thus preventing premature fetus rejection. On the other hand, RLX might be useful in order to maintain and restore a Th1-oriented response that would be required for the delivery. A local imbalance in the concentration of the two hormones (in favor of RLX) in the early phase of gestation might impair the Th2 shift, thus allowing the production of high concentrations of IFN-γ and TNF-β, and therefore the premature rejection of the conceptus. Thus, the Th1/Th2 paradigm once more reveals its usefulness for the understanding of important pathophysiologic processes. Furthermore, the fact that hormonal influences seem to play a role in determining the predominance of one or the other cytokine pathway provides an excellent frame of reference to test additional hypotheses on the physiology of the immune system, as well as on its relationship with the endocrine system.

PRIMARY IMMUNODEFICIENCIES

HYPER-IgE SYNDROME

Selective defects or imbalances of lymphokine production have been reported in some primary immunodeficiencies. Circulating T cells from patients with the hyper-IgE syndrome were found to produce significantly reduced IFN-γ concentrations in response to stimulation with mitogens, calcium ionophores and phorbol ester.[735,736] A clonal analysis revealed that patients with hyper-IgE syndrome had markedly lower proportions of circulating T cells able to produce IFN-γ and TNF-α in comparison with controls.[735] Since IFN-γ inhibits the synthesis of IgE and both IFN-γ and TNF-α play an important role in inflammatory reactions, it has been suggested that reduced IFN-γ production may primarily account for hyperproduction of IgE and the combined defect of IFN-γ and TNF-α may contribute to deficiency of cell-mediated and nonspecific immunity observed in patients suffering from this syndrome.[735] A large drop in serum IgE was indeed observed in hyper-IgE patients following injection of IFN-γ[737] or IFN-α,[738] associated in some cases with clinical improvement of skin lesions.[738]

OMENN'S SYNDROME

Omenn's syndrome (OS) is a rare and severe combined immuno-deficiency, characterized by hypereosinophilia and increased serum levels of IgE. Defective production of IFN-γ and IL-2 and increased production of IL-4, IL-5 and IL-10 have been described in a 17-month-old girl suffering from this disease.[56] Interestingly, in this patient a therapeutic trial with IFN-γ induced not only amelioration of the clinical status and normalization of eosinophil count but also downregulated the in vivo expression of Th2-type cytokines.[56] Subsequent studies on three children with OS and one child with Omenn's-like syndrome showed high expression of CD30 in lymph node and skin-infiltrating T cells (Fig. 8.1), as well as high serum levels of sCD30.[55] T cell cloning of sorted CD30+ T cells from the peripheral blood of one of these children resulted in the development of virtually all these cells into Th2/Th0 clones, whereas the great majority of CD30- T cells developed in vitro into Th1-like clones.[55] Measurement of sCD30 in the serum of one of these children after successful bone marrow transplantation (BMT) revealed a dramatical decrease of its values in comparison with pretreatment values.[55]

Profound defects of IL-2, IFN-γ or IL-4 production upon activation with mitogens have been reported in patients with common variable hypogammaglobulinemia (CVH).[739-741] However, the possibility that alterations of distinct subsets of lymphokine-producing T cells are involved in different CVH patients has not yet been fully explored.

ATOPIC ALLERGY

Atopic allergy is a genetically determined disorder characterized by an increased ability of B lymphocytes to form IgE antibodies to certain groups of ubiquitous antigens that can activate the immune system after inhalation or ingestion, and perhaps after penetration through the skin (allergens). IgE antibodies are able to bind to high affinity (type I) Fcε receptors (FcεRI) present on the surface of mast cells/basophils and allergen-induced FcεRI crosslinking triggers the release of vasoactive mediators, chemotactic factors and cytokines that are responsible for the allergic cascade. In addition to IgE-producing B cells and IgE-binding mast cells/basophils, eosinophils also appear to be involved in the pathogenesis of allergic reactions, since these cells usually accumulate in the sites of allergic inflammation and the toxic products they release significantly contribute to the induction of tissue damage.

PATHOGENIC ROLE OF ALLERGEN-SPECIFIC TH2-LIKE CELLS

The mechanisms accounting for the joint involvement of IgE-producing B cells, mast cells/basophils and eosinophils in the pathogen-

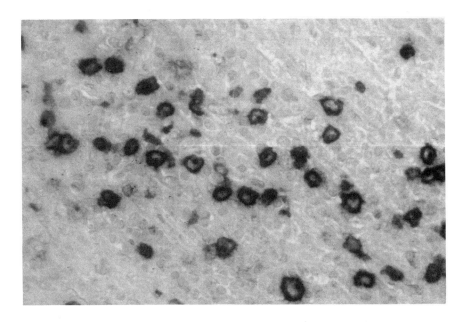

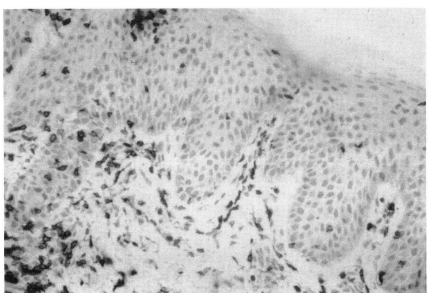

Fig. 8.1. Detection by immunohistochemistry of high numbers of CD30⁺ T cells in a lymph node (top) and in the skin (bottom) of a patient with Omenn's syndrome. LSAB-immunoperoxidase. Courtesy of Dr. M. Chilosi, Department of Pathology, University of Verona.

esis of allergic reactions have remained unclear until the existence of Th1 and Th2 cells was discovered. Because of its ability to produce IL-3, GM-CSF, IL-4, IL-5 and IL-10, the allergen-specific Th2 cell represents indeed an excellent candidate to explain why the mast cell/eosinophil/IgE-producing B cell triad is involved in the pathogenesis of allergy. IL-3, IL-4 and IL-10 are growth factors for mast cells; IL-3, GM-CSF and IL-5 favor the differentiation, the activation and the in situ survival of eosinophils. Moreover, IgE antibody synthesis results from the collaboration between Th2 cells and B cells. To this end, Th2 cells provide B cells with at least two signals: the former is delivered by IL-4;[742] the latter is represented by a T cell-to-B cell physical interaction, occurring between the CD40L expressed on the activated Th cell and the CD40 molecule constitutively expressed on the B cell.[743] The Th2 cell-derived IL-4 induces germ line ε expression on the B cell, whereas the CD40L/CD40 interaction is required for the expression of productive mRNA and for the synthesis of IgE protein. Another cytokine, IL-13, is also able to induce germ line ε expression, but its production is not restricted to the Th2 subset.[326] On the other hand, Th1 cells that produce IFN-γ but not IL-4, as well as Th0 cells that produce high concentrations of IFN-γ in addition to IL-4 and/or IL-13, are unable to support but rather suppress the IL-4-dependent IgE synthesis[742] (Fig. 8.2).

Strong evidence supports the concept that atopic allergic reactions are initiated by a Th2-type response: (1) allergens preferentially expand Th2-like cells in atopic subjects;[16,17] (2) Th2-like cells accumulate in the target organs of allergic patients;[744-748] (3) allergen-challenge results in the local activation and recruitment of allergen-specific Th2-like cells[749,750] and (4) successful specific immunotherapy associates with upregulation of Th1 cells or downregulation of allergen-reactive Th2 cells.[751-754] Allergen-reactive Th2-like cells expressing membrane CD30 are present in the circulation of allergic patients during seasonal allergen exposure.[48] Moreover, some CD30+ T cells are present in the lesional skin, and high levels of soluble CD30 are detectable in the serum of patients with atopic dermatitis.[54]

MECHANISMS RESPONSIBLE FOR THE DEVELOPMENT OF ALLERGEN-SPECIFIC T CELLS INTO TH2 CELLS IN ATOPIC SUBJECTS

The mechanisms responsible for the preferential activation of allergen-specific Th2 cells in atopic subjects are not yet clear. It is highly probable that LC present in the skin, as well as dendritic cells that are localized in the respiratory mucosa, represent the primary point of contact between the immune system and allergens coming into contact with the skin or the respiratory airways, respectively. Skin LC and mucosal dendritic cells are probably involved in allergen transport to regional lymph nodes where allergen presentation to allergen-specific CD4+ T cells

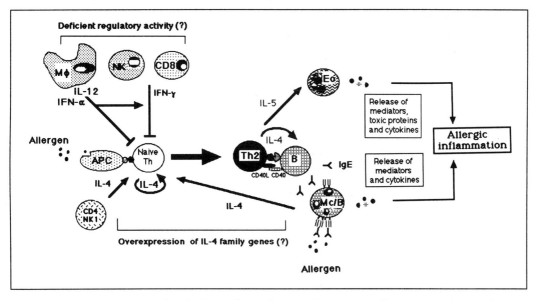

Fig. 8.2. Role of allergen-specific Th2-like cells in allergic inflammation. Allergens stimulate preferential development of Th2-like T cells in genetically determined individuals showing overexpression of IL-4 family genes at the level of Th cells (and/or CD4+NK.1+ cells and/or cells of the mast cell/basophil lineage) and/or deficient regulatory activity by cells (macrophages, NK cells, CD8+ T cells) producing Th2-inhibitory cytokines (IL-12, IFN-γ, IFN-α). Allergen-specific Th2 cells produce IL-4 (which promotes IgE switching in B cells), and IL-5 (which induces differentiation, activation and promotes in situ survival of eosinophils). Crosslinking by allergen of IgE bound to Fcε receptors on mast cells/basophils promotes the release of mediators and cytokines, including IL-4 which in turn may amplify the Th2 response. Mediators, toxic proteins, and cytokines released by both eosinophils and mast cell/basophils initiate and all together sustain the allergic inflammation in the target organ (eye, nose, bronchi, skin).

occurs. Some data suggest that atopic patients with asthma may have higher numbers of intraepithelial DC than nonasthmatic subjects and that these cells in the presence of allergen molecules can induce T cell activation and production of IL-4 and IL-5.[755] However, the actual role played by APC in driving the development of allergen-reactive Th2-like cells remains to be elucidated. Although evidence for the pivotal role of specific Vβ-expressing T cell subsets in the stimulation of IgE production and increased airway responsiveness induced by ragweed allergen has been reported,[254] the role of TCR repertoire in determining the development of Th1 or Th2-type responses is controversial (see above). However, it cannot be excluded that the recognition of allergen by the TCR provides a signal or sets of signals that drive the T cells in a certain direction, e.g., to produce IL-4 or alternatively, IFN-γ. So far, however, the most dominant factor in determining the likelihood for Th2-cell polarization appears to be IL-4 produced at the time of T cell activation.[183-185] The cell sources possibly responsible for the early IL-4 production, which is required in order to favor the Th2-cell development, have been discussed in a previous paragraph.

Mast cells, basophils, and eosinophils have been shown to release stored IL-4 in response to FcεR triggering.[191-202] However, allergens would be unable to crosslink these receptors prior to a specific immune response that had produced allergen-specific IgG and IgE antibodies. A possible role of CD4⁺ NK1⁺ T cells in providing early IL-4 required for the Th2-cell development has also been suggested.[216] In this respect, it is of note that SJL mice, which are unable to produce IgE, also lack CD4⁺NK1⁺ T cells.[220] However, these cells appear to be present in similar proportions in both nonatopic and atopic human donors (unpublished results). A final possibility is that early IL-4 is provided by the allergen-specific naive Th cell itself.[226-229] In this case, the fact that allergens induce Th2-type responses only in selected people suggests that the genetic background of atopic individuals, rather than environmental conditions, is essential in favoring the development of allergen-reactive Th2 cells. This means that atopic subjects would have genetic disregulation in the production of IL-4 and/or of cytokines exerting regulatory effects on the development and/or function of Th2 cells (Fig. 8.2).

POSSIBLE GENETIC ALTERATIONS FAVORING ALLERGEN-SPECIFIC TH2 RESPONSES IN ATOPIC SUBJECTS

The possibility that atopic subjects have a genetic dysregulation at the level of IL-4 produced by Th cells is supported by several observations. First, CD4⁺ T cell clones from atopic individuals are able to produce noticeable amounts of IL-4 and IL-5 in response to bacterial antigens, such as PPD and streptokinase, that usually evoke responses with a restricted Th1-like cytokine profile in nonatopic individuals.[756] Second, T cell clones generated from cord blood lymphocytes of newborns with atopic parents produce higher IL-4 concentrations than neonatal lymphocytes of newborns with nonatopic parents.[757] Moreover, large panels of *Parietaria officinalis* group 1 (Par O 1)-specific T cell clones were generated from donors with low or high serum IgE levels and assessed for their profile of cytokine production and reactivity to two immunodominant Par O 1 peptides (p92 and p96). Interestingly, both p92- and p96-specific T cell clones generated from 'high IgE' donors produced remarkable amounts of IL-4 and low IFN-γ. In contrast, T cell clones generated from 'low IgE' donors showed a different profile of cytokine production: the majority of those specific for p96 produced high amounts of both IL-4 and IFN-γ, whereas most p92-specific T cell clones showed a Th1-like profile (high IFN-γ and low IL-4) (P. Parronchi et al, manuscript in preparation). Taken together, these data strongly suggest that allergen peptide ligand can influence the cytokine profile of Th cells; however, mechanisms underlying noncognate regulation of IgE responsiveness are overwhelming.

Regarding the role of the allergen peptide ligand, several studies have underlined the potential importance of MHC class II haplotype[758] but the data remain controversial. A gene (or genes) in the TCRα/δ complex has been described to influence the development of a specific IgE response in allergic subjects,[759] and a restricted usage of Vα13 by T cell clones specific for *Lolium perenne* group 1 (Lol p 1), as well as an intra- and interindividually restricted TCR-Vβ usage in both Lol p 1- and *Poa pratensis* group 9 (Poa p 9)-specific T cell lines, was also reported.[255] On the other hand, the evidence for a linkage of overall IgE to markers in chromosome 5q31.1, especially to the IL-4 gene,[760] suggests that one or more polymorphisms exist in a coding region or, more probably, a regulatory region of the IL-4 gene. Several studies have identified potential mechanisms governing the IL-4 gene expression in human and murine T cells. Transcription of IL-4 gene is stringently regulated by multiple promoter elements acting together[312-316] (Fig. 8.3). More recently, the existence of a polymorphism at the level of the IL-4 gene promoter has been directly demonstrated.[318] Thus, the more likely possibility is that atopic subjects have an altered regulation at the level of the IL-4 gene. However, numerous genes map within 5q31.1, including IL-13, which might influence IgE production. Other possible candidates are IRF1, whose gene product upregulates IFN-α, which in turn can downregulate IgE production and inhibit Th2 cell development[177,179] and IL12B, which encodes the β chain of IL-12, a known inducer of IFN-γ production by CD4+ and CD8+ T cells and by NK cells,[146] as well as a powerful inducer of Th1 responses.[147,153] In this respect, it is noteworthy that the depletion of a subpopulation of IFN-γ-producing CD8+ T cells with a sublethal dose of ricin results in a massive increase in serum IgE.[761] More importantly, IFN-γ released by MHC class I-restricted CD8+ γδ+ T cells prevents the development of Th2-like cells in response to nonreplicating antigens presented at mucosal surfaces.[762,763] Recent experiments suggest a possible role of CD8+ T cells in controlling the allergen-specific Th2 response in humans, as well. First, the Par O 1 peptide 92 (see above) expanded higher numbers of CD8+ T cell clones in "low" than in "high" IgE producers. In addition, lactalbumin expanded higher numbers of CD8+ T cell clones in nonatopic than in atopic milk-sensitive donors (P. Parronchi et al, unpublished results), suggesting that allergen-specific CD8+ T cells may play an important role (via IFN-γ production?) in shifting the response of CD4+ Th cells to the same allergen from Th2 to Th1.

Thus, either alterations of molecular mechanisms directly involved in the regulation of IL-4 gene expression, or deficient regulatory activity of cytokines responsible for inhibition of Th2-cell development (such as IFN-α/γ and IL-12), or both, may account for the preferential Th2-type response towards environmental allergens in atopic people. An overexpression of other cytokine genes (IL-3, IL-5, GM-CSF and IL-9), located together with IL-4 and IL-13 within the same cluster of chromosome 5, may also be present. The overexpression of the above genes can account for the preferential development of Th2 cells in response to allergens, as well as for the production by Th2 cells and even by other cell types of the cytokines involved in the allergic inflammation and therefore explain the persistent histological, pathophysiological and clinical aspects of allergic disorders[764] (Fig. 8.2).

VERNAL CONJUNCTIVITIS

The first description of the cytokine profile of T cells from tissue in allergic disease was in vernal conjunctivitis, a condition of papillary hyperthrophy of the conjunctiva with eosinophil and lymphocyte infiltration and associated high serum IgE. T cell clones were made from tissues by initial expansion with PHA followed by IL-2. Clones from the conjunctival tissue of three patients were mostly CD4$^+$ and produced IL-4 but little IFN-γ. These clones supported IgE synthesis in vitro.[24] Interestingly, an allergic-like blepharitis (inflammation of the eyelid) with a mononuclear cell infiltrate was observed in a cohort of IL-4 transgenic mice expressing IL-4 at the level of B lymphocytes.[765]

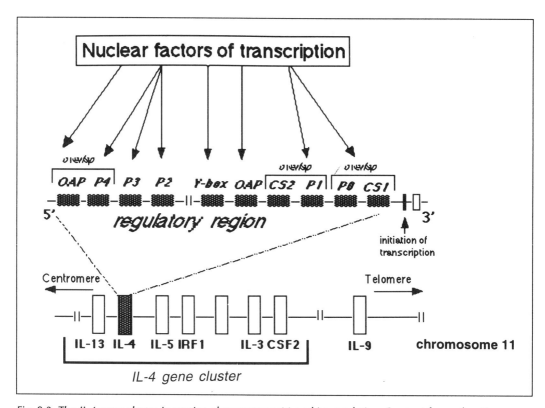

Fig. 8.3. The IL-4 gene cluster in murine chromosome 11 and its regulation. See text for explanations.

ALLERGIC RHINITIS

Nasal allergen provocation, followed by nasal mucosa biopsy 24 hours after allergen challenge, in patients with allergic rhinitis is associated with a cellular infiltrate, in which CD4⁺ T cells and eosinophils are pre-eminent.[766] By use of the complementary techniques of immuno-

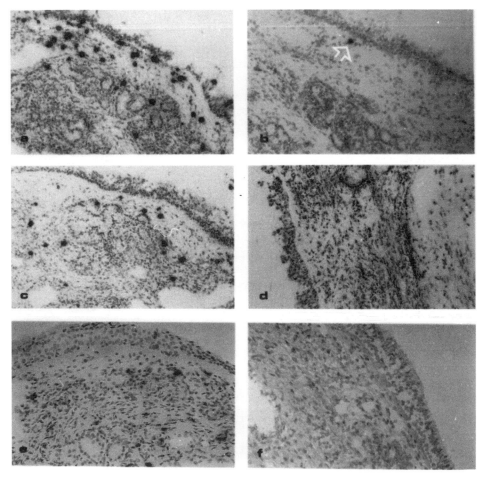

Fig. 8.4. Presence of IL-4 and IL-5 expressing cells and of eosinophils in the nasal mucosa of an allergic patient.
(a) and (b): autoradiographs of cryostat sections of nasal biopsies from allergen- and control-challenged sites. Sections were hybridized with a labeled antisense IL-5 probe.
(c) and (d): autoradiographs of sections from allergen-challenged sites hybridized with ³⁵S-labeled anti-sense and sense IL-4 probes
(e) and (f): cellular infiltration by EG2⁺ eosinophils at allergen-challenged sites compared with control sites (after challenge with the allergen diluent). Sections were immunostained using the alkaline phosphatase-anti-alkaline phosphatase method.
Courtesy of Dr. A.B. Kay, Department of Allergy and Clinical Immunology, National Heart and Lung Institute, London.

histology and in situ hybridization an increase in cytokine mRNA expression for IL-3, IL-4, IL-5 and GM-CSF was found, which correlated with the degree of local eosinophilia[766] (Fig. 8.4). Accordingly, CD4+ T cell clones generated from the nasal mucosa after allergen challenge, many of which were specific for the allergen used in the challenge test, showed a prevalent Th2 profile.[749] However, in another study performed on patients with perennial allergic rhinitis a complete lack of any cytokine immunoreactivity localized to tissue lymphocytes was found. Mast cells accounted for >90% of IL-4- and IL-6- and >50% of IL-5-immunoreactive cells.[38] These findings leave open the question of whether allergic inflammation in the mucosa of patients with allergic rhinitis is initiated by Th2 cells that do not accumulate cytokines in sufficient concentrations to be consistently detected by immunohistochemical methods, or by mast cells which may be able to secrete Th2 cytokines rapidly and in high concentrations.

ALLERGIC ASTHMA

Animal models

Antigen challenge to the lungs of sensitized mice produces an intense influx of eosinophils into the BAL fluid and lung tissue. Bronchial hyperreactivity is an important feature of asthmatic airways and can be demonstrated in sensitized mice following repeated exposure to antigen.[767] There is also increased expression of IL-4 and IL-5 mRNA, as well as IL-4 and IL-5 protein levels, but not significant increases in IFN-γ in the lungs of allergic mice, with the main source coming from T cells.[768-770] Administration of anti-IL-4 antibodies or soluble IL-4 receptors inhibits IgE and IgG$_1$ production, as well as airway hyperreactivity, but not eosinophilia, in sensitized mice,[771,772] whereas administration of anti-IL-5 antibody at levels that suppressed eosinophils to less than 1% of recruited cells had no effect on the subsequent airway response.[773] The possibility that IL-4 can induce tissue inflammation has been demonstrated by injection of murine Th2 cells into the footpad of naive animals. Th2 cells induced swelling that peaked at 6 hours and lasted about 48 hours and was completely blocked by anti-IL-4 antibody or soluble IL-4 receptors.[774] However, the majority of data suggest that airway hyperreactivity is also IL-5-dependent. First, antibodies to IL-5 inhibit both pulmonary eosinophilia and hyperreactivity in allergic mice.[775] More importantly, in IL-5-deficient mice, the eosinophilia, lung damage and airway hyperreactivity normally resulting from allergen challenge are abolished.[776] The role of Th2-type cytokines in the induction and maintenance of the allergic inflammation is supported by the observation that administration of recombinant IFN-α, induction of endogenous IFN-α/β by Poly I-Poly C, or administration of IL-12 (which downregulate Th2 responses) inhibit

antigen-induced eosinophil infiltration in the murine trachea and airways hyperreactivity.[770,777] The inhibitory effect of IL-12 on antigen-
induced airway hyperresponsiveness was dependent on IFN-γ activity,
whereas depletion of eosinophils was only partially IFN-γ dependent.[770]
Parenteral administration of IFN-γ also failed to decrease IgE production
and to normalize airway function, but treatment regimens of sensitized mice with nebulized IFN-γ caused a decrease in cutaneous reactivity and normalization of airway responsiveness.[778] The possible role
of increased numbers of IFN-γ producing CD8⁺ T cells in this process
was suggested.[779] Finally, mice lacking the IFN-γ receptor have an impaired ability to resolve lung eosinophilic inflammatory reactions
associated with Th2 responses.[780]

Bronchial hyperresponsiveness and eosinophil infiltration into lung
tissue and BAL are also a characteristic feature of antigen challenge to
the airways of sensitized guinea pigs. Treatment with antibodies to
IL-5 inhibits these pulmonary responses.[781] Furthermore, administration of murine IL-5 to normal guinea pig lungs induces a small but
significant increase in bronchoconstrictor reactivity and an increase in
the number of inflammatory cells in the BAL fluid.[782] IL-5 is also
involved in the development of eosinophilic lung inflammation and
bronchial hyperresponsiveness in monkeys, because treatment with an
anti-IL-5 antibody inhibits both eosinophil influx into the airways and
early and late phase bronchoconstriction and bronchial hyperresponsiveness in antigen-challenged *Ascaris Suum*-sensitive cynomolgus
monkeys. Interestingly, inhibition of the pulmonary eosinophilia and
bronchial hyperresponsiveness by the anti-IL-5 antibody were seen to
persist for at least three months after a single treatment.[783] These results demonstrate the importance of Th2 cytokines, especially of IL-5,
in the induction of allergic pulmonary inflammation and airway
hyperreactivity in both rodents and nonhuman primates.

Human asthma

Astma in humans is a complex disorder characterized by intermittent, reversible airway obstruction, and by airway hyperresponsiveness
and inflammation. Although its causes remain unknown, we now recognize that asthma is a syndrome whose common pathologic expression is inflammation of the airways.[784] Based on clinical and labora-
tory findings, asthma may be divided into allergic (extrinsic) and
nonallergic (intrinsic) forms. Allergic asthma usually starts during child-
hood and is characterized by allergen-dependent, often seasonal symptoms with positive skin tests to allergens and elevated total and allergen-specific serum IgE. In contrast, nonallergic asthma usually begins
in adulthood, is perennial and more severe, has no elevation in serum
IgE, and is often associated with sinusitis and nasal polyposis. Both
allergic and intrinsic asthma are characterized by infiltration of the

bronchial mucosa with large numbers of activated eosinophils and the presence of elevated concentrations of eosinophil-derived proteins, such as major basic protein and the eosinophil cationic protein.[785]

By specific immunostaining of bronchial mucosal biopsies obtained via the fibrotic bronchoscope, a significant increase in the number of IL-2 receptor-positive (activated T cells) in the airways of mild, steady-state asthmatics was observed.[786] Using in situ hybridization technique, cells showing mRNA for Th2, but not Th1, lymphokines were found at the site of late phase reactions in skin biopsies from atopic patients,[744] and in mucosal bronchial biopsies or BAL of patients with atopic asthma.[747,748] By use of immunomagnetic separation the majority of IL-4 and IL-5 mRNA in BAL cells from asthmatic subjects were shown to be associated with CD2$^+$ T cells[748] (Fig. 8.5). Interestingly, corticosteroid treatment in asthma resulted in downregulation of BAL cells expressing mRNA for IL-4 and IL-5, whereas the number of cells expressing mRNA for IFN-γ was increased.[787] GCS, as well as the immunosuppressants FK506 and cyclosporin A, also suppress IL-5 production by PBMC from mite-sensitive atopic asthmatics.[788] In contrast, no effect on the number of BAL cells expressing mRNA for IL-4 and IL-5 was observed, suggesting that steroid-resistant asthma may be associated with a dysregulation in the expression of the genes encoding for Th2/Th1 cytokines in airway cells.[789] In order to assess whether the T cell response to inhaled allergens induced activation and recruitment of allergen-specific Th2 cells in the airway mucosa of patients with respiratory allergy, T cell clones were generated from biopsy specimens of bronchial mucosa of patients with grass pollen-induced asthma or rhinitis, taken 48 hours after a positive bronchial provocation test with the relevant allergen. As control, T cell clones were also derived from biopsy specimens taken from the bronchial mucosa of patients with toluene diisocyanate (TDI)-induced asthma 48 hours after positive bronchial provocation test with toluen TDI. Proportions ranging from 14-22% of CD4$^+$ clones derived from stimulated mucosae of grass-allergic patients were specific for grass allergens and most of them exhibited a definite Th2 profile and induced IgE production by autologous B cells in the presence of the specific allergen.[749] In contrast, none of the T cell clones derived from the bronchial mucosa of patients with TDI-induced asthma were specific for grass allergens and the majority of them were CD8$^+$ T cells producing IFN-γ and IL-2 or IFN-γ, IL-2 and IL-5, but no IL-4.[749] Likewise, allergen inhalation challenge resulted in the activation of CD4$^+$ T cells, increased Th2-type cytokine mRNA expression, and eosinophil recruitment in BAL of patients with atopic asthma.[787,790]

Because many studies addressing abnormalities of T lymphocyte cytokine secretion in asthma have been performed on subjects who are also atopic, the question of whether disordered cytokine synthesis by T lymphocytes in asthmatics simply reflects the existence of atopy or

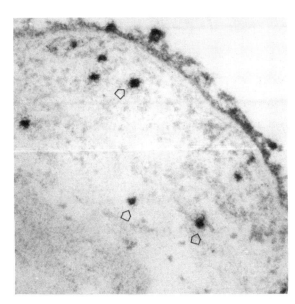

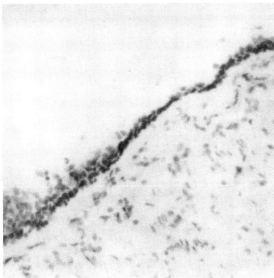

Fig. 8.5. Autoradiograph of bronchial asthma mucosa of a patient with symptomatic asthma. In situ hybrydization was performed under high-stringency conditions with a ^{32}P-labeled cRNA probe coding for IL-5 mRNA. Arrows indicate the IL-5 mRNA positive cells. On the bottom: the section was hybridized with IL-5 cRNA antisense probe. Courtesy of Dr. A.B. Kay, Department of Allergy and Clinical Immunology, National Heart and Lung Institute, London.

implies a role in asthma pathogenesis is still unsolved. In a recent study, PBMC from atopic and nonatopic asthmatic children were stimulated with PHA in vitro and concentrations of both IL-4 and IFN-γ released into cell supernatants were measured. Although stimulated PBMC from the atopic asthmatics secreted significantly more IL-4 and significantly less IFN-γ than those from both the nonatopic asthmatics and the normal controls, no significant differences were observed in the secretion of both cytokines by cells from the nonatopic asthmatics and the normal controls,[791] suggesting that the imbalance in cytokine secretion relates to the atopic state rather than specifically to the presence of asthma and that "intrinsic" asthma is a distinct immunopathological entity.[792] Indeed, while increased levels of IL-4 and IL-5 were measured in the BAL of allergic asthmatics, in nonallergic asthmatics IL-2 and IL-5 predominated.[793] Accordingly, CD8[+] T cell clones producing IFN-γ and IL-5, but not IL-4, were generated from the bronchial mucosa of nonatopic patients with TDI-induced asthma.[749] Moreover, CD4[+] and CD8[+] T cell lines generated from the BAL of asthmatics secreted significantly higher quantities of IL-5 and GM-CSF than lines from the atopic and nonatopic controls.[794] Taken together, these data suggest that elevated IL-4 synthesis by T lymphocytes is a feature of the atopic state and is not a prerequisite for the development of asthma, whereas elevated secretion of IL-5 is a feature of asthmatic patients and may occur in asthmatic patients in the absence of elevated IL-4 secretion. Thus, the Th1/Th2 model does not appear sufficiently flexible to account for the behavior of T cells in the pathogenesis of asthma. The picture is further complicated by the accumulating evidence showing that IL-4 and IL-5 may originate not only from activated Th2-like cells, but also from mast cells, basophils and eosinophils present in the bronchial mucosa and BAL of asthmatics.

ATOPIC DERMATITIS

Atopic dermatitis (AD) is the cutaneous disorder of atopic allergy due to chronic skin inflammation which results from the exposure to foreign proteins. The majority of patients with AD (>80%) have positive intracutaneous skin test reactions to one or more environmental allergens and elevated serum IgE levels, which represent antibodies specific to the allergens concerned. The histological appearance of lesional AD skin is characterized by dermal perivascular infiltrates of mononuclear cells, mainly consisting of CD4[+] T cells and eosinophils.[795,796] However, the relationship between allergy and the pathogenesis of the skin lesions in AD is still unclear. By using the RT-PCR technique, spontaneous mRNA IL-4 expression was found in PBMC from AD patients,[797] whereas IL-13, another IgE-switching cytokine, was not produced.[798] IFN-γ mRNA expression was also increased in PBMC from AD patients, but IFN-γ production was reduced, suggesting a posttranscriptional defect of IFN-γ secretion.[799] IFN-γ production by PBMC from AD patients was found to be deficient in response to stimulation with toxic shock syndrome toxin-1 (TSST-1) or IL-12, whereas both IL-12 production and IL-12 receptor (IL-12R) expression in the same patients were normal.[800] However, neutralization of IL-4, and even more of IL-10, activity caused a great augmentation of IFN-γ production. These data suggest that PBMC from AD patients, despite normal levels of IL-12 production and IL-12R expression, are unable to generate normal IL-12-induced IFN-γ responses, which may be related to the excess production of IL-4 and IL-10.[800]

High proportions of Der p-specific Th2-like CD4$^+$ T cell clones were obtained from the skin lesions of patients with AD, indicating accumulation or expansion of these T cells in lesional skin.[746,801] Interestingly, Der p-specific Th2-like clones were also derived from biopsy specimens of intact skin taken after contact challenge with Der p, suggesting that percutaneous sensitization to aeroallergens may play a role in the induction of skin lesions in patients with AD.[746,802] More recent data partially confirm both the Der p-specificity and the Th2-type profile of high proportions of T cell clones derived from Der p-induced patch test lesions of AD patients. However, the majority of T cell clones derived from the lesional skin of patients with AD had a mixed (Th0-like) phenotype and only a minority of them were specific for Der p. Interestingly, Der p-specific T cell clones generated from the skin of AD patients usually have a more polarized Th2 cytokine profile than those obtained from the peripheral blood of the same patients and consistently produce IL-10 in addition to IL-4 and IL-5.[803] In some patients, most T cell clones derived from lesional skin exhibited high IFN-γ production and a few of them appeared to be specific for bacterial antigens. More importantly, the presence of both Der p-specific and Th2-like cells in the skin of AD patients did not correlate with the presence in the serum of Der p-specific IgE antibody or the serum levels of IgE protein.[804] By using the RT-PCR technique, overexpression of IL-10, but not of IL-4, was found in AD lesions in comparison with allergic contact dermatitis lesions and tuberculin reactions.[805] Moreover, by assessing the kinetics of T cell-derived cytokine production, it was found that in the initiation phase IL-4 production is predominant over IFN-γ production. This is in line with the recent demonstration that epicutaneous exposure of protein antigens can induce a predominant Th2-like response with high IgE production in mice.[81] In the late and chronic phase (lesional skin) the situation may be reversed and IFN-γ production predominates over IL-4 production. Taken together, these data suggest that Th2-like responses against Der p or other allergens at skin level are involved in the initiation of skin lesions, but there is a subsequent influx of Th1 cells, which may be responsible for the aggravation of the inflammation. However, the relationship between aeroallergen sensitization and pathogenesis of AD still remains unclear.

CONTACT DERMATITIS

Contact allergens, in contrast to atopic allergens, are small chemicals that passively cross the epidermis and can induce dermatitis after repeated exposure. The reaction is based on a chronic DTH. Mouse model experiments have stressed the importance of both CD4$^+$ and CD8$^+$ T cells in contact hypersensitivity,[806] as well as the role of TNF-α as a critical mediator.[807,808] However, a number of other cytokines are produced in the skin after the application of antigens for contact hypersensitivity, including IFN-γ, GM-CSF, IL-1α, IL-1β and IL-10.[809]

The response typically peaks at 24 hours, with some reduction at 48 hours, and by 72 hours the area can return to normal size despite the continuous presence of antigen, suggesting that Th1-type cytokines (IFN-γ, TNF-α) are responsible for the inflammatory response and other cytokines promote its downregulation. Accordingly, injection of an anti-IL-12 antiserum inhibited both IFN-γ production by about 55% and significantly reduced ear swelling responses by 85%, thus almost completely preventing contact sensitization.[810,811] Evidence has also been provided to suggest that IL-10 is the main mediator in the natural control of contact hypersensitivity responses.[812] Injection of mice with IL-10 shortly before sensitization with trinitro cholorbenzene (TNCB) induced anergy[813] and administration of IL-10 before rechallenge diminished the recall response.[812,814] In contrast, the infusion of mice with IL-4 reduced the magnitude of the recall response, but failed to inhibit the sensitization step.[815] Likewise, IL-10-deficient mice exhibit an exaggerated contact hypersensitivity response to irritant crotton oil, whereas responses of IL-4-deficient mice did not differ from wildtype controls.[816] These data suggest that IL-10, but not IL-4, is the natural suppressant of Th1-mediated contact hypersensitivity responses, and it limits immunopathologic damage in the skin. More recent data, however, provide evidence that CD is not always a Th1-dominated pathology. In BALB/c mice, both 2,4-dinitrofluorobenzene (DNFB) and fluorescein isotiocyenate (FITC) induce CD. However, the DNFB response is Th1-predominant, while the FITC response is Th2 predominant.[817] Interestingly, however, depletion of CD8+ T cells before sensitization of BALB/c mice with DNFB or oxazolone resulted in low or abrogated contact hypersensitivity response, whereas depletion of CD4+ T cells resulted in increased and prolonged response, indicating CD4+ T cells as negative regulators of the response. DNFB sensitization induced CD8+ T cells producing IFN-γ and no IL-4 or IL-10, whereas DNFB-induced CD4+ T cells produced IL-4 and IL-10 and no or little detectable IFN-γ. Moreover, epicutaneous exposure of protein antigen has recently been found capable of inducing a predominant Th2-like response with high IgE production.[88]

About 10% of the human population is sensitized to the contact allergen nickel. Most of the nickel-specific T cell clones generated from PBMC of patients with contact dermatitis were common CD4+ T cells that produced high concentrations of TNF-α, IL-2, granulocyte/macrophage-colony-stimulating factor (GM-CSF) and IFN-γ, but not IL-4 and IL-5, thus revealing a restricted Th1-like profile.[819] Since IFN-γ is an important mediator in the DTH reaction, IFN-γ secretion by nickel-specific T cell clones may be a crucial feature of the pathogenesis. However, it is intriguing that nickel-specific Th1-type clones could be isolated from the peripheral blood of both nickel-allergic and nonallergic donors, suggesting that the DTH reaction in nickel-allergic patients is not due to a basic abnormality in lymphokine secretion.[820] In addition, nickel-specific T cell clones generated from the site of inflammation in one nickel-sensitive patient were found to express a Th2/Th0-like phenotype, suggesting that in addition to IFN-γ, the Th2 cytokines IL-4 and IL-5 may be involved in the immunopathogenesis of contact dermatitis.[820]

AUTOIMMUNE DISORDERS

Several findings indicate that autoimmune diseases develop as a result of abnormalities in the immune response mediated by activated T cells and T cell-derived lymphokines. Strong evidence deriving from both studies in animal models and investigation in human disease suggests that Th1-type lymphokines are involved in the genesis of organ-specific autoimmune diseases. In contrast, a less restricted lymphokine pattern is emerging from experimental studies on systemic autoimmune diseases. Accordingly, data so far available in human diseases are in favor of a prevalent Th1 lymphokine profile in target organs of patients with organ specific autoimmunity, such as Hashimoto's thyroiditis, multiple sclerosis (MS) and type 1 insulin-dependent diabetes mellitus (IDDM), whereas a less restricted lymphokine pattern is detectable in patients with rheumatoid arthritis (RA) and Sjögren's syndrome or even a prevalent Th2 pattern in patients with systemic lupus erythematosus (SLE) and systemic scleroderma (SSc) (Table 8.1).

AUTOIMMUNE THYROID DISEASES

Autoimmune thyroid diseases include Hashimoto's thyroiditis (HT) and Graves' disease (GD). HT is an organ-specific autoimmune disease that is characterized by massive infiltration of lymphoid cells in the thyroid gland and parenchimal destruction leading to hypothyroidism. GD is another autoimmune disorder of the thyroid gland with similar histologic picture, but distinguishable from HT by associated

Table 8.1. Spectrum of autoimmune disorders according to their prevalent Th cell cytokine profile

Th1	Th0	Th2
Multiple sclerosis		
Insulin-dependent diabetes mellitus		
Uveoretinitis		
Hashimoto's thyroiditis		
	Graves' disease	
	Rheumatoid arthritis	
	Sjögren's syndrome	
		Systemic lupus erythematosus
		Systemic sclerosis

ophtalmopathy and production of thyroid-stimulating antibodies leading to hyperthyroidism.

Experimental autoimmune thyroiditis

An experimental autoimmune thyroiditis (EAT) can be induced by immunization of susceptible mice with thyroglobulin in CFA, which results in strong activation of thryoidal antigen-specific T cells.[821] Autoreactive T cell clones can indeed transfer a disease very similar to that induced by immunization.[822] Transfer of the disease can be achieved with both CD4+ and CD8+ specific T cell lines and clones specific for thyroid epithelial cells that exhibit a clear-cut Th1 pattern of cytokine production.[823,824] Moreover, IL-12 and IFN-γ play a major role in the expression of thyroiditis in the BioBreeding (BB) rat, in whose inflammatory lesions Th1 lymphocytes predominate over Th2 lymphocytes.[825] By contrast, in vitro incubation of thyroglobulin-specific effector cells with IL-10 reduced lymphocytic infiltrations of the recipient thyroid glands, whereas incubation with IL-4 had no effect on lymphocytic infiltrations, but significantly reduced the levels of anti-thyroglobulin antibodies into recipient mice,[826] thus supporting the view that experimental autoimmune thyroiditis is generally a Th1-mediated disorder. However, when T cells were cultured in the presence of anti-IFN-γ antibody or anti-IL-2 receptor antibody another histological form of thyroiditis could be induced,[827,828] suggesting that under these conditions Th0 or even Th2 cells are activated and determine a distinct form of autoimmune process.

Hashimoto's thyroiditis and Graves' disease

Although the precise etiology of HT remains largely unknown, there is general consensus that infiltrating T lymphocytes play an essential role in the destruction of target organs. Several studies have shown that T cells from lymphocytic thyroid infiltrates of patients with HT or GD exhibit both a restricted Th1 lymphokine profile with production of high TNF-α and IFN-γ concentrations, and strong cytolytic potential.[23,829-834] A prevalent Th1-like cytokine profile was also observed by RT-PCR in the thyroid gland of patients with HT. A quite homogenous Th1 phenotype was also observed in CD4+ T cell clones derived from retroorbital infiltrates of patients with Graves' ophtalmopathy.[835] Similar results were obtained by analyzing cytokine gene expression by RT-PCR in intrathyroidal lymphocytes from six patients with GD. IL-2, IFN-γ and TNF-α, but not IL-4, mRNA were found, suggesting clear predomination of Th1 responses.[836] In contrast, by using the same technique, other authors found a more heterogenous cytokine profile in both the thryoid gland and retroorbital infiltrates of patients with GD.[837-840] The reason for these discrepancies may be explained with the different cytokine profile of thyroid antigen-specific T cells. Indeed, the majority of thyroid peroxidase (TPO)-specific clones showed a Th1 profile, whereas the cytokine profile of clones specific for thyroid-stimulating hormone receptor (TSHR) was more characteristic of Th0 or Th2 cells.[841] Thus, it is possible that the thyroid microenvironment allows the expansion not only of autoreactive T cells able to release IFN-γ, but also of other clones which secrete IL-4 and IL-10, and therefore are more active in promoting the synthesis of pathogenic autoantibodies.

AUTOIMMUNE DEMYELINIZATING DISEASES

Multiple sclerosis (MS) is considered a prototypic autoimmune disorder of the central nervous system (CNS). Active lesions in the brains of MS patients are characterized by lymphocytes (mainly CD4+ T cells) and macrophage infiltration, which associate with a progressive demyelinizing process. Although the etiology of the disease is still unclear, the pathogenesis clearly involves an autoimmune reaction against myelin antigens, such as MBP, PLP and possibly other proteins.[842]

Experimental allergic encephalomyelitis

There is a primary animal model for MS showing clinical and pathological similarities to the human disease, which is named experimental allergic encephalomyelitis (EAE).[843] EAE can be induced by immunization with different CNS-related proteins emulsified in CFA, including myeline basic protein (MBP) and proteolipiol protein (PLP). This results in the activation of peptide-specific CD4+ T cells which in turn can adoptively transfer the disease in naive animals. The majority of T cell clones derived from mice immunized with MBP or PLP peptides, when analyzed on the basis of IFN-γ/IL-2 production versus IL-4/IL-10 production, exhibit a restricted Th1 phenotype.[844-848] Production of TNF-α and TNF-β, which are known to kill oligodendrocytes in vitro,[849,850] also strongly associates with EAE induction. Moreover, at the peak of disease, perivascular infiltrates within the CNS stain positive for the macrophage-derived cytokines, IL-1, IL-6, IL-8, TNF-α and the Th1-derived cytokines, IL-2 and IFN-γ. By contrast, disease recovery associates with the appearance of TGF-β1 and IL-4[851] (Fig. 8.6). Finally, treatment of EAE with IL-4 or IL-4-inducing chemicals results in the induction of MBP-specific Th2 cells, diminished demyelinization, inhibition of the synthesis of inflammatory cytokines in the CNS, and improvement of clinical manifestations.[852,853] Administration of TGF-β or IL-10 also prevents EAE relapses, whereas anti-IL-10 antibody increases both the incidence and the severity of such relapses.[854] Accordingly, selective suppression of Th1, but not Th2, cytokines by the phosphodiesterase inhibitor pentoxifylline or by activation of CD4+ T cells in the presence of a nondepleting antibody to CD4 prevents induction of EAE in Lewis rats.[116,855] The expression of IL-4 in the brains of animals recovering from EAE suggests that remission of the disease might be related to the presence of antigen-specific Th2 cells. This hypothesis is also supported by the following observations: (1) transfer of Th2 cells does not induce EAE, but rather ameliorates the disease; (2) most MBP-specific CD4⁺ T cell clones gener-ated from SJL/J mice fed and immunized with MBP secrete TGF-β1 and/or IL-4 and IL-10 and protect actively immunized animals from EAE[10] and (3) PLP-specific Th2 clones, that produce high amounts of IL-4 and IL-10, suppress the induction of EAE if transferred at the time of active immunization, or at the onset of clinical symptoms.[109] Thus, it is likely that myelin peptide-specific Th1 cells are involved in the pathogenesis of EAE, whereas Th2 cells play a protective role in this disease. The occurrence of a Th1 response in mice affected by EAE is probably due to both the genetic background and the emulsi-fication of the immunizing peptide with CFA. Susceptibility to EAE varies indeed according to the mouse strain, although the genes which control this process have not yet been identified. Several findings sug-gest that autoantigenic stimulation requires high affinity binding to MHC class II molecules.[856,857] However, EAE-resistant BALB/c mice may have highly encephalitogenic MBP-specific T cell clones that rec-ognize a MBP peptide with high affinity for MHC class II.[858] Of note is that among SJL mice, males are significantly more resistant to EAE induction than age-matched female mice, suggesting a possible influ-ence of hormonal regulation.[859] Furthermore, adoptive transfer of mac-rophages from EAE-susceptible female mice followed by immuniza-tion with self-antigen results in the induction of EAE in the disease-resistant male mice, suggesting that macrophage APC popula-tions in EAE-resistant mice are deficient in either a costimulatory molecule or secretion of cytokine(s) required for Th1-cell priming.[859] The role for costimulatory molecules in the differential activation of Th1/Th2 development pathways has been demonstrated using anti-B7 antibodies. Administration of anti-B7-1 antibodies reduced the inci-dence of disease, while anti-B7-2 increased disease severity by altering the T cell cytokine profile.[109,853] Administration of anti-B7-1 at immu-nization promoted the prevalent generation of Th2 clones, whose transfer not only prevented induction of EAE, but also abolished established disease. Moreover, cotreatment with anti-IL-4 antibody prevented dis-ease improvement, clearly suggesting that the protective effects of anti-B7-1 antibody result from the activation of the Th2 pathway.[109] In this respect, it is also of note that the blockade of CD28-B7 interac-tions by injecting soluble CTLA4-Ig prevented the appearance of EAE by inducing a shift in the response toward the Th2 function.[860-862] On the other side, induction of active EAE as a consequence of emulsifi-cation of myelin antigen with CFA probably reflects the stimulation of macrophage IL-12 production by components of the mycobacterial cell wall, with subsequent increase in IFN-γ production. Indeed, in vitro stimulation of antigen-primed lymph node cells with PLP-primed mice and recombinant IL-12 enhances their subsequent encephalitogenicity,[852] whereas inhibition of endogenous IL-12 in vivo after lymph node cell transfer prevented paralysis, suggesting that endogenous IL-12 plays a pivotal role in the pathogenesis of EAE.[863] Furthermore, administration of anti-IFN-γ antibody at the time of immunization inhibits EAE development.[852] Other important factors are the route of antigen administration, as well as the dose and the structure of antigen. The role of the antigen route is exemplified by studies of oral tolerance to myelin antigens. EAE can be suppressed by the oral administration of MBP, which also induces a profound decrease in MBP-reactive, IL-2 and IFN-γ secreting lymphocytes relative to control animals. Such a reduction is probably related to the induction of a state of clonal anergy.[864] At high antigen concentrations deletion by apoptosis may be indeed the predominant tolerizing mechanism, but, at lower antigen doses, the induction of T cells that produce Th2 cytokines IL-4 and IL-10 and also cells which secrete TGF-β and protect SJL/J mice from the induction of EAE by MBP and PLP, are demonstrable.[10] The mechanisms by which cells producing IL-4, IL-10 and TGF-β are induced have not yet been clearly defined. Low-dose feeding appears capable of inducing prominent secretion of IL-4, IL-10 and TGF-β, whereas minimal secretion of these cytokines was observed with high-dose feeding.[87] Of note is also that epitopes of MBP that trigger TGF-β release after oral tolerization are distinct from encephalitogenic epitopes and mediate epitope-driven bystander suppression.[865] Studies performed in EAE induced with PLP 139-151 by altering single amino acids also suggest an important role for the structure of the ligand. These altered peptides are able to protect from disease induced with the native peptide because they activate antigen-specific T cells which are crossreactive, but produce Th2-type cytokines on activation. Interestingly, this change in phenotype occurs despite immunization being carried in the presence of CFA.[866] In vivo tolerization of a T cell clone specific for the MBP epitope p87-99 and capable of inducing EAE with an analog of p87-99 resulted in reversion of established paralysis, as well as regression of brain inflammatory infiltrates. Of note is that an antibody raised against IL-4 reversed the tolerance induced by the altered peptide ligand.[867] It should also be remembered that some studies are not consistent with the critical role of IFN-γ in the pathogenesis of EAE and with the protective function of Th2 cells in Th1-induced EAE. First, mice with a disrupted IFN-γ gene are still susceptible to the induction of EAE.[868] Moreover, neuroantigen-specific Th2 cells were inefficient suppressors of EAE induced by effector Th1 cells.[869]

Multiple sclerosis

Several studies in human disease suggest a role for TNF-α and IFN-γ in the pathogenesis of MS. First, high levels of TNF-α are present in the cerebrospinal fluid (CSF) of patients with chronic progressive MS.[870,871] Determination of TNF-α in both plasma and CSF may predict

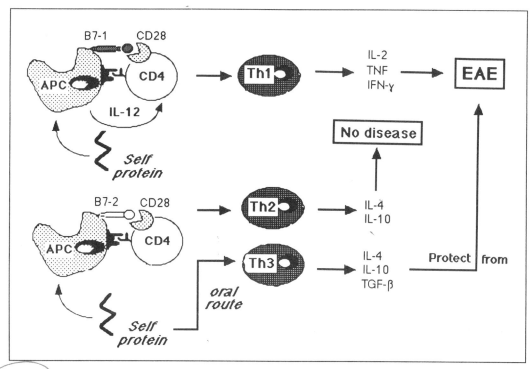

Fig. 8.6. Schematic view of the possible role of Th1/Th2 cells in EAE. Presentation of myelin autoantigens to CD4⁺ Th cells by B7-1-expressing, IL-12-producing, APC results in the development of myelin-specific Th1 cells. The Th1 cytokines TNF-α and β and IFN-γ are responsible for the CNS damage. In contrast, presentation of myelin autoantigens by B7-2-expressing APC (in the absence of IL-12 production) promote the development of Th2 cells, whose cytokines (IL-4 and IL-10) are not dangerous for CNS. Administration of the same autoantigen for oral route also induces the development of Th effectors producing IL-4, IL-10, and TGF-β (Th3), which are protective against the Th1-induced disease.

relapses in MS patients.[872] By using RT-PCR, high levels of TNF-α mRNA were also found in PBMC from MS patients[873] and increased TNF-α expression appeared to precede relapses by 4 weeks in patients with relapsing remitting MS, whereas IL-10 and TGF-β expression was decreased at the same time.[874] Most clones derived from both PBMC and CSF of patients with MS showed a Th1 profile,[875,876] and increased numbers of IFN-γ-secreting T cells, which produced IFN-γ upon activation by several myelin antigens and several MBP peptides were found in the CSF of MS patients.[877] T cell clones specific for PLP peptides generated from MS during an acute attack showed a clear-cut Th1 profile, whereas during remission in the same patients a more heterogenous cytokine profile was found. These clones produced significantly higher levels of both IL-10 and TGF-β than clones isolated during acute attacks.[878] High levels of LAG-3 expression and sLAG-3 production by T cell clones generated from the CSF were also found. Moreover, high levels of sLAG-3 were detected in the serum of patients with relapsing remitting MS.[58] Using immunohistochemistry, both TNF-α and TNF-β were identified in acute and chronic active MS lesions, but not in spleens or PBMCs from MS patients. TNF-β expression was associated with T lymphocytes, whereas TNF-α was associated with astrocytes in all areas of the lesion.[879] By using semiquantitative RT-PCR and immunohistochemistry, the costimulatory molecules B7-1, B7-2 and the cytokine IL-12p40 were found to be upregulated in acute MS plaques from early disease cases. The differences in cytokine mRNA expression were specific for IL-12p40, whereas no differences were observed for other cytokines, suggesting that an early event in the initiation of MS involved upregulation of costimulatory molecules and IL-12.[880] These probably represent the conditions that maximally stimulate T cell activation and induce Th1-type immune responses. Finally, the antagonistic effects of treatments with IFN-γ and IFN-β on the course of the clinical outcome of the disease provide further indirect support for a pathogenic role of Th1 cells in MS. In some clinical trials, it has been shown that IFN-γ administration induces relapses of MS,[881] probably because it upregulates MHC class II expression by microglial cells and APC-like macrophages and stimulates the secretion of potentially myelinotoxic mediators, such as TNF-α from macrophages. In contrast, fibroblast- and leukocyte-derived IFN-β, which inhibits IFN-γ-induced MHC class II expression, has been shown to reduce the rate of relapse in MS.[882] In conclusion, although studies of the T cell immune response in MS are not yet so clear as studies of EAE, there is convincing evidence to suggest that Th1 cells play a critical pathogenic role in this disease.

Autoimmune Uveites

Experimental autoimmune uveoretinitis

Immunization with retinal antigens (S antigen) in CFA induces an experimental autoimmune uveoretinitis (EAU) in susceptible rat strain LEW and (LEW x BN)F1 hybrids.[883,884] This disease is mediated by T lymphocytes and is probably a Th1-mediated disease, inasmuch as it can be transferred by S antigen-specific Th1-like T cell lines.[885] Furthermore, administration of $HgCl_2$, which triggers IL-4 production in (LEW x BN)F1 hybrids, protects the animals from the development of EAU.[886] Other findings, however, argue against the possibility that EAU is a Th1- mediated disorder. For example, it is surprising that administration of IFN-γ given at the initiation of the disease is capable of preventing the induction of EAU.[887]

Behçet disease

Behçet's disease (BD) is a chronic, relapsing-remitting systemic vasculitis, whose manifestations include orogenital ulcers, synovitis, trombophlebitis, uveitis and other symptoms related to the CNS.[888,889]

The uveitis in Behçet disease may be a human equivalent of the EAU. In fact, T cell clones specific for the bovine S antigen have been generated from PBMC of patients with BD.[890] Histopathological studies have revealed cellular infiltration consisting of lymphocytes, plasma cells and polimorphonuclear neutrophils. In these patients, increased serum levels of IL-1β and IFN-γ and spontaneous production of TNF-α, IL-6, IL-8 and IFN-γ from cultured T lymphocytes have been observed.[891-893] Recently, large series of T cell clones, generated from the CSF of patients with neuro-BD, showed the ability to produce both IFN-γ and IL-4 in response to stimulation with PMA plus anti-CD3 antibody; however the amounts of IFN-γ produced by the majority of these clones were exceptionally high (unpublished results).

TYPE 1 OR INSULIN-DEPENDENT DIABETES MELLITUS

The development of insulin-dependent diabetes mellitus (IDDM) in humans and in the spontaneous animal models, the BB rat and the nonobese diabetic (NOD) mouse, is the result of a cellular autoimmune process that selectively destroys the pancreatic islet beta cells.[894-897] A common histopathological feature associated with the development of IDDM is insulitis, characterized by the presence within and around the islets of T lymphocytes and to a lesser degree of macrophages.[898] Moreover, treatments such as neonatal thymectomy, administration of cyclosporin A or administration of anti-T lymphocyte antibodies, which suppress cellular autoimmunity, prevent development of diabetes.[899-900]

IDDM in BB and NOD mice

Evidence suggesting a role for Th1 cells in the pathogenesis of IDDM is supported by studies on BB and NOD mice. In BB mice, both IL-12 p40 chain and IFN-γ mRNA are present in the inflammatory lesions, whereas mRNA for IL-2 and IL-4 is minimal or undetectable.[825] All NOD mice spontaneously develop insulitis early in life (between 2 and 4 weeks of age), but it is not until 10-20 weeks later that this insulitis progresses to diabetes in about 80% of the female mice and in only 20% of the male mice. There is extensive infiltration of the islets by CD4+ and CD8+ T cells, B cells and macrophages, as it occurs in human IDDM. Although it is possible that CD8+ T cells can cause diabetes in NOD mice in the absence of CD4+ T cells,[901] Th1 cells play the major role in the induction of diabetes. IFN-γ-producing Th1-like clones cause IDDM after transfer into neonatal NOD mice,[902,903] and transfer of T cell clones that secrete IFN-γ and IL-2 precipitates diabetes in recipient NOD mice.[904,905] By contrast, Th2 clones are unable to transfer diabetes[904,905] (Fig. 8.7). NOD mice produce large amounts of IFN-γ in response to glutamic acid decarboxylase (GAD), a key β-cell antigen recognized by both T cells and B cells.[906,907] Administration of anti-IFN-γ antibodies can prevent the development of diabetes induced in NOD mice either by cyclophosphamide or adoptive transfer of diabetogenic cells.[908,909] The expression of IFN-α in the β cells of transgenic mice leads to a hypoinsulinemic diabetes associated with mixed inflammation centered in the islets.[910] Injection of IL-12 also induces massive Th1-cell infiltration in the pancreatic islets and accelerates IDDM development in NOD mice,[911-913] although intermittent IL-12 administration was surprisingly found to delay the IDDM development.[914] Moreover, IL-12 p40 knockout mice on NOD background, which produce no or very low IFN-γ, showed almost no insulitis at any age tested and their spontaneous IDDM incidence was very low. Diabetes incidence was also much lower in these mice than in control littermates in a model of cyclophosphamide-accelerated IDDM.[915] Finally, systemic administration of IL-4 prevents diabetes in NOD females.[916] This latter finding suggests a possible protective role of Th2 cells in the development of IDDM in NOD mice. Such a protective role was recently demonstrated by using double transgenic mice in which the majority of CD4+ T cells express a TCR that is MHC I-A^d-restricted and hemagglutinin (HA)-specific and also express HA as a neo-autoantigen in β-islet cells (HNT-TCR x Ins-HA mice). These mice had no thymic or peripheral clonal deletion, or inactivation, but exhibited two very distinct phenotypes depending on the genetic background of the strain to which they were backcrossed. On a BALB/c background, double transgenic mice secreted high levels of IFN-γ and IL-4 and did not develop diabetes, whereas on a B10.D2 background they produced high levels of IFN-γ, but low and transient levels of IL-4 and developed early spontaneous diabetes.[917] Since the Th2-promoting activity of IL-4 is dominant over the Th1-promoting cytokines IL-12 and IFN-γ, a genetic predisposition towards the Th2 differentiation (as it is in BALB/c mice) confers resistance to spontaneous autoimmune diabetes. This possibility is further supported by the observation that in BALB/c double transgenic mice homozygous for a disrupted IL-4 gene there is a significant increase in the incidence and severity of insulitis.[918] Interestingly, transgenic NOD mice carrying an I-A^g allele that had been mutated at positions 56 and 57 were protected from both diabetes and insulitis.[907] They produced autoantibodies mainly belonging to IgG1 and IgE classes and their T cells failed to proliferate and to produce IFN-γ in response to β-antigens in vitro, but could inhibit the adoptive transfer of diabetes. Moreover, the prevention of diabetes was shown to be at least in part due to the production of IL-4 and/or IL-10 by T cells.[918,919] The results of other studies do not agree, however, with this view. First, pancreatic expression of IL-10 actually promotes disease in NOD mice.[920] Moreover, transfer of Th1 or Th2 cells induced destruction of β cells or nondestructive perislet insulitis, respectively,[904] but destructive insulitis induced by Th1 cells was not prevented even in the presence of a nine-fold excess of Th2-like cells.[905] Moreover, administration of anti-B7-1 and anti-B7-2 antibodies, which prevent

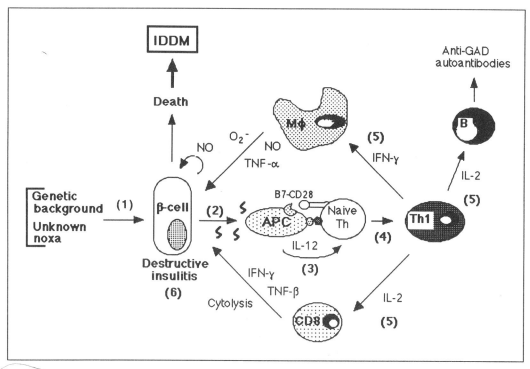

Fig. 8.7. Schematic view of the possible role of Th1 cells in the development of the autoimmune response in IDDM. A still unknown noxa in genetically predisposed individuals (1) can allow the presentation of β-cell antigens (2) by the APC to the naive Th cell under conditions (high IL-12/low or no IL-4 production) (3) that favor its development into a Th1-like effector cell (4). Autoantigen-specific Th1 cells stimulate the secretion of autoantibodies by B cells and the activation of CD8+ CTL (via the production of IL-2) (5) and activate macrophages (Mφ) (via the production of IFN-γ) (5). CTL, their cytokines, as well as cytokines and toxic products of activated macrophages contribute to the destructive insulitis, death of the β-cell, and development of IDDM.

and worsen EAE, respectively (see above), had an opposite effect on IDDM of NOD mice. Female NOD mice treated at the onset of insulitis with an anti-B7-2 antibody did not develop diabetes. By contrast, administration of anti-B7-1 antibodies significantly accelerated the development of disease in female mice and, most interestingly, induced diabetes in normally resistant male mice.[111] Thus, the dichotomy between insulitis mediated by Th1 ('destructive') and Th2 ('benign') cells appears to be too simple to account for all observations.

Human type 1 diabetes

There are a few contributions to a characterization of the inflammatory cell infiltrate in the insulitis lesion in human type 1 diabetes. Such studies had to be largely confined to autopsies on patients who died of recent onset of diabetes where the pancreatic tissue had been formalin-fixed. Thus, the combined problems of autolysis, due to the interval between death and autopsy, and protein denaturation, due to fixation, have severely limited the knowledge in this field. However, it appears that the cell infiltrate is composed of both lymphocytes and macrophages (ratio 7-9:1) and that high proportions of lymphocytes (about 40%) contain IFN-γ.[921] Autoreactive T cell clones generated from newly onset patients with IDDM exhibited a predominant Th1 profile, whereas those derived from a prediabetic patient were prevalently Th2.[922]

RHEUMATOID ARTHRITIS

Rheumatoid arthritis (RA) is an autoimmune chronic synovitis which often leads to joint destruction.[923]

Collagen-induced arthritis

A murine collagen-induced arthritis, which requires immunization with the antigen type II collagen (CII) emulsified with CFA, has been used as a major model for RA. Studies performed by using this model have clearly shown that CD4$^+$ T cells are involved in the induction phase, whereas their role in the effector phase of the inflammatory reaction is still unclear. For example, injection of anti-CD4 antibody can prevent the induction of arthritis in DBA/1 mice if administered around the time of immunization with CII, but appears to be ineffective in animals with established disease.[924] Anti-CD4 antibody treatment can halt disease progression only if combined with anti-Thy-1 antibody.[925] Accordingly, treatment with anti-TCR antibody completely blocked the induction of arthritis when administered around the time of collagen immunization, but it led to a simple reduction in disease severity when given after the onset of arthritis.[926] The pro-inflammatory cytokines mainly produced by macrophages and other accessory cells are also heavily involved in the pathogenesis of arthritis. Administration of either an anti-TNF-α antibody or recombinant soluble TNF-receptor after the onset of symptoms reduced the clinical and histological severity of arthritis.[927,928] Similar effects were also obtained by the injection of anti-IL-1α and anti-IL-1β antibodies,[929] whereas the administration of anti-TGF-β antibody antagonized the development of polyarthritis in susceptible rats and prevented the induction of CII-induced arthritis in DBA/1 mice.[930,931] Interestingly, the combined injection of anti-CD4 and anti-TNF-α antibodies acted synergistically in improving established collagen-induced arthritis.[932] Upon stimulation with CII in vitro, spleen cells from immunized mice synthesize IFN-γ.[933] In addition, IL-12 in combination with CII can replace *Mycobacteria* in causing severe arthritis of DBA/1 mice and this effect correlates with a 3- to 10-fold increase in the production of IFN-γ by antigen-stimulated T cells.[934] More importantly, neutralization of IFN-γ in vivo prevented the development of arthritis in collagen-immunized and IL-12-treated mice.[935] Finally, in agreement with EAE model,[87] oral administration of an immunodominant human collagen peptide modulates collagen-induced arthritis.[936] These data clearly suggest that a Th1-type autoimmune reaction is responsible for the collagen-induced arthritis in DBA/1 mice. However, other findings do not fit with this interpretation. When high amounts of IFN-γ were injected into DBA/1 mice immunized with CII in CFA, the onset of arthritis was delayed and the severity reduced.[937] Accordingly, high doses of IL-12 inhibited the development of joint disease in DBA/1 mice immunized with CII in CFA.[938] The mechanisms responsible for these apparently paradoxical effects are still unclear.

Human disease

It is well-established that proinflammatory cytokines, such as TNF-α, IL-1, GM-CSF and IL-6,[939-944] as well as chemokines, such as IL-8, RANTES and MIP-1,[945] are produced by the synovial membrane in RA and play an important role in the pathophysiology of the disease. In fact, these cytokines can both induce bone resorption and cartilage destruction, and can stimulate PGE_2 release and collagenase production.[946] In contrast to the abundance of monocyte-derived cytokines, T cell-derived cytokine proteins have often been difficult to detect in RA synovium,[947,948] despite the fact that synovial membrane-infiltrating T cells appear phenotypically activated.[949] This has led to the suggestion that the pathogenesis of RA is mediated solely by macrophages and their effector cytokines.[950] An alternative view is that T cell cytokines may be important, but are expressed at levels too low for detection by conventional methods.[951] In favor of this possibility is the observation that mRNA for IFN-γ and IL-2 can be demonstrated by either PCR or in situ hybridization in synovial tissue of RA patients, whereas IL-4 mRNA is detectable only in a few cases;[952-954] moreover, most T cell clones derived from the RA synovium are of the Th1 type,[955,956] even if some rheumatoid inflammatory T cell clones exhibit a Th0-like profile.[956] On the other hand, in addition to proinflammatory cytokines, a compensatory anti-inflammatory response has also been observed in RA synovial membranes. Thus, there is expression of high levels of IL-1RA, soluble TNF-receptors (of both the 55 and 75 kD receptor), TGF-β and IL-10 in the RA synovium,[944,948,957] which suggests that homeostatic mechanisms exist in the rheumatoid joint by which the immune system attempts to contain inflammation and limit joint destruction. Moreover, elevated Th1- or Th0-like cytokine mRNA was found in peripheral circulation,[958] and high levels of sCD30 were detected in the joint fluid[959] of RA patients. IL-10 may function as an endogenous regulatory molecule in rheumatoid synovium.[960] Indeed, blocking IL-10 in synovial membrane cultures resulted in increase of both TNF-α and IL-1β.[957] Due to the powerful inhibitory activity of IL-10 on Th1 cytokine production,[25,28] it is reasonable to suggest that IL-10 represents the (or one of the) reason(s) of the "elusiveness" of

Th1-derived cytokines in RA. However, the questions of whether increased production of proinflammatory cytokines in RA is secondary to Th1 cell activation or represents a primary phenomenon, as well as the existence of a less restricted Th-cell cytokine profile, still remain unclear. Recently, a possible role for IL-15 in T cell migration and activation in RA has also been suggested.[961]

SJÖGREN SYNDROME

Sjögren syndrome (SS) is a chronic autoimmune disease clinically defined by the simultaneous presence of keratoconjunctivitis sicca and xerostomia, and immunologically by a hyperactivity expressed by hypergammaglobulinemia, multiple organ and nonorgan-specific autoantibodies and focal lymphocytic infiltration of the exocrine glands, in patients not full-filling criteria for any other chronic inflammatory connective tissue disease.[962,963] Although not yet conclusive, the results of different studies suggest a predominant activation of Th1 cells in patients with SS. First, the cytokines IL-1, IL-6, TNF-α and IFN-γ were identified in labial salivary gland specimens from patients with SS.[964,965] Second, increased levels of IL-6 and IFN-γ have been found in the serum of SS patients.[966] Finally, spontaneous IFN-γ mRNA in freshly isolated unstimulated T cells from SS patients has been observed.[967] Increased production of IL-10 by stimulated, and spontaneous IL-10 mRNA expression by freshly isolated, PBMC from SS patients has also been observed,[967,968] which may reflect the attempt to downregulate the inflammatory reaction induced by Th1 cytokines. Recently, however, a SS-like lymphoproliferation associated with high levels of anti-nuclear autoantibodies has been observed in TGF-β1 knockout mice.[969] These mice produced high amounts of IL-2, IL-6 and IL-10, without showing a predominance of Th1- or Th2-type cytokines,[969] suggesting that in this disease, as in some forms of SLE, a general defect of suppressor mechanisms rather than a prevalence in Th1 or Th2 responses may play the major pathogenic role.

SYSTEMIC LUPUS ERYTHEMATOSUS

Systemic lupus erythematosus (SLE) is an autoimmune disorder characterized by over-production of a wide range of autoantibodies and immune complexes and a constellation of pathologic abnormalities involving the kidney, skin, brain, lungs and other organs.[970] In theory, a prevalent production of Th2 cytokines may be critical to disease induction by contributing to the increased B cell activation characteristic of SLE patients, and also to disease perpetuation.[971,972]

Experimental lupus induced by allogeneic reactions or chemicals

It is well-established that autoimmune alterations observed in the context of allogeneic reactions and following exposure to some chemicals, such as gold salts and mercurials, are Th2-mediated disorders.[973] In both the chronic graft versus host disease (GVHD) reaction (see also below) and the model of neonatal tolerance to alloantigens, also called HVG reaction, CD4[+] T cells are induced which recognize MHC class II molecules on B cells leading to B cell polyclonal activation. In both conditions, the alloreactive T cells produce IL-4 and IL-10 but not IL-2 or IFN-γ.[973,974] On the other hand, susceptible rats (Brown Norway) given $HgCl_2$, gold salts or *D*-penicillamine also exhibit CD4[+] T cells that recognize normal syngeneic MHC class II molecules and produce Th2 cytokines.[265,973] The mechanism of induction of Th2 cells probably relies on the ability of these chemicals to directly trigger IL-4 production by a population of T cells in genetically susceptible animals.[265] This property can also account for the ability of these agents to switch an autoimmune response from pathogenic Th1 response to a nonpathogenic Th2 one.[266]

Lupus-prone mice

Results presently available in lupus-prone mice suggest that both Th1-type and Th2-type cytokines or cells showing no restricted cytokine profile may play a pathogenic role. For example, administration of anti-IFN-γ antibody attenuates the severity of the disease in (NZB x NZW),[975] but continuous administration of anti-IL-10 antibodies also delays onset of autoimmunity, whereas IL-10 accelerates the onset of autoimmunity in (NZB x NZW)F_1 mice.[976] Autoreactive T cell lines producing both IL-4 and IFN-γ have been derived from MRL lpr/lpr mice, which manifest autoimmune disease state such as massive systemic lymphoadenopathy, autoantibody production, arthritis, nephritis, and tissue infiltration by CD4[+] and double negative (CD4[-]CD8[-]) T cells; these lines trigger a nephritis which is prevented by administration of anti-IFN-γ antibody.[977] However, the lupus disease is also blocked by anti-IL-10 treatment and accelerated by IL-6 administration.[976,978] Analysis of cytokine gene expression by RT-PCR revealed that IL-1, IL-5, IL-6, IFN-γ, TNF-α, TNF-β and TGF-β were transcribed by various T cell subsets.[979] IFN-γ was most markedly augmented in MRL/l mice, IL-1 was most severely overexpressed in BXSBm mice, while IL-10 was equally increased in both strains.[980] When MRL mice with accelerated development of lupus-like autoimmune disease (MRL.Yaa) were compared with those showing prolonged survival (MRL-lpr/lpr.ll), an enhanced expression of IFN-γ versus IL-4 and IL-10 mRNA in CD4[+] T cells was found.[981] IL-12 and NO play also an important role in the development of spontaneous autoimmune disease in MRL/MP-lpr/lpr mice.[982] Taken together, these data suggest that both Th1 and Th2 cells, or perhaps more heterogenous Th cell subsets, may be activated, but an imbalance towards Th1 predominance plays a significant role in the acceleration of lupus-like autoimmune disease in lupus-prone mice.

Human SLE

SLE patients have significantly fewer cells producing Th1 cytokines, IFN-γ and IL-2, but significantly more cells secreting Th2 cytokines, IL-6 and IL-10, than normal controls.[983,984] SLE patients also have excess IL-4 production and increased numbers of IL-4 secreting cells,[983-986] as well as increased serum levels of sCD30, which correlate with disease activity.[987] However, the major abnormalities seem to involve IL-6 secretion and IL-6/IL-6 receptor interactions.[966,988-990] Moreover, abnormal production of both IL-6 and IL-10 in SLE seem to be due to macrophages and B cells[968,983,984,991] rather than to T lymphocytes. Thus, the predominant activation and pathogenic role of Th2 cells in SLE still remains to be established. A general defect in suppressor activity, as shown in TGF-β1 knockout mice, which exhibit high levels of IL-2, IL-6 and IL-10, as well as of anti-nuclear autoantibodies,[969] rather than the occurrence of a Th1- or Th2-dominated response, may be suggested.

SYSTEMIC SCLEROSIS

Systemic sclerosis (SSc) is a disorder characterized by inflammatory, vascular and fibrotic changes of the skin (scleroderma) and a variety of internal organs, such as the gastrointestinal tract, lungs, heart and kidney. In the skin, a thin epidermis overlies compact bundles of collagen, which lie parallel to the epidermis. Increased numbers of T cells are present in skin lesions, as well as in other organs, in the early stages of the disease.[992,993] Several soluble factors secreted by T cells or other cells of the immune system may modulate fibrosis or promote vascular damage in SSc. They include IL-1α and IL-1β, IL-6, TNF-β and TGF-β, which have been shown to be able to alter various fibroblast activities, such as growth, production of extracellular matrix components, production of collagenase or PGs.[994] IL-4 also induces human fibroblasts to synthesize elevated levels of extracellular matrix proteins, as well as to stimulate the growth of subconfluent fibroblasts and induce chemotaxis of these cells.[995-997] Interestingly, PBMC from patients with SSc produce higher amounts of IL-2 and IL-4 than controls.[998] Likewise, IL-2, IL-4 and IL-6, but not IFN-γ, were each found more frequently in sera from SSc patients than in sera from normal individuals.[999,1000] More recently, the analysis by RT-PCR of spontaneous cytokine and CD30 gene expression by PBMC from SSc patients showed spontaneous IL-4, IL-5 and CD30, but no IFN-γ or IL-10, mRNA expression. T cell clones generated from the skin cellular infiltrates were in great majority Th2 and high proportions of them appeared to be autoreactive (topoisomerase-specific). Accordingly, large numbers of CD4+ T cells present in the perivascular infiltrates of skin biopsy specimens were CD30+ and high levels of sCD30 were found in the serum of most SSc patients, especially those showing active disease (Mavilia et al, submitted). These data strongly suggest a predominant activation of Th2 cells in SSc and support the view that abnormal

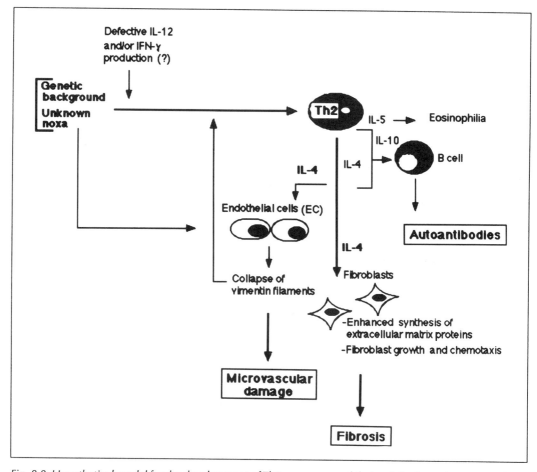

Fig. 8.8. Hypothetical model for the development of Th2 responses and their role in the pathogenesis of SSc. Unknown noxa(e) induce cytoskeletal alterations of endothelial cells and evoke Th2 responses in predisposed individuals (defective production of IFN-γ and/or IL-12 ?) or, alternatively, the changes in endothelial cells occur in response to IL-4 production by Th2 cells, resulting in microvascular damage. IL-4 also promotes enhanced synthesis of extracellular matrix proteins by fibroblasts, as well as their growth and chemotaxis, thus accounting for fibrosis. IL-4 and IL-10 produced by Th2 cells also stimulate autoantibody production by B cells; IL-5 production is responsible for eosinophilia.

and persistent IL-4 production by the activated Th2 cells may play an important role in the genesis of fibrosis and, therefore, in the pathogenesis of the disease (Fig. 8.8).

OTHER CHRONIC INFLAMMATORY DISORDERS

HELICOBACTER PILORI-RELATED GASTRODUODENAL PATHOLOGIES
Colonization of the mucosa of the stomach and the duodenum by *Helicobacter pilori* (Hp) is thought to be the major cause of acute and

chronic gastroduodenal pathologies in humans. These include gastric and duodenal ulcer, as well as gastric carcinoma and lymphoma of the mucosa associated lymphoid tissue (MALT). The great majority of patients with duodenal ulcer disease harbor Hp infection in the gastric antrum and exhibit an associated chronic antral gastritis, characterized by a mucosal infiltrate of polymorphonuclear and mononuclear leukocytes. Evidence for a role of Hp infection in the pathogenesis of ulcer disease comes from the clinical observation that removal of Hp speeds up ulcer healing, prevents duodenal and gastric ulcer relapse, and reduces ulcer complication. However, a direct cause-effect relationship between Hp colonization of gastric antrum and ulcer disease is not yet clearly proven.[1001,1002]

A gastric pathology resembling human disease was observed in infections with Hp strains expressing a vacuolating cytotoxin (VacA), which induces vacuole formation in epithelial cells, and an immunodominant cytotoxin-associated antigen (CagA), but not with noncytotoxic strains.[1003] Of note is that mice infected with *Helicobacter felis* showed a Th1 response with local and systemic production of IFN-γ and undetectable levels of IL-4 and IL-5. In vivo neutralization of IFN-γ resulted in a significant reduction of gastric inflammation.[1004] Very recently, we have analyzed the pattern of cytokines that are produced by the immunologically active cells within the mucosa from antral biopsies of Hp-infected patients with duodenal ulcer and Hp-negative dyspeptic controls by using RT-PCR and immunohistochemistry. T cell clones were also generated from parallel samples of the antral mucosa of the same Hp-infected patients and assessed for their reactivity with Hp antigens, profile of cytokine production and effector functions. Antral biopsies from all Hp-infected patients with duodenal ulcer showed IL-12, IFN-γ, TNF-α and IL-12, but not IL-4, mRNA expression, as well as the presence of IFN-γ-containing CD4⁺ T cells (Fig. 8.9), whereas neither cytokine mRNA signal nor cytokine-containing mononuclear cells were found in the mucosa of Hp-negative controls. When assayed for responsiveness to a Hp lysate, 24 of 163 CD4⁺ clones (15%) exhibited marked proliferation in response to Hp lysate. Eleven clones reacted with Cag-A, two with Vac-A and one with Ure-B. Upon stimulation with the specific antigen, the great majority of Hp-reactive clones (20/24) produced IFN-γ but not IL-4 or IL-5 (Th1-like), whereas four clones produced both IFN-γ and IL-4 or IL-5 (Th0-like). Under the same experimental conditions, all Hp-reactive clones produced high concentrations of TNF-α. These results demonstrate that Hp-specific T cells showing Th1-like profile of cytokine production and related effector functions are present in the gastric antral mucosa of patients with peptic ulcer. These cells may play a role in the pathogenesis of both peptic ulcer and gastric malignancies associated with Hp infection.

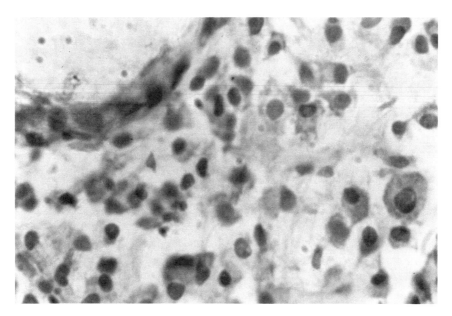

Fig. 8.9. Detection by immunohistochemistry of IFN-γ production by T cells infiltrating the gastric antral mucosa in a H. pilori-infected patient. For explanations, see legend of Fig. 2.6. Courtesy of Dr. P. Romagnani, Department of Physiopathology, Endocrinology Unit, University of Florence.

CHRONIC INFLAMMATORY BOWEL DISEASES

The idiopathic inflammatory bowel diseases (IBD) comprise a spectrum of disorders that are marked by the presence of chronic inflammation of the gastrointestinal tract which cannot be ascribed to a specific pathogen.[1005] At one end of the spectrum is ulcerative colitis (UC), a disease that affects the large bowel exclusively, at the other is Crohn's disease (CD) that, in contrast to ulcerative colitis, can affect any part of the alimentary canal, from the mouth to the rectum, but most commonly involves the terminal ileum and the ascending colon. The etiology of both UC and CD is unknown. Insults from microbial agents have been suspected, but there is no definite proof for the infective theory. Much circumstantial evidence, however, supports the concept that immunologic mechanisms are responsible for the pathogenesis of both UC and CD.

Experimental models of IBD

In the last few years, an impressive number of different model of IBD in mice and rats have been described. An IBD-like picture develops in mice with alterations in T cell subpopulations and T cell selection (TCR-α chain-deficient mice, TCR-β chain-deficient mice, MHC class II-deficient mice),[1006] with targeted disruption of cytokine genes

(IL-2, IL-10 and TGF-β deficient mice),[1007-1010] with lacking signaling proteins (G protein subunit Gα2-deficient mice),[1011] as well as in mice subject to rectal application of the hapten reagent 2,4,6-trinitrobenzene sulfonic acid (TNBS).[1012] Data from a number of these models indicate that a subpopulation of T cells plays a critical role in the normal regulation of intestinal immune responses. Moreover, evidence is accumulating suggesting that cytokines are involved in the pathogenic and regulatory pathways.[1013] The Th1-derived cytokines IFN-γ and TNF-α appear to be responsible for the pathogenesis of colitis in SCID mice restored with memory CD4+ T cells, as disease was prevented by the administration of anti-IFN-γ antibody and significantly reduced in severity by anti-TNF antibody.[1014] Moreover, antibodies to IL-12 abrogated established experimental colitis induced in mice by rectal application of the hapten reagent TNBS.[1012] Taken together, these data suggest a pivotal role of IL-12 and Th1 cytokines in the induction of murine chronic intestinal inflammation. On the other hand, IL-10 and TGF-β certainly play an important role in the regulation of pathogenic inflammatory responses, as IL-10-deficient mice develop colitis,[1009] and TGF-β1-deficient mice also develop inflammatory lesions in a number of organs, including the gastrointestinal tract.[1010] Development of colitis in IL-2-deficient mice[1007] suggests that IL-2 is somehow involved in the immunoregulatory pathway. In contrast, data presently available argue against a prominent role for IL-4 in the regulation of experimental IBD, as IL-4-deficient mice do not develop colitis[1008] and systemic administration of IL-4 had no effect on colitis development in T cell-restored SCID mice.[1015]

Crohn's disease

Increased levels of IL-1, IL-6, IL-8, TNF-α, as well as of IL-2 and IL-2 receptor, have been found in the intestinal mucosa and/or serum of patients with IBD,[1016-1023] suggesting activation of macrophages and perhaps of Th1-like cells. Moreover, increased expressions of mRNA for IL-2, IFN-γ and IL-10 are present in the mucosa of patients with active CD, whereas IL-4 mRNA expression was frequently below the detection limits.[1024] In a recent study, it was found that T cell clones generated from the colonic mucosa of patients with CD are able to produce higher levels of IFN-γ, but significantly reduced levels of IL-4 and IL-5, in comparison with T cell clones derived from the colonic mucosa of patients with noninflammatory bowel disorders.[1149] In contrast, no differences in the production of IL-10 between the two groups of clones were found, suggesting that a defect in the regulatory role of IL-4 rather than of IL-10 may be operating in human IBD. IL-10, however, is not a selective Th2 product in human beings, but is also produced by Th1 and Th0 cells and even more by B cells and macrophages.[21,25,991] Thus, a possible concomitant defect in IL-10 production

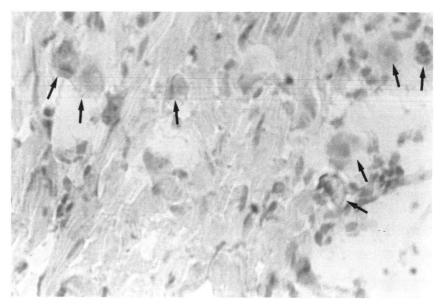

Fig. 8.10. Detection by immunohistochemistry of IL-12-producing macrophages in the intestinal muscularis propria of a patient with Crohn's disease. Parformaldehyde (4%)-fixed sections were incubated with anti-IL-12 mouse monoclonal antibody, followed by biotinylated anti-mouse IgG antibody and the avidin-biotin-peroxidase complex. Sections were then counterstained with Gill's hematoxylin. Arrows indicate IL-12-expressing cells. Courtesy of Dr. P. Romagnani, Department of Physiopathology, Endocrinology Unit, University of Florence.

by non-T cells from IBD patients cannot be excluded. More recently, the possible pathogenic role of Th1-dominated responses was further supported by the results of immunohistochemical studies. High numbers of activated CD4+ T cells showing CD26, LAG-3 and IFN-γ reactivity, as well as of IL-12-containing macrophages, were found to infiltrate the muscularis of gut from patients with Crohn's disease, but not of controls (Fig. 8.10). In addition, culturing IL-2-conditioned T cells from the mucosa of CD patients in the presence of anti-IL-12 antibody had an inhibitory effect on the development of IFN-γ producing T cells, suggesting that constitutive IL-12 production plays a critical role in the development of Th1 cells at the intestinal level (Fig. 8.11).

CHRONIC INFLAMMATORY LUNG DISEASES

Some chronic interstitial lung diseases share common features, including an unknown etiology, intense inflammatory response and end-stage fibrosis. Although the sequence of events in the pathology of these diseases is not clearly established, the role of cytokines produced by both immune and nonimmune cells, such as epithelial cells, endothelial cells and fibroblasts, has been implicated in the pathogenesis of these disorders.

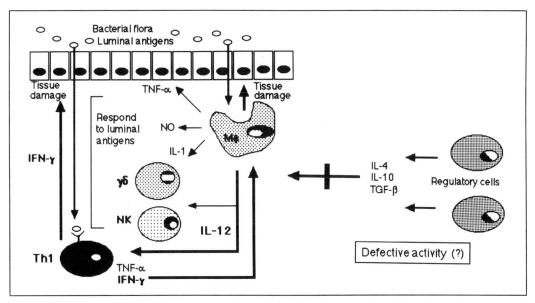

Fig. 8.11. Hypothetical model for the development of Th1 responses and their role in the pathogenesis of Crohn's disease. Bacterial flora antigens coming from the intestinal lumen are usually challenged at mucosal level by macrophages, NK cells and T cells. Excessive production of IL-12 and/or defective activity of regulatory cells producing TGF-β, IL-10, and IL-4 favor the development of antigen-specific Th1 responses, which result via IFN-γ production in high and persistent activation of macrophages, continuous release of toxic products (TNF-α, NO, IL-1) and subsequent tissue damage.

Idiopathic pulmonary fibrosis

Pulmonary fibroblasts are essential for the evolution of interstitial fibrosing lung diseases, as they are able to synthesize both cytokines and extracellular matrix. Recent findings, however, suggest that the degree of inflammation and subsequent fibroblast activation is dependent upon a balance between Th1 and Th2 cytokines, which are expressed during disease development. First, IFNs (especially IFN-γ) have profound suppressive effects on the production of extracellular matrix proteins, such as collagen and fibronectin.[1025,1026] More importantly, IL-4 is a potent stimulus for the production of fibroblast-derived extracellular matrix,[996-997] as well as a chemotactic factor for directed movement of fibroblasts.[995] Additional studies have also shown that IL-4 can efficiently communicate with fibroblasts via a single class of high affinity IL-4 receptors.[1027,1028] Fibroblasts posses not only a membrane-bound IL-4 receptor, but also a secreted form of the IL-4 receptor, which may function either as an IL-4-binding protein with antagonistic activity or as a carrier of IL-4 with its biological properties left intact.[1028] This is the reason why strong and persistent IL-4 production, as occurring in schistosoma egg-induced granuloma formation,[650] chronic GVHD[1029] and SSc (Mavilia et al, submitted), is consistently associated with extensive fibrotic processes. It is of note that eosinophilia has also been demonstrated in chronic inflammatory disorders in which fibrosis occurs,[1030,1031] and eosinophils are in turn capable of releasing factors which stimulate human lung fibroblasts to undergo replication and synthesize extracellular matrix.[1032] Thus, a persistent activation of Th2 cells at the lung level may provide the basis for a potential fibrotic network, leading to end-stage pathology in idiopathic pulmonary fibrosis. Recent data strongly support such a hypothesis as a Th2 cytokine phenotype appears to predominate in the pulmonary interstitium of idiopathic pulmonary fibrosis.[1033]

Sarcoidosis

Sarcoidosis is a multisystem granulomatous disease but with preferential localization at lung level, of unknown etiology, characterized by the expansion of activated oligoclonal CD4+ T cells and macrophages at sites of disease. Using semiquantitative PCR, elevated mRNA and protein levels of IFN-γ, but not of IL-4, were found in sarcoid lung cells and fluids compared with those in normal samples. Moreover, higher mRNA expression of the IL-12 p40 subunit, but not of IL-10, were present in sarcoid compared with normal lung cells. Sarcoid alveolar macrophages produced greater amounts of IL-12 than normal alveolar macrophages when cultured in vitro.[1034] These data suggest that sarcoidosis is a Th1-mediated disorder driven by a chronic, dysregulated, production of IL-12 at sites of disease.

ATHEROSCLEROSIS

In atherosclerotic plaques strong expression of IFN-γ, but not of IL-4, mRNA has been found compared to normal arteries. IL-12 p40 mRNA and IL-12 p70 protein were also found to be abundant in atherosclerotic plaques. Interestingly, IL-12 was induced in monocytes in vitro in response to highly oxidized low density lipoproteins (LDL), but not minimally modified LDL. IL-10 was also expressed in some atherosclerotic lesions and exogenous IL-10 was found to inhibit LDL-induced IL-12 release.[1035] Taken together, these data suggest that atherosclerosis may be a chronic inflammatory reaction in which the balance between IL-12 and IL-10 production determines the level of Th1-mediated tissue injury.

TRANSPLANTATION REJECTION AND TOLERANCE

GRAFT REJECTION

Allograft rejection results from the coordinated activation of alloreactive T cells and APCs. T cell activation begins when T cells recognize intracellularly processed fragments of foreign proteins embedded with the groove of the MHC proteins expressed on the surface of APCs. Some T cells of the recipient directly recognize the allograft, i.e., donor antigen(s) presented on the surface of donor APCs, while other T cells recognize the donor antigen after it is processed and presented by the self APCs. Alloreactive T cells include both MHC class II-restricted CD4[+] T cells and MHC class I-restricted CD8[+] T cells, but CD4[+] T cells are critical for the rejection process.[1036,1037] It appears that some Th1-dependent effector mechanisms, such as DTH and CTL activity, play a central role in acute allograft rejection.[1036,1037] Proteins and/or transcripts for intragraft IL-2, IFN-γ and the CTL specific marker, granzyme B, have consistently been detected in rejecting allografts. IFN-γ is believed to recruit macrophages into the graft, cause macrophage activation, enhance CTL activation, and amplify the ongoing immune response by upregulating the expression of both MHC and costimulatory molecules (e.g., B7) upon graft parenchimal cells and APCs. IL-2 stimulates proliferation of CD4[+] cells in an autocrine fashion and leads to the paracrine activation of CD8[+] CTLs.[1036,1037] Cytokines are probably involved in the genesis of the main anatomo-pathological lesions characteristic of allograft rejection. Several authors reported increased serum or plasma TNF-α, IL-1 and IL-6 values, as well as overexpression of these cytokines at the rejecting allograft level, at the time of acute rejection episodes.[1038-1040] It has also been shown that CD4[+] and CD8[+] T cell clones derived from rejected kidney grafts expressed a predominant Th1 lymphokine profile in comparison with T cell clones derived from the peripheral blood[1041] and that Th1 cytokines are prominently expressed in human renal allografts prior to or during rejection.[1042-1044] However, IL-4 and IL-5 mRNA was also detected in 80% of biopsies of rejecting renal allografts, whereas IL-2 mRNA was found in only 20% of the cases.[1045]

TRANSPLANTATION TOLERANCE

Transplantation tolerance can be defined as the inability of the organ graft recipient to express a graft destructive immune response.[1036,1037] In animal models, therapies which block optimal APC-T cell interactions or directly target the T cell are capable of precluding T cell activation and allograft rejection. In the absence of continuous exposure to antigen, however, tolerance is lost.[1036,1037] This means that in order for enduring tolerance to develop the immune system of the recipient must continually 'see' the alloantigen, albeit in a setting of dampened T cell activation. The production of Th2-type cytokines may be central to the induction and maintenance of allograft tolerance. Several in vivo studies that examined the pattern of cytokine expression during tolerance induction have consistently shown a dramatic decrease in the expression of IL-2 and IFN-γ, while increased levels of IL-4 and IL-10 transcripts are manifest.[1046-1050] Moreover, in an interesting set of experiments, Maeda et al[1051] developed a class II-reactive CD4[+] T cell clone that was able, upon adoptive transfer into naive mice, to inhibit the generation of antigen-specific CTL responses and, therefore, to prolong skin graft survival in an antigen-specific fashion. This clone produced IL-4 and IL-10, but not IL-2 or IFN-γ, upon stimulation with antigen.[1051] Accordingly, both prior *N. brasiliensis* infection and prior treatment with a soluble worm product significantly delayed kidney allograft rejection in rats, probably due to the crossregulatory suppression of Th1 activity by nematode-induced Th2 cytokines.[1052] A subset of γδTCR-positive cells was found to be the major source of Th2 cytokines responsible for inhibition of graft rejection in C3H/HeJ mice receiving B10.BR skin grafts following portal or lateral tail vein infusion of irradiated B10.BR spleen cells.[1053] Thus, although its validity is not yet proven, the Th1/Th2 paradigm may represent the basis for understanding the mechanisms of rejection and tolerance in transplantation.[1036,1037] Other findings, however, do not agree with this possibility. Very low levels of transcripts for all cytokines tested (IL-2, IFN-γ, IL-4, IL-10 and IL-13) or even decreased IL-4 levels were found within the heart or liver allografts of tolerant animals.[1054-1056] Moreover, a study of pig proislet xenograft transplantation indicated that rejection, in this setting, associates with activation of Th2 cells and tolerance with lack of IL-4 expression. Reversal of tolerance to islet grafts was accompanied by a selective increase in IL-4 transcripts.[1057] Isolated graft-infiltrating lymphocytes from irreversibly rejected human renal allografts had a high frequency of IL-10-decreting cells, suggesting that IL-10 did not inhibit rejection.[1058] Comparable levels of IL-10 mRNA were noted in tolerant and rejecting hepatic grafts in rats and in acute and chronic rejection in human liver transplants.[1059,1060] In addition, two different studies suggest that a prolonged administration of IL-10 actually has a detrimental effect on graft survival.[1061,1062] Finally, when cells transfected with IL-4 or IL-10 cDNAs were introduced into the graft recipient, conflicting results were obtained. In a mouse skin graft model, neither IL-4- nor IL-10-producing cells had an effect on graft survival, even though graft survival was prolonged by an anti-IFN-γ antibody.[1063] However, in a heterotopic cardiac graft model, IL-4-transfected cells prolonged graft survival.[1064] In another model in which plasmid or viral-based constructs were used to transfect organs at the time of or before grafting, IL-10 was able to prolong significantly allograft survival while TGF-β, although beneficial, has a less marked effect.[1065] The possibility has also been suggested that Th2 cytokines may evoke allograft rejection by recruitment of alternate effector mechanisms, but their deleterious effect on allograft survival may be prevented by the inhibitory activity of donor-reactive CD8+ CTL which, therefore, favor a Th1-dominated response.[1066] The overall picture from these recent studies is, therefore, not a simple one of associated expression of Th1 cytokines with rejection and of Th2 cytokines with tolerance.

GRAFT VS. HOST REACTION

EXPERIMENTAL GVHR

A single inoculation of parental cells from DBA mice into an unirradiated, immunocompetent F_1 recipient, or lethal irradiation of recipient mice and reconstitution with donor bone marrow containing

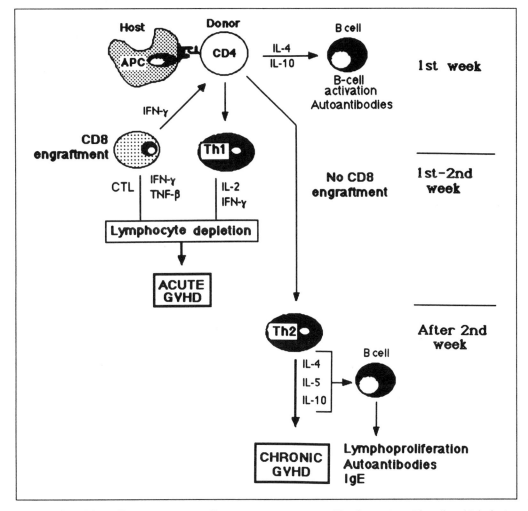

Fig. 8.12. Th1/Th2 cells in GVHD. Host alloantigens are recognized by donor CD4+ Th cells, which during the first week usually produce Th2-type cytokines such as IL-4 and IL-10 that favor intense B cell activation, proliferation, and autoantibody production. Between the first and the second week two possibilities may occur: (1) if there is CD8+ T cell engraftment, a strong Th1 response develops, which results in lymphocyte depletion and acute GVHD; (2) if there is no CD8+ T cell engraftment, a chronic Th2 response occurs, which results in strong lymphoproliferation, autoantibody production and high IgE levels (chronic GVHD).

mature T cells, induces profound defects in the host immune response, which are known as graft versus host reaction (GVHR). Depending on both MHC disparity and non-MHC-linked loci, GVH disease (GVHD) can be found in acute and chronic form. Interestingly, both acute and chronic GVHD are initially characterized by increased Th2 cytokine (IL-4 and IL-10) production and evidence of B cell activation, such as increased B cell expression of MHC class II molecules, increased numbers of splenic B cells, elevated serum IgG anti-ssDNA antibody levels, which persist until the second week (Fig. 8.12). Divergence of acute and chronic GVHD occurs during the second week after cell transfer, at which time chronic GVHD continues to exhibit lymphoproliferation, B cell activation and autoantibody production, whereas acute GVHD mice develop reduced numbers of host lymphocytes and reduced serum autoantibody levels. However, the factors that determine which form of GVHD will subsequently develop following the initial GVHR are still unclear.

Acute GVHD

The acute GVRD results in a complete abrogation of immune reactivity and in the repopulation of the host spleen with donor T cells.[1067,1068] The earliest distinguishing features of acute GVHD were detectable between day 5 and 7 of the disease and consisted of an expansion of donor CD8+ T cells and increased IFN-γ production by donor CD4+ and CD8+ T cells. Despite the decline in cell numbers, acute GVHD mice continue to exhibit evidence of B cell activation and elevated levels of IL-4 and IL-10 mRNA during the second week of the disease. The subsequent transition from B cell activation to lymphocytopenia is critically related to the successful engraftment of donor CD8+ T cells. In addition to their role as cytotoxic effectors that mediate the cytopenic features of acute GVHD, the donor CD8+ T cells also exert a regulatory role in the development of acute GVHD by virtue of their ability to influence cytokine secretion by donor CD4+ T cells, in part through their production of IFN-γ.[1069] Thus, established acute GVHD is characterized by a predominant production of Th1 cytokines, as shown by the increased expression of IFN-γ mRNA and the ability of anti-IL-2 antibody in vivo to block acute GVHD development.[1070,1071] NK-like cytotoxicity mediated by γδ+ T cells is probably also involved in the pathogenesis of acute GVHD.[1072] Finally, recent work indicates that IL-12 plays a central role in the Th1 polarization, since in vivo neutralization of endogenous IL-12 ameliorates acute GVHD, in association with reduced splenic NK cell activity, IFN-γ production, immunosuppression, weight loss and mortality. Conversely, the administration of exogenous IL-12 exacerbates the disease and converts the chronic GVHD into a lethal acute GVHD-like syndrome.[1073] It is of note that both polarized CD4+ and CD8+ Th2 alloreactive donor T cells generated in vitro from mature T cell populations can function in vivo to inhibit Th1 responses and such inhibition attenuates the systemic morbidity of GVHD after bone marrow transplantation across both MHC class I or class II barriers in mice.[1074]

Chronic GVHD

Chronic GVRD is characterized by a less severe form of immunodeficiency than acute GVHD, consisting of a selective loss of CD4+ Th functions and IL-2 production, associated with hyperactivation of B cell functions, which leads to the production of autoantibodies, antibody-mediated glomerulonephritis and hypergammaglobulinemia (including a significant increase in serum IgE levels), which can be completely prevented by the early administration of an anti-IL-4 antibody.[1075] In addition, IL-4 and IL-10 mRNA can be detected in the spleens of mice with chronic GVHD, whereas IL-2 and IFN-γ production are defective.[974] Lastly and more importantly, anti-IL-4 antibody treatment prevents immunodysfunction including T cell differentiation in the thymus or the spleen and autoimmune symptoms, strongly supporting the view that chronic GVHD results from predominant activation of Th2 cells.[1076] Since in DBA/F₁ mice these changes occur in the absence of significant expansion of donor CD8+ T cells or detectable anti-host CTL activity, the possibility that chronic GVHD is caused by an underlying defect in DBA CD8+ T cells has been postulated.[1069] The demonstration that treatment with IL-12 stimulates the development of acute GVHD in mice that normally would develop chronic GVHD[1077] provides additional support to this possibility.

GVHD AFTER ALLOGENEIC BONE MARROW TRANSPLANTATION

Although allogeneic BMT is the therapy of choice for a number of diseases, GVHD remains the major complication and the major barrier of this type of treatment to a variety of diseases. T cells in the donor bone marrow recognize and react against host alloantigens and thereby initiate GVHD. Activated donor T cells proliferate indeed and differentiate into effector cells. It is generally thought that when the principal T cell response is a Th1 response (mainly IL-2 and IFN-γ) these cytokines activate host mononuclear cells and macrophages to secrete pro-inflammatory cytokines, such as IL-1 and TNF-α, as well as active NO, which induce tissue injury. The overall result is the acute or "suppressive" form of GVHD. When the principal T cell response is a Th2 response, IL-4 and IL-10 predominate, the overall result is the chronic or "stimulatory" form of GVHD, with increased IgE synthesis and exaggerated lymphoproliferation.[1078]

TH1/TH2 CELLS AND TUMORS

TUMORS OF TH2 CELLS

Sézary syndrome

Patients with Sézary syndrome (SS), a leukemic form of cutaneous T cell lymphoma, characterized by malignant atypical CD4+ CD45RO+ lymphocytes (Sézary cells) in the skin and peripheral blood exhibit, in addition to erythroderma, an array of immunologic abnormalities that parallel the in vitro activities of Th2 cytokines, particularly IL-4 and IL-5, such as eosinophilia and increased levels of IgE and IgA.[1079,1080] Accordingly, PBMC from patients with SS showed increased IL-4 production and decreased IL-2 and IFN-γ production,[1081] and highly purified T cells from SS patients also exhibited marked an upregulation of IL-4 mRNA expression.[1082] In addition, skin specimens from patients with SS had demonstrable mRNA for IL-4 and/or IL-5.[1083] Finally, it has been shown that PBMC from patients with SS have a significantly decreased ability to produce IL-12 in response to stimulation with *Staphylococcus aureus* or LPS, whereas pretreatment of PBMC with IL-12 reverted cytokine and immune abnormalities of patients with this syndrome.[1084]

In contrast to SS, Mycosis fungoides (MF), a localized form of cutanous T cell lymphoma, has been found to have a predominant Th1-like profile or an undefined profile.[1085] However, whether this pathway is due to the neoplastic cell itself or rather to the reactive cells present in the neoplastic lesions is still unclear. It is noteworthy that intralesional injection of IFN-γ after chemotherapy appeared to be successful in the treatment of MF tumors.[1086]

Clonal Th2-cell proliferation in the hypereosinophilic syndrome

A clonal proliferation of Th2 cells has also been observed in a subject with idiopathic hypereosinophilic syndrome. The clone was CD4+CD3−, secreted massive concentrations of IL-4 and IL-5 and very low amounts of IL-2 and IFN-γ. The serum levels of IL-5 dropped dramatically with steroid treatment and eosinophilia was reduced after the initiation of IFN-α-2b therapy.[1087]

ROLE OF TH1 AND TH2 CELLS AGAINST TUMORS

It is generally believed that the immune response against malignantly transformed cells requires the elaboration of cytokines produced by T cells. For example, cytokines appear to be essential for the activation of CD8+ CTL to lyse tumor targets.[1088] The importance of CD4+ T cells in the generation of anti-tumor immunity has also been documented in several animal models, in which the CD4+ subset appears to be crucial in determining the rejection of established local and disseminated tumors.[1089,1090] Although IL-4 has been found to posses anti-tumor effects,[1091-1093] which seem to be mainly mediated by eosinophil activation,[1092,1093] in the great majority of models CD4+ T cells producing Th1 cytokines appear to be protective, whereas those producing Th2-cytokines seem rather to favor tumor growth. First, splenic T cells from mice bearing renal cell carcinoma or colon carcinoma preferentially produced Th2 cytokines (i.e., IL-4) upon activation and showed a marked decrease in Th1 cytokine (particularly IFN-γ) production compared with production observed in normal splenic T cells.[1094] Likewise, splenocytes from plasma cell tumor-bearing mice demonstrated reduced proliferation and production of Th1 cytokines (IL-2 and IFN-γ) without alterations in the production of Th2 cytokines (IL-4 and IL-10).[1095] Both T cell anergy and reduced production of IFN-γ have been attributed, at least in part, to the production of IL-10 by noncytotoxic CD8+ T cells.[1096] This finding is consistent with the observation that cessation of IL-10 secretion, as a consequence of low-dose L-phenylalanine mustard, restored the ability of splenic cells from mice bearing MOPC-315 tumor to produce IFN-γ.[1097] TGF-β contributes to the shift toward Th2-type responses in tumor-bearing mice through direct and IL-10-mediated pathways.[1098]

In agreement with the results obtained in experimental animal models, Th1 cytokines appear in general to be more protective than Th2 cytokines against human neoplasias. The local cytokine response to basal cell carcinoma appeared to be Th2-like, whereas the response towards a benign growth was Th1-like, suggesting that the type 2 lymphokine response can induce immunosuppression at the tumor site and in this way contributes to the tumor development.[1099] The majority of CD4+ T cell clones generated from tumor-infiltrating lymphocytes (TILs) of patients with melanoma exhibited a Th0-like profile,[1100] and supernatants from these Th0 or Th1 clones, as well as IL-2, enhanced cytotoxicity by CD8+ CTL, whereas both Th2 clone supernatants and IL-4 decreased killing compared with control CTL.[1101] Recently, we have observed high proportions of CD8+ T cells showing an unusual Th2-like phenotype in the Kaposi's sarcoma lesions of patients with AIDS, whose number was significantly reduced in the same skin areas after successful therapy with IFN-α.[65] Accordingly, the presence of autologous tumor-specific Th2 cells was found among melanoma TILs.[1102] These findings suggest that the knowledge of factors influencing the selective activation of Th1 or Th2 responses to benign and malignant tumors is still unclear, but it may be fundamental to our understanding of the immune response to cancer.

The role of Th1 cytokines in favoring the generation of tumor-reactive cells has raised several attempts aimed at utilizing and/or potentiating their effects. When tumor cells were heat-shocked, the cytotoxicity by specific Th1 clones was significantly enhanced[1103] When murine carcinoma cell lines were transfected with IL-2 and IFN-γ, rejection was increased to at least 10,000-fold above the parental cells.[1104]

Intravescical instillation of BCG induced IFN-γ and TNF-α, but not IL-4, mRNA expression in the bladder wall and was highly effective in eliminating bladder tumors.[1105] Likewise, staphylococcal enterotoxin A-reactive CD4[+] Th1-like T cells, specifically targeted to c-*erbB*-2 positive human colon cancer cells using SEA-conjugated-anti-c-*erbB*-2 monoclonal antibody, resulted in the augmentation of cytotoxicity against c-*erbB*-2-positive tumor cells.[1106] Finally and most importantly, IL-12 administration has been shown to be more efficacious than IL-2 in several murine tumour models.[1107] It appears clear that the anti-tumor function of IL-12 treatment depends upon the induced expression of IFN-γ by T cells and/or NK cells, the amplification of the immune response mediated by IFN-γ-induced expression of chemoattractant chemokines, and the IL-12-dependent potentiation of the cytolytic effector function of recruited CD8[+] T cells.[1108-1110] Accordingly, the antitumor therapeutic efficacy of peptide-pulsed dendritic cells appeared to be mainly related to the induced secretion of IL-12, thereby driving a CD4[+] Th1-associated immune response.[1111] It is noteworthy that, whereas in vivo neutralization studies clearly supported the requirement of endogenous IL-12 for rejection of P815 tumor variants,[1112] as well as for the effectiveness of dendritic cell-tumor peptide-based therapy,[1111] no additional significant advantage was observed in this latter condition with systemic coadministration of recombinant IL-12, suggesting that dendritic cell-based therapies elicit sufficient endogenous IL-12 for clinical impact.[1111]

======= CHAPTER 9 =======

POSSIBLE THERAPEUTIC IMPLICATIONS OF THE TH1/TH2 PARADIGM

It is now clear that the nature of human specific immune responses against offending agents is determined by the set of lymphokines produced by T cells. The human T cell response is heterogenous, but under some in vitro and even in vivo conditions T cell stimulation can result in the development of a restricted Th1-type or Th2-type pattern of lymphokine production. The understanding of fine tuning of events occurring as a consequence of matching between antigen profile and host genetic background allows to hypothesize new therapeutic strategies not only for control of infectious diseases but also for the manipulation of immunopathological reactions.

DEVELOPMENT OF NEW VACCINES AGAINST INFECTIOUS AGENTS

VACCINES BASED ON THE USE OF SELECTED PEPTIDES

T cells recognize antigen epitopes in the form of peptides 8-12 amino acids long bound to the groove of MHC class I or class II molecules on the surface of APCs. As a rule, CD8$^+$ CTL recognize peptides in connection with MHC class I determinants derived from endogenously de novo-synthesized proteins, while CD4$^+$ T cells respond to MHC class II-associated peptides generated from phagocytized proteins entering the lysosomal pathway. Epitopes recognized by T cells under these conditions can be mimicked by synthetic peptides. These peptides on delivery in appropriate adjuvants such as CFA or liposomes can bind to empty cell surface-expressed MHC determinants and in consequence trigger an immune response, suggesting that synthetic peptides might be suitable as vaccines. Peptide vaccines have several advantages over traditional vaccines: they are safe; they can be synthesized with high reproducibility and exquisite purity in large quantities; and they can be designed to induce well-defined monofunctional immune responses.

Selected peptides may be obtained from antigens that induce preferential Th1 responses; this is the case of the recombinant 403 aminoacid protein from *L. braziliensis* homologous to ribosomal protein eIF-4A[139] and of the promastigote surface antigen 2 from *L. major*.[367] Peptides can also be opportunely modified, since it is clear that changes as little as those concerning single amino acid residues,[77,140,141] as well as selection of ligands with various class binding affinity,[144] can deviate the ability of the T cell epitopes to the induction of a different cytokines profile.

SELECTED ADJUVANTS INCLUDING CYTOKINES

The antigen can also be manipulated to favor Th1 responses and therefore the induction of CMI. Antigen manipulations include polymerization,[127,128] incorporation into immune complexes,[132] coupling to oxidized mannan,[133] or its injection together with components of the mycobacterial cell wall, in view of their ability to stimulate the production of IL-12 by both macrophages and dendritic cells. Recombinant *M. bovis* (BCG) strains have also been proposed as optimal adjuvants for the induction of Th1 responses against *L. major*,[1113] *M. tuberculosis*,[1114] and measles virus.[1115] Orally administered live recombinant *Salmonella* also elicites dominant antigen-specific Th1-type responses in both mucosal and systemic tissues, in the absence of expression of Th2 cytokines Il-4 and IL-5.[498]

Several studies indicate that the administration of cytokines boosts both the humoral and cellular immune responses greatly[1116] and improves the ability of a vaccine to confer protective immunity in disease models. In particular, IL-12 has an adjuvant effect in a vaccine against *L. major* by shifting the cytokine pattern from a Th2 type to a Th1 type,[165] and improves vaccine immunogenicity against *L. monocytogenes*[1117] and RSV.[558] Coadministration of eggs from *S. mansoni* plus IL-12 prevents fibrosis induced by schistosome infection,[660] whereas administration of IL-12 as an adjuvant in conjunction with a soluble lung-stage *S. mansoni* larval antigen preparation induces a Th1 cell-mediated protective immunity to *S. mansoni*.[1118] Thus, manipulation of the cytokine response in this way may represent an important advance in vaccine research.[1119]

PLASMID DNA IMMUNIZATION (NAKED DNA VACCINES)

Another revolutionary approach, originally developed for gene therapy, is based on vaccination with plasmid vectors. These genetic vaccines are commonly called naked DNA or polynucleotide vaccines. In current techniques of gene transfer, the DNA is packaged into recombinant viral vectors, such as retroviruses, vaccinia-virus or adenovirus, or attached to cationally charged molecules, such as liposomes or calcium salts. By contrast, naked DNA consists of a desired gene inserted into a plasmid which can enter and remain episomally in cells close to the injection site, where it is subsequently transcribed and translated, causing expression of the gene product.[1120,1121] There are three major advantages to this technique. First, naked-DNA vaccines could bypass the numerous problems associated with other vectors, such as immune responses against the delivery vectors and concern about safety related to the use of any viral vector. Second, they could induce the expression of antigens that resemble native epitopes more closely than do standard live attenuated and killed vaccines where the process of manufacturing can alter the structure of protein and thus lower the antigenicity of the vaccine. Third, they may be constructed so that genes from several different pathogens are included on the same plasmid, thus potentially decreasing the number of vaccinations required for children. Finally and most importantly, the gene protein enters the cells' MHC class I pathway since only proteins that originate inside a cell are processed by this pathway. This results in the stimulation of CD8[+] cytotoxic T cells and evokes CMI, thus challenging the escape attempts of the infectious agent from the humoral system, a striking phenomenon in chronic infections with agents (HCV and HIV), in which many mutations in the envelope genes are often found in the viruses from a single infected patient.[1122,1123] Accordingly, the results of a recent study suggest that intradermal immunization of BALB/c mice with naked plasmid DNA encoding for *E. coli* β-galactosidase (β-gal) induces a Th1 immune response, as demonstrated by a highly restricted IgG2a antibody response to β-gal together with IFN-γ, but not IL-4 or IL-5, secretion by in vitro β-gal-stimulated splenic CD4[+] T cells, whereas immunization with the corresponding protein, β-gal, in saline or alum induces a Th2 response.[1124]

DEVIATION OF ESTABLISHED TH1 OR TH2 RESPONSES

One major issue of the Th1/Th2 paradigm is whether it is possible to manipulate established Th1 or Th2 responses. The initial studies suggested that once naive T cells were committed to Th1 or Th2 patterns of cytokine secretion, their memory populations would secrete identical arrays of cytokines upon antigen restimulation.[182,188] More recent data indicate that regardless of prior commitment, memory CD4[+] cells may retain the capacity to be further influenced by IL-4, IFN-γ or IL-12 during effector cell development to become subsets that are at least temporarily polarized to have a particular pattern of cytokine secretion.[156,157] These findings confirm previous studies on human Th subsets suggesting that memory cells may be previously committed to either Th1 or Th2 patterns of cytokine secretion, but can be induced to produce cytokines of the opposite phenotype when T cell lines are derived from primed populations in the presence of IL-4 or IFN-γ, respectively.[121,177] Once established, the Th2 phenotype appears to be more stable than the Th1 phenotype in both mice[1125] and humans.[154,251] Stimulation of human Th1 clones in the presence of progesterone results in IL-4 production,[251] whereas stimulation of Th2 clones in the presence of IL-12 promotes only transient IFN-γ mRNA expression.[154] Reversibility of both Th1 and Th2 cell populations is lost after long-term stimulation.[1126]

Evidence is accumulating suggesting the plasticity in the cytokine secretion capacity of preexisting memory cells, at the level of individual cells or the population, even in vivo.[96,375,660] It is not known if any of these phenomena involve the actual switching of cytokine production by partially or fully differentiated T cells or the replacement of one T cell population by another. In any case, this condition is certainly advantageous for defense against infections that progress through intracellular as well as extracellular stages, engendering different sets of conditions of antigen presentation and requirements for successful elimination during the course of the response. Thus, mutability of cytokine secretion by memory CD4⁺ cells may enable rapid adjustment of the relative contributions of Th1 and Th2 cytokines under conditions in which the infectious process is not only changing, but being quickly resolved by the memory response. The plasticity of cytokine secretion by memory CD4 effector cells, combined with the ability to use selected adjuvants or exogenous cytokines to develop distinct subsets in vitro, may be exploited therapeutically not only in situations in which either Th1 or Th2 cells are necessary for protection against a particular pathogen, but also in conditions in which harmful Th1 or Th2 responses develop against environmental antigens or autoantigens, such as allergic or autoimmune disorders.

STRATEGIES FOR THE TREATMENT OF ALLERGIC DISEASES

Induction of Th2/Th1 class switch

The possibility to switch the allergen-specific Th2 response toward a less dangerous pathway appears of primary importance in the development of novel efficient forms of allergen-specific immunotherapy for allergic disorders. This might be achieved by downregulating established allergen-specific Th2 responses, i.e., by acting at the level of memory T cells. Indeed, although several studies in the animal models had previously shown a failure to tolerize Th2 clones,[351,352] more recent data have demonstrated tolerance induction in both the Th1- and Th2-like subpopulations.[357,360] A potentially more successful approach should be the upregulation of allergen-specific Th1 responses, which is directed to prime naive T cells in manner which selects for prevalent Th1 phenotype. Predominant secretion of Th1-type cytokines in response to allergen will not only result in development and recruitment of different effector responses (IgG production, macrophage activation instead of IgE and eosinophil activation), but will also probably inhibit the function of established Th2 responses, as a result of crossregulatory circuits. Indeed, although in vitro generated Th2 cells could not be converted into IFN-γ producers, inasmuch as they lose their sensitivity to IL-12,[1125] compelling evidence that established Th2 responses can be shifted in vivo to Th1-like responses has been provided in both mice[375] and humans.[751-754] Upregulation of allergen-specific Th1 responses has already been achieved both in vitro and in vivo by using cytokines, such as IFN-γ or α[177,179] and IL-12.[153] An alternative way to upregulate Th1-type responses to allergens may be the use of recombinant *Mycobacteria* or other adjuvants, APCs that select for the Th1 phenotype, or plasmid DNA (allergen epitope plus cytokine) gene therapy (see above).

Antagonizing Th2 cytokines

Other potentially efficient therapeutic strategies are based on targeting the effector molecules produced as a consequence of activation of Th2 cells (nonallergen-specific immunotherapy). This approach has become conceptually available after evidence was accumulated suggesting that probably Th2 responses are not critical for survival and protection. First, IL-4-deficient mice which do not develop Th2 responses are better protected against the great majority of infections than wild animals.[189] Th2 responses are more protective than Th1 responses only in infections sustained by some gastrointestinal nematodes which do not represent a major problem, at least in well-developed countries. IL-4 activity may be antagonized by soluble IL-4 receptors[772] or more effectively by a human IL-4 mutant protein.[1127] Interestingly, this protein also antagonizes the biological activity of IL-13, as well as the IL-4-driven differentiation of Th2 cells in vitro.[1128] IL-5 activity may be antagonized by humanized antibodies to IL-5, which appeared to be capable of inhibiting eosinophil infiltration and normalizing airway hyperreactivity in monkeys challenged with *Ascaris suum* [775,1129] or by a IL-5 specific gene transcription inhibitor.[1130]

STRATEGIES FOR THE TREATMENT OF AUTOIMMUNE DISORDERS

Oral tolerance

Oral tolerance may be defined as a specific reduction in the immune response brought about by feeding an antigen. It can occur by two distinct mechanisms according to the antigen dosage and frequency of feeding. With multiple low doses of antigen the following mode of action has been proposed: the antigen passes from the lumen of the gut across multifold-cells lying under Peyer's patches, and hence into APCs within the patches. APCs then activate a local population of T cells which, in the absence of inflammatory and costimulatory molecules, specializes in the secretion of TGF-β and IL-4. These cells have been named Th3 cells.[10] The inhibitory cytokines produced by Th3 cells suppress the activity of neighboring disease-inducing Th1 cells.[1131] By contrast, feeding a single high dose of antigen induces anergy of antigen-specific Th1 lymphocytes with intact Th2 responses or minimal secretion of IL-4, IL-10 and TGF-β.[87] It has been suggested that oral induction of anergy might depend on the systemic dissemination of antigen (or its fragments) absorbed from the gut.[1132] Experiments in animal models of human autoimmune diseases have shown that it is not necessary to use the primary antigen responsible for disease induction. Antigens implicated in secondary immune phenomenon can act similarly by means of the so-called "bystander suppression."[865,1135] Modulation of EAE[864,1134] collagen-induced arthritis,[936] uveitis[1135] and experimental autoimmune myasthenia gravis[1136] has been obtained by oral administration of organ-specific antigens. Of interest is that nasal administration of glutamate decarboxylase (GAD65) peptides was also capable of inducing Th2 responses and preventing murine IDDM.[1137] For diseases such as MS and RA, candidate antigens for desensitization are already available. Oral myelin tolerization of relapsing-remitting MS patients resulted in fewer attacks, as compared to a placebo-fed group.[86] The frequency of TGF-β1-secreting T cell lines after MBP and PLP stimulation in fed patients was greater than that of nonfed patients.[1138] A number of patients with RA also responded to treatment with oral type II collagen.[1139]

Cytokine-induced immune deviation

An increasing amount of data indicate the dominant suppressor activity of IL-4 and IL-10 on inflammatory reactions, sustained by strong and prolonged activation of Th1-type immune responses (see above). This suppression is due to the crossregulatory activity of IL-4 and IL-10 on the development and function of Th1 cells but even more to their potent downregulatory effect on mediators of inflammation released by macrophages, such as TNF-α, IL-1 and reactive oxygen/nitrogen. This is the reason why IL-10 not only inhibits cytokine production, vascular leakage, and swelling during Th1-induced DTH reactions,[1140] but is also capable of protecting mice from lethal endotoxemia.[1141,1142] Accordingly, administration of IL-4, IL-10, or a combination of both, has been found to be effective in improving or preventing EAE, IDDM and collagen-induced arthritis,[852,854,911,916] as well as to prevent and reverse cartilage degradation in RA.[1143] Therefore, administration of IL-4 and/or IL-10 may be a promising therapeutic approach for human diseases characterized by autoreactive or exaggerated DTH responses. The induction of autoreactive Th2 cells by immune deviation with selected autoantigens might also prove to be promising approach for vaccination against inflammatory autoimmune diseases.[1144] Thus far, little is known about the effects and side effects of IL-4 on the human immune system in vivo, whereas therapeutic regimens with IL-10 are well-tolerated,[1145] suggesting their quick utilization for the therapy of Th1-mediated disorders.

REFERENCES

1. Romagnani S. Th1 and Th2 subsets of CD4⁺ T lymhocytes. Science & Medicine 1994; 1:68-77.
2. Parish CR. The relationship between humoral and cell-mediated immunity. Transplant. Rev. 1972; 13:35-66.
3. Mosmann TR, Cherwinski H, Bond MW, Giedlin MA, Coffman RL. Two types of murine T cell clone. I. Definition according to profiles of lymphokine activities and secreted proteins. J. Immunol. 1986; 136:2348-2357.
4. Mosmann TR, Coffman RL. TH1 and TH2 cells: different patterns of lymphokine secretion lead to different functional properties. Ann. Rev. Immunol. 1989; 7:145-73.
5. Romagnani S, Maggi E. Th1 versus Th2 responses in AIDS. Curr. Opin. Immunol. 1994; 6:616-622.
6. Romagnani S. Biology of human Th1 and Th2 cells. J. Clin. Immunol. 1995; 15:121-129.
7. Street NE, Schumaker JH, Fong TAT, Bass H, Fiorentino DF, Leverah JA, Mosmann TR. Heterogeneity of mouse helper T cells. Evidence from bulk cultures and limiting dilution cloning for precursors of Th1 and Th2 cells. J. Immunol. 1990; 144:1629-1639.
8. Maggi E, Del Prete GF, Macchia D, Parronchi P, Tiri A, Chretien I, Ricci M, Romagnani S. Profiles of lymphokine activites and helper function for IgE in human T cell clones. Eur. J. Immunol. 1988; 18:1045-1050.
9. Paliard X, de Waal Malefijt R, Yssel H, Blanchard D, Chretien I, Abrams J, de Vries EJ, Spits H. Simultaneous production of IL-2, IL-4, and IFN-γ by activated human CD4⁺ and CD8⁺ T cell clones. J. Immunol. 1988; 141:849-855.
10. Chen Y, Kuchroo VK, Inobe J, Hafler DA, Weiner HL. Regulatory T cell clones induced by oral tolerance: suppression of autoimmune encephalomyelitis. Science 1994; 265:1237-1240.
11. Mosmann TR, Sad S. The expanding universe of T-cell subsets: Th1, Th2 and more. Immunol. Today 1996; 17:138-146.
12. Openshaw P, Murphy EE, Hosken NA et al. Heterogeneity of intracellular cytokine synthesis at the single-cell level in polarized T helper 1 and T helper 2 populations. J. Exp. Med. 1995; 182:1357-1367.
13. O' Garra A, Murphy KM. Role of cytokines in the development of Th1 and Th2 cells. Chem. Immunol. 1996; 63:1-13.
14. Kelso A. Th1 and Th2 subsets: paradigm lost? Immunol. Today 1995; 16:374-379.
15. Bucy RP, Karr L, Huang G-Q, Li J, Carter D, Honjo K, Lemons JA, Murphy KM, Weaver CT. Single cell analysis of cytokine gene coexpression during CD4⁺ T-cell phenotype development. Proc. Natl. Acad. Sci. USA 1995; 92:7565-7569.
16. Wierenga EA, Snoek M, de Groot C, Chretien I, Bos JD, Jansen HM, Kapsenberg ML. Evidence for compartmentalization of functional subsets of CD4⁺ T lymphocytes in atopic patients. J. Immunol. 1990; 144:4651-4656.

17. Parronchi P, Macchia D, Piccinni M-P, Biswas P, Simonelli C, Maggi E, Ricci M, Ansari AA, Romagnani S. Allergen- and bacterial antigen-specific T-cell clones established from atopic donors show a different profile of cytokine production. Proc. Natl. Acad. Sci. USA 1991; 88:4538-4542.

18. Del Pret GF, De Carli M, Mastromauro C et al. Purified protein derivative of Mycobacterium tuberculosis and excretory-secretory antigen(s) of Toxocara canis expand in vitro human T cells with stable and opposite (type 1 T helper or type 2 T helper) profile of cytokine production. J. Clin. Invest. 1991; 88:346-351.

19. Romagnani S. Human T_H1 and T_H2: doubt no more. Immunol. Today 1991; 12:256-57.

20. Haanen JBAG, de Waal Malefijt R, Res PCM, Kraakman EM, Ottenhoff THM, de Vries RRP, Spits H. Selection of a human T helper type 1-like T cell subset by Mycobacteria. J. Exp. Med. 1991; 174:583-592.

21. Yssel H, Shanafelt MC, Soderberg C, Schneider PV, Anzola J, Peltz G. *Borrelia burgdorferi* activates a T helper type 1-like T cell subset in Lyme arthritis. J. Exp. Med. 1991; 174:593-601.

22. Salgame P, Abrams JS, Clayberger, Goldstein H, Convitt J, Modlin RL, Bloom BR. Differing lymphokine profiles and functional subsets of human CD4[+] and CD8[+] T cell clones. Science 1991; 254:279-281.

23. Del Prete GF, Tiri A, Mariotti S, Pinchera A, Ricci M, Romagnani S. 1987. Enhanced production of gamma-interferon by thyroid-derived T cell clones from patients with Hashimoto's thyroiditis. Clin. Exper. Immunol. 1987; 69:323-331.

24. Maggi E, Biswas P, Del Prete GF, Parronchi P, Macchia D, Simonelli C, Emmi L, De Carli M, Tiri A, Ricci M, Romagnani S. Accumulation of Th2-like helper T cells in the conjunctiva of patients with vernal conjunctivitis. J. Immunol. 1991; 146:1169-1174.

25. Del Prete GF, De Carli M, Almerigogna F, Giudizi M-G, Biagiotti R, Romagnani S. Human IL-10 is produced by both type 1 helper (Th1) and type 2 helper (Th2) T cell clones and inhibits their antigen-specific proliferation and cytokine production. J. Immunol. 1993; 150:1-8.

26. Romagnani S. Lymphokine production by human T cells in disease states. Annu. Rev. Immunol. 1994; 12:227-257.

27. de Waal-Malefyt R, Abrams JS, Zurawski SM, Lecron JC, Mohan-Peterson S, Sanjanwala B, Bennett B, Silver J, de Vries JE, Yssel H. Differential regulation of IL-13 and IL-4 production by human CD8[+] and CD4[+] Th0, Th1 and Th2 T cell clones and EBV-transformed B cells. Int. Immunol. 1995; 7:1405-1416.

28. Fiorentino DE, Bond MW, Mosmann TR. Two types of mouse T helper cell. IV. Th2 clones secrete a factor that inhibits cytokine production by Th1 clones. J. Exp. Med. 1989; 150:1-8.

29. Del Prete GF, De Carli M, Ricci M, Romagnani S. Helper activity for immunoglobulin synthesis by Th1 and Th2 human T-cell clones: the help of Th1 clones is limited by their cytolytic capacity. J. Exp. Med. 1991; 174:809-813.

30. Del Prete GF, De Carli M, Lammel RM, D'Elios MM, Daniel KC, Giusti B, Abbate R, Romagnani S. Th1 and Th2 T-helper cells exert opposite regulatory effects on procoagulant activity and tissue factor production by human monocytes. Blood 1995; 86:250-257.

31. Moretta A, Pantaleo G, Moretta L, Cerottini JC, Mingari MC. Direct demonstration of the clonogenic potential of every human peripheral blood T cell. Clonal analysis of HLA-DR expression and cytolytic activity. J. Exp. Med. 1983; 157:743-753.

32. Del Prete GF, De Carli M, D'Elios MM, Maestrelli P, Ricci M, Fabbri L, Romagnani S. Allergen exposure induces the activation of allergen-specific Th2 cells in the airway mucosa of patients with allergic respiratory disorders. Eur. J. Immunol. 1993; 23:1445-1449.

33. Kawasaki ES. Amplification of RNA. In: Innis, ed. PCR Protocols, a Guide to Methods and Applications. Academic Press, Inc., 1991:21-27.

34. Dirks RW. Development and application of in situ hybridization procedures for the localization of mRNA. Dept. of Cytochemistry and Cytometry. The Netherlands: Leiden University Press, 1992.

35. Klinman DM, Nutman TB. Elispot assay to detect cytokine-secreting human cells. In: Shevach E, ed. Current Protocols In Immunology. New York: Gree Publishing Associated and Wiley Interscience, 1994.

36. Jung T, Schauer U, Heusser C, Neumann C, Rieger C. Detection of intracellular cytokines by flow cytometry. J. Immunol. Methods 1993; 159:197-207.

37. Assenmacher M, Schmitz J, Radbruch A. Flow cytometric determination of cytokines in activated murine T helper lymphocytes: expression of interleukin 10 in interferon-gamma and in interleukin-4 expressing cells. Eur. J. Immunol. 1994; 24:1097-1101.

38. Bradding P, Feather IH, Wilson S, Bardin PG, Heusser CH, Holgate ST, Howarth PH. Immunolocalization of cytokines in the nasal mucosa of normal and perennial rhinitic subjects: the mast cells as a source of IL-4, IL-5, and IL-6 in human allergic mucosal inflammation. J. Immunol. 1993; 151:3853-3860.

39. Bottomly K, Luqman M, Greenbaum L, Carding S, West J, Pasqualini T, Murphy DB. A monoclonal antibody to murine CD45R distinguishes CD4 T cell populations that produce different cytokines. Eur. J. Immunol. 1989; 19:617-623.

40. Lee WT, Vitetta ES. Changes in expression of CD45R during the development of Th1 and Th2 cell lines. Eur. J. Immunol. 1992; 22:1455-1459.

41. Seder RA, Paul WE. Acquisition of lymphokine-producing phenotype by CD4+ T cells. Ann. Rev. Immunol. 1994; 12:635-673.

42. Ebel F, Schmitt E, Peter-Katalinic J, Kniep B, Muhlradt PF. Gangliosides: differentiation markers for murine T helper lymphocyte subpopulations Th1 and Th2. Biochemistry 1992; 31:12190-12197.

43. Pernis A, Gupta S, Gollob KJ, Garfein E, Coffman RL, Schindler C, Rothman P. Lack of interferon γ receptor β chain and the prevention of interferon γ signalling in Th1 cells. Science 1995; 269:245-247.

44. Scheel D, Richter E, Toellner K-M, Reiling N, Key G, Wacker H-H, Ulmer AJ, Flad HD, Gerdes J. Correlation of CD26 expression with Th1-like reactions in granulomatous diseases. In: Schlossmann SF, Boumsell L, Gilks W, eds. Leukocyte Typing V "White Cell Differentiation Antigens". Oxford: Oxford University Press, 1995:1111-1114.

45. Kanegane H, Kasahara Y, Niida Y, Yachie A, Sugii S, Takatsu K, Taniguchi N, Miyawaki T. Expression of L-selectin (CD62L) discriminates Th1- and Th2-like cytokine-producing memory CD4+ T cells. Immunology 1996; 87:186-190.

46. Assenmacher M, Scheffold A, Schmitz J, Segura Checa JA, Miltenyi S, Radbruch A. Specific expression of surface interferon-γ on interferon-γ-producing T cells from mouse and man. Eur. J. Immunol. 1996; 26:263-267.

47. Smith CA, Gruss H-J, Davis T et al. CD30 antigen, a marker for Hodgkin's lymphoma, is a receptor whose ligand defines an emerging family of cytokines with homology to TNF. Cell 1993; 73:1349-1360.

48. Del Prete G-F, De Carli M, Almerigogna F et al. Preferential expression of CD30 by human CD4+ T cells producing Th2-type cytokines. FASEB J. 1995; 9:81-86.

49. Bengtsson A, Johansson C, Tengvall Linder M, Hallden G, van der Ploeg I, Scheynius A. Not only Th2 cells but also Th1 and Th0 cells express CD30 after activation. J. Leuk. Biol. 1995; 58:683-689.

50. Hamann D, Hilkens CMU, Grogan JL, Lens SMA, Kapsenberg ML, Yazdanbakhsh M, van Lier RAW. CD30 expression does not discriminate between human Th1- and Th2-type T cells. J. Immunol. 1996; 156:1387-1391.

51. Seitzer U, Flad H-D, Gerdes J. Within the spectral forms of leprosy cell bound CD30 cannot be regarded as an operational marker for a Th2-like reaction. J. Leukoc. Biol. 1996; 59:311-311.

52. Del Prete G-F, De Carli M, D'Elios MM et al. CD30-mediated signalling promotes the development of human Th2-like T cells. J. Exp. Med. 1995; 182:1-7.

53. McDonald PP, Cassatella MA, Bald A et al. CD30 ligation induces nuclear factor-kB activation in human T cell lines. Eur. J. Immunol. 1995; 25:2870-2876.

54. Romagnani S. Th1 and Th2 in human diseases. Clin. Immunol. Immunopathol. 1996; 80:225-235.

55. Chilosi M, Facchetti F, Notarangelo LD et al. CD30 cell expression and abnormal soluble C5-D30 serum accumulation in Omenn's syndrome. Evidence for a Th2-mediated condition. Eur. J. Immunol. 1996; 26:329-334.

56. Schandené L, Ferster A, Mascart-Lemone F et al. T helper type 2-like cells and therapeutic effects of interferon-γ in combined immunodeficiency with hypereosinophilia (Omenn's syndrome). Eur. J. Immunol. 1993; 23:56-60.

57. Triebel F, Jitsukawa S, Baixeras E et al. LAG-3, a novel lymphocyte activation gene closely related to CD4. J. Exp. Med. 1990; 171:1393-1405.

58. Annunziato F, Manetti R, Tomasevic L, Giudizi M-G, Biagiotti R, Giannò V, Germano P, Mavilia C, Maggi, Romagnani S. Expression and release of LAG-3-associated protein by human CD4+ T cells are associated with IFN-γ. FASEB J. 1996; 10:767-776.

59. Fong TA, Mosmann TR. Alloreactive murine CD8+ T cell clones secrete the Th1 pattern of cytokines. J. Immunol. 1990; 144:1744-1752.

60. Seder RA, Boulay J-L, Finkelman F et al. CD8+ T cells can be primed in vitro to produce IL-4. J. Immunol. 1992; 148:1652-1656.

61. Erard F, Wild M-T, Garcia-Sanz JA, Le Gros G. Switch of CD8 T cells to noncytolytic CD8-CD4- cells that make Th2 cytokines and help B cells. Science 1993; 260:1802-1805.

62. Sad S, Marcotte R, Mosmann TR. Cytokine-induced differentiation of precursor mouse CD8+ T cells into cytotoxic CD8+ T cells secreting Th1 or Th2 cytokines. Immunity 1995; 2:271-279.

63. Croft M, Carter L, Swain SL, Dutton RW. Generation of polarized antigen-specific CD8 effector populations: reciprocal action of interleukin (IL)-4 and IL-12 in promoting type 2 versus type 1 cytokine profiles. J. Exp. Med. 1994; 180:1715-1728.

64. Coyle AJ, Erard F, Bertrand C, Walti S, Pircher H, Le Gros G. Virus-specific CD8+ cells can switch to interleukin 5 production and induce airway eosinophilia. J. Exp. Med. 1995; 181:1229-1233.

65. Romagnani S, Del Prete G-F, Maggi E, Parronchi P, De Carli M, Manetti R, Piccinni M-P, Almerigogna F, Giudizi M-G, Biagiotti R, Sampognaro S. Human Th1 and Th2 cells: regulation of development and role in protection and disease. In: Gergely J et al, eds. Progress In Immunology VIII. Springer Hungarica, 1993:239-246.

66. Maggi E, Giudizi M-G, Biagiotti R et al. Th2-like CD8+ cells showing B cell helper function and reduced cytolytic activity in human immunodeficiency virus type 1 infection. J. Exp. Med. 1994; 180:489-495.

67. Paganelli R, Scala E, Ansotegui IJ, Ausiello CM, Halapi E, Fanales-Belasio E, D'Offizi G, Mezzaroma I, Pandolfi F, Fiorilli M, Aiuti F. CD8+ T lymphocytes provide helper activity for IgE synthesis in human immunodeficiency virus-infected patients with hyper-IgE. J. Exp. Med. 1995; 181:423-428.

68. Wassenaar A, Reinhardus C, Abraham-Inpijin L, Kievits F. Type-1 and type-2 CD8+ T-cell subsets isolated from chronic adult periodontitis tissue differ in surface phenotype and biological functions. Immunology 1996; 87:113-118.

69. Birkhofer A, Rehbock J, Fricke H. T lymphocytes from the normal human peritoneum contain high frequencies of Th2-type CD8+ T cells. Eur. J. Immunol. 1996; 26:957-960.

70. Cronin DC, Stack R, Fitch FW. IL-4-producing CD8+ T cell clones can provide B cell help. J. Immunol. 1995; 154:3118-3127.

71. Sad S, Mosmann TR. Interleukin (IL)-4, in the absence of antigen stimulation induces an anergy-like state in differentiated CD8+ TC1 cells: loss of IL-2 synthesis and autonomous proliferation but retention of cytotoxicity and synthesis of other cytokines. J. Exp. Med. 1995; 182:1505-1515.

72. Seder RA, Le Gros G. The functional role of CD8+ T helper type 2 cells. J. Exp. Med. 1995; 181:5-7.

73. Manetti R, Annunziato F, Biagiotti R, Giudizi M-G, Piccinni M-P, Giannarini L, Sampognaro S, Parronchi P, Vinante F, Pizzolo G, Romagnani S. CD30 expression by CD8+ T cells producing type 2 helper cytokines. Evidence for large numbers of CD8+CD30+ T cell clones in human immunodeficiency virus infection. J. Exp. Med. 1994; 180:2407-2412.

74. Ferrick DA, Schrenzel MD, Mulvania T, Hsieh B, Ferlin WG, Lepper H. Differential production of interferon-γ and interleukin-4 in response to Th1- and Th2-stimulating pathogens by T cells. Nature 1995; 373:255-257.

75. Rosat JP, Conceiçao-Silva F, Waanders GA, Beermann F, Wilson A, Owen MJ, Hayday AC, Huang S, Aguet M, MacDonald HR. Expansion of gammadelta+ T cells in BALB/c mice infected with *Leishmania major* is dependent upon Th2-type CD4+ T cells. Infect. Immun. 1995; 63:3000-3004.

76. Rocken M, Muller KM, Saurat JH. Lectin-mediated induction of IL-4-producing CD4+ T cells. J. Immunol. 1991; 146:577-584.

77. Evavold BD, Williams SG, Hsu BL, Buus S, Allen PM. Complete dissection of the Hb (64-76) determinant using T helper 1 and T helper 2 clones and T cell hybridomas. J. Immunol. 1992; 148:347-53.

78. Seder R, Paul WE, Davis MM, Fazekas de St. Groth B. The presence of interleukin 4 during in vitro priming determines the lymphokine-producing potential of CD4+ T cells from T cell receptor transgenic mice. J. Exp. Med. 1992; 176:1091-1098.

79. Hsieh C-S, Heimberger AB, Gold JS, O'Garra A, Murphy KM. Differential regulation of T helper phenotype development by interleukins 4 and 10 in an alpha-beta-T-cell-receptor transgenic system. Proc. Natl. Acad. Sci. USA 1992; 89:6065-6069.

80. Swain SL. Regulation of the development of distinct subsets of CD4+ T cells. Res. Immunol. 1991; 142:14-18.

81. Kamogawa Y, Minasi LE, Carding SR, Bottomly K, Flavell RA. The relationship of IL-4- and IFN-γ-producing T cells studied by lineage ablation of IL-4-producing cells. Cell 1993; 75:985-995.

82. Renz H, Smith HR, Henson JE, Ray BS, Irvin CG, Gelfand EW. Aerosolized antigen exposure without adjuvant causes increased IgE production and air-

ways hyperresponsiveness in the mouse. J. Allergy Clin. Immunol. 1992; 89:1127-1138.

83. Xu-Amano J, Kiyono H, Jackson RJ, Staats HF, Fujiashi K, Burrows PD, Elson CO, Pillai S, McGhee JR. Helper T cell subsets for immunoglobulin A responses: oral immunization with tetanus toxoid and cholera toxin as adjuvant selectively induces Th2 cells in mucosa associated tissues. J. Exp. Med. 1993; 178:1309-1320.

84. Marinaro M, Staats HF, Hiroi T, Jackson RJ, Coste M, Boyaka PN, Okahashi N, Yamamoto M, Kiyono H, Bluethmann H, Fujihashi K, McGhee JR. Mucosal adjuvant effect of cholera toxin in mice results from induction of T helper 2 (Th2) cells and IL-4. J. Immunol. 1995; 155:4621-4629.

85. Jain SL, Barone KS, Michael JG. Activation patterns of murine T cells after oral administration of an enterocoated soluble antigen. Cell Immunol. 1996; 167:170-175.

86. Weiner HL, Maklin GA, Matsui M, Orav EJ, Khoury SJ, Dawson DM, Hafler DA. Double-blind pilot trial of oral tolerization with myelin antigens in multiple sclerosis. Science 1993; 259:1321-1324.

87. Chen Y, Inobe J-I, Kuchroo VK, Baron JL, Janeway CA, Weiner HL. Oral tolerance in myelic basic protein T-cell receptor transgenic mice: suppression of autoimmune encephalomyelitis and dose-dependent induction of regulatory cells. Proc. Natl. Acad. Sci. USA 1996; 93:388-391.

88. Wang L-F, Lin J-Y, Hsieh K-H, Lin R-H. Epicutaneous exposure of protein antigen induces a predominant Th2-like response with high IgE production. J. Immunol. 1996; 156:4079-4082.

89. Williams JR, Unanue ER. Costimulatory requirements of murine Th1 clones. The role of accessory cell-derived signals in responses to anti-CD3 antibody. J. Immunol. 1990; 145:85-93.

90. Magilavy DB, Fitch FW, Gajewski TF. Murine hepatic accessory cells support the proliferation of Th1 but not Th2 helper T lymphocyte clones. J. Exp. Med. 1989; 170:985-990.

91. Gajewski TF, Pinnas M, Wong T, Fitch FW. Murine Th1 and Th2 clones proliferate optimally in response to distinct antigen-presenting cell populations. J. Immunol. 1991; 146:1750-1758.

92. Beck L, Roth R, Spiegelberg HL. Comparison of monocytes and B cells for activation of human T helper cell subsets. Clin. Immunol. Immunopathol. 1996; 78:56-60.

93. Schmitz J, Assenmacher M, Radbruch A. Regulation of T helper cell cytokineexpression: functional dichotomy of antigen-presenting cells. Eur. J. Immunol. 1993; 23:191-199.

94. Stockinger B, Zal T, Zal A, Gray D. B cells solicit their own help from T cells. J. Exp. Med. 1996; 183:891-899.

95. Fabry Z, Sandor M, Gajewski TF, Herlein JA, Waldschmidt MM, Lynch RG, Hart MN. Differential activation of Th1 and Th2 CD4⁺ cells by murine brain microvessel endothelial cells and smooth muscle/pericytes. J. Immunol. 1993; 151:38-47.

96. Finkelman FD. Relationships among antigen presentation, cytokines, immune deviation, and auotimmune disease. J. Exp. Med. 1995; 182:279-282.

97. Hans R, Freeman GJ, Wolf ZB, Gimmi CD, Benacerraf B, Nadler LM. Murine B7 antigen provides an efficient costimulatory signal for activation of murine T lymphocytes via the T cell receptor/CD3 complex. Proc. Natl. Acad. Sci. USA 1992; 89:271-275.

98. Tan P, Anasetti C, Hansen JA, Melrose J, Brunvand M, Bradshaw J, Ledbetter JA, Linsley PS. Induction of alloantigen-specific hyporesponsiveness in hu-

man T lymphocytes by blocking interaction of CD28 via its natural ligand B7/BB1. J. Exp. Med. 1993; 177:165-173.

99. Lu P, di Zhou X, Chen S-J, Moorman M, Morris SC, Finkelman FD, Linsley P, Urban JF, Gause WC. CTLA-4 ligands are required to induce an in vivo interleukin 4 response to a gastrointestinal nematode parasite. J. Exp. Med. 1994; 180:693-698.

100. Lu P, di Zhou X, Chen S-J, Moorman M, Shoneveld A, Morris S, Finkelman FD, Claassen E, Gause WC. Requirement of CTLA-4 counter receptors for IL-4 but not IL-10 elevations during a primary systemic in vivo immune response. J. Immunol. 1995; 154:1078-1087.

101. Corry DB, Reiner SL, Linsley PS, Locksley RM. Differential effects of blockade of CD28-B7 on the development of Th1 or Th2 effector cells in experimental leishmaniasis. J. Immunol. 1994; 153:4142-4148.

102. King CL, Stupi RJ, Craighead N, June CH, Thyphronitis G. CD28 activation promotes Th2 subset differentiation by human CD4+ cells. Eur. J. Immunol. 1995; 25:587-595.

103. Webb LMC, Feldmann M. Critical role of CD28/B7 costimulation in the development of human Th2 cytokine-producing cells. Blood 1995; 86: 3479-3486.

104. Brinkmann V, Kinzel B, Kristofic C. TCR-independent activation of human CD4+45RO- T cells by anti-CD28 plus IL-2: induction of clonal expansion and priming for a Th2 phenotype. J. Immunol. 1996; 156:4100-4106.

105. Kawamura T, Furue M. Comparative analysis of B7-1 and B7-2 expression in Langerhans cells: differential regulation by T helper type 1 and T helper type 2 cytokines. Eur. J. Immunol. 1995; 25:1913-1917.

106. With-Dreese FA, Dellemijin TAM, Majoor D, de Jong D. Localization in situ of the co-stimulatory B7.1, B7.2, CD40 and their ligands in normal human lymphoid tissue. Eur. J. Immunol. 1995; 25:3023-3029.

107. Ozawa H, Aiba S, Nakagawa S, Tagami H. Interferon-γ and interleukin 10 inhibit antigen presentation by Langerhans cells for T helper type 1 cells by suppressing their CD80 (B7.1) expression. Eur. J. Immunol. 1996; 26:648-652.

108. Freeman GJ, Boussiotis VA, Anumanthan A, Bernestein GM, Ke X-Y, Rennert PD, Gray GS, Gribben JG, Nadler LM. B7-1 and B7-2 do not deliver identical costimulatory signals, since B7-2 but not B7-1 preferentially costimulates the initial production of IL-4. Immunity 1995; 2:523-532.

109. Kuchroo YK, Prabhu Das M, Brown A, Ranger AM, Zamvil SS, Sobel RA, Weiner HL, Nabavi N, Glimcher LH. B7-1 and B7-2 costimulatory molecules activate differentially the Th1/Th2 developmental pathways: application to autoimmune disease therapy. Cell 1995; 80:707-718.

110. Linsley PS, Greene JL, Brady W, Bajorath J, Ledbetter JA, Peach R. Human B7-1 (CD80) and B7-2 (CD86) bind with similar avidities but distinct kinetics to CD28 and CTLA-4 receptors. Immunity 1994; 1:793-801.

111. Lenschow DJ, Ho SC, Sattar H, Rhee L, Nabavi N, Herold KC, Bluestone JA. Differential effects of anti-B7-1 and anti-B7-2 on the development of diabetes in the nonobese diabetic mouse. J. Exp. Med. 1995; 181:1145-1155.

112. Lanier LL, O'Fallon S, Somoza C, Philips JH, Linsley PS, Okumura K, Ito D, Azuma MJ. CD80 (B7) and CD86 (B70) provide similar costimulatory signals for T cell proliferation, cytokine production, and generation of CTL. Immunol. 1995; 154:97-105.

113. Natesan M, Razi-Wolf Z, Reiser H. Costimulation of IL-4 production by murine B7-1 and B7-2 molecules. J. Immunol. 1996; 156; 2783-2791.

114. Faith A, O'Heir RE, Malkovsky M, Lamb JR. Analysis of the basis of resistance and susceptibility of CD4+ T cells to HIV-gp120 induced anergy. Immunology 1992; 76:1-8.

115. Brostoff SW, Mason DW. Experimental allergic encephalomyelitis: a successful treatment in vivo with a monoclonal antibody that recognizes T helper cells. J. Immunol. 1984; 133:1938-1942.

116. Stumbles P, Mason D. Activation of CD4+ T cells in the presence of a nondepleting monoclonal antibody to CD4 induces a Th2-type response in vitro. J. Exp. Med. 1995; 182:5-13.

117. Lamb JR, Faith A, Higgins JA, Verhoef A, Schneider P, Yssel H, O'Heir RE. Clonal analysis of CD4 mediated accessory function on the effector activity of human CD4+ T cell subsets. Clin. Exper. Allergy 1995; 25:839-847.

118. Stuber E, Strober W, Neurath M. Blocking the CD40L-CD40 interaction in vivo specifically prevents the priming of T helper 1 cells through the inhibition of interleukin 12 secretion. J. Exp. Med. 1996; 183:693-698.

119. Kennedy MK, Picha KS, Fanslow WC, Grabstein KH, Alderson MR, Clifford KN, Chin WA, Mohler KM. CD40/CD40 ligand interactions are required for T cell-dependent production of interleukin 12 by mouse macrophages. Eur. J. Immunol. 1996; 26:370-378.

120. Blotta MH, Marshall JD, DeKruyff RH, Umetsu DT. Cross-linking of the CD40 ligand on human CD4+ T lymphocytes generates a costimulatory signal that up-regulates IL-4 synthesis. J. Immunol. 1996; 156:3133-3140.

121. Maggi E, Parronchi P, Manetti R, Simonelli C, Piccinni M-P, Santoni-Rugiu F, De Carli M, Ricci M, Romagnani S. Reciprocal regulatory role of IFN-γ and IL-4 on the in vitro development of human Th1 and Th2 cells. J. Immunol. 1992; 148:2142-2147.

122. Dransfield I, Buckle A-M, Hogg N. Early events of the immune response mediated by leukocyte integrins. Immunol. Rev. 1990; 114:29-44.

123. De Fougerolles AR, Stacker SA, Schwarting R, Springer TA. Characterization of ICAM-2 and evidence for a third counter receptor for LFA-1. J. Exp. Med. 1991; 174:253-255.

124. Faith A, Higgins JA, O'Heir R, Lamb JR. Differential dependence of Th0, Th1 and Th2 CD4+ T cells on co-stimulatory activity provided by the accessory molecule LFA-1. Clin. Exper. Allergy 1995; 25:1163-1170.

125. Heufler C, Koch F, Stanzl U, Topar G, Wysocka M, Trinchieri G, Enk A, Steinman RM, Romani N, Schuler G. Interleukin-12 is produced by dendritic cells and mediates Th1 development as well as IFN-γ production by Th1 cells. Eur. J. Immunol. 1996; 26:659-668.

126. Kang K, Kubin M, Cooper KD, Lessin SR, Trinnchieri G, Rook AH. IL-12 synthesis by human Langerhans cells. J. Immunol. 1996; 156:1402-1407.

127. HayGlass KT, Stefura W. Antigen-specific modulation of murine IgE and IgG2a responses with glutaraldehyde-polymerized allergen is independent of MHC haplotype and IgH allotype. Immunology 1991; 73:24-30.

128. Gieni RS, Yang X, HayGlass KT. Allergen-specific modulation of cytokine synthesis patterns and IgE responses in vivo with chemically modified allergen. J. Immunol. 1993; 150:302-310.

129. Gieni RS, Yang X, HayGlass KT. Limiting dilution analysis of CD4 T-cell cytokine production in mice administered native versus polymerized ovalbumin: directed induction of T-helper type 1-like activation. Immunology 1996; 87:119-126.

130. Janeway C, Carding S, Jones B et al. CD4+ T cells: specificity and function. Immunol. Rev. 1988; 101:39-80.

131. Forsthuber T, Yip HC, Lehmann PV. Induction of Th1 and Th2 immunity in neonatal mice. Science 1996; 271:1728-1730.

132. Villacres-Eriksson M. Antigen presentation by naive macrophages, dendritic cells and B cells to primed T lymphocytes and their cytokine production

following exposure to immunostimulating complexes. Clin. Exp. Immunol. 1995; 102:46-52.

133. Apostolopoulos V, Pietersz GA, Loveland BE, Sandrin MS, McKenzie IFC. Oxidative/reductive conjugation of mannan to antigen selects for T1 or T2 immune responses. Proc. Natl. Acad. Sci. 1995; 92:10128-10132.

134. Bretscher PA, Wei G, Menon JN, Bielefeldt OH. Establishment of stable, cell-mediated immunity that makes "susceptible" mice resistant to *Leishmania major*. Science 1992; 257:539-542.

135. Constant S, Pfeiffer C, Pasqualini T, Bottomly K. Extent of T cell receptor ligation can determine the functional differentiation of naive CD4⁺ T cells. J. Exp. Med. 1995; 182:1591-1596.

136. Hosken NA, Shibuya K, Heath AW, Murphy KM, O'Garra A. The effect of antigen dose on CD4⁺ T helper cell phenotype development in a T cell receptor-αβ-transgenic model. J. Exp. Med. 1995; 182:1579-1584.

137. Reiner SL, Wang Z-E, Hatam F, Scott P, Locksley RM. Th1 and Th2 cell antigen receptors in experimental leishmaniasis. Science 1993; 259:1457-1460.

138. Liew FY, Millott SM, Schmidt JA. A repetitive peptide of Leishmania can activate T helper type 2 cells and enhance disease progression. J. Exp. Med. 1990; 172:1359-1365.

139. Skeiky JAW, Gauderian JA, Benson DR et al. A recombinant Leishmania antigen that stimulates human peripheral blood mononuclear cells to express a Th1-type cytokine profile and to produce interleukin 12. J. Exp. Med. 1995; 181:1527-1537.

140. Soloway P, Fish S, Passmore H et al. Regulation of the immune response to peptide antigens: differential induction of immediate-type hypersensitivity and T cell proliferation due to changes in either peptide structure or major histocompatibility complex haplotype. J. Exp. Med. 1991; 174:847-858.

141. Racioppi L. Ronchese F, Matis LA, Germain RN. Peptide-major histocompatibility complex class II complexes with mixed agonist/antagonist properties provide evidence for ligand-related differences in T cell receptor-dependent intracellular signaling. J. Exp. Med. 1993; 177:1047-1060.

142. Pfeiffer C, Murray J, Madri J, Bottomly K. Selective activation of Th1 and Th2 like cells in vivo. response to human collagen IV. Immunol. Rev. 1991; 123:65-84.

143. Pfeiffer C, Stein J, Southwood S et al. Altered peptide ligands can control CD4 T lymphocyte differentiation in vivo. J. Exp. Med. 1995; 181:1569-1574.

144. Kumar V, Bhardwaj V, Soares L et al. Major histocompatibility complex binding affinity of an antigenic determinant is crucial for the differential secretion of interleukin 4/5 or interferon by T cells. Proc. Natl. Acad. Sci. USA 1995; 92:9510-9514.

145. Murray JS, Kasselman JP, Schountz T. High-density presentation of an immunodominant minimal peptide on B cells is MHC-linked to Th1-like immunity. Cell. Immunol. 1995; 166:9-15.

146. Chehimi J, Trinchieri G. Interleukin-12: a bridge between innate resistance and adaptive immunity with a role in infection and acquired immunodeficiency. J. Clin. Immunol. 1995; 14:149-161.

147. Hsieh C-S, Macatonia SE, Tripp CS et al. Development of TH1 CD4⁺ T cells through IL-12 produced by *Leisteria*-induced macrophages. Science 1993; 260:547-49.

148. Macatonia SE, Hosken NA, Litton M et al. Dendritic cells produce IL-12 and direct the development of Th1 cells from naive CD4⁺ T cells. J. Immunol. 1995; 154:5071-5079.

149. Goodman RE, Nestle F, Naidu YM, Green JM, Thompson CB, Nickoloff BJ, Turka LA. Keratinocyte-derived T cell costimulation induces preferential production of IL-2 and IL-4 but not IFN-γ. J. Immunol. 1994; 152:5189-5198.

150. Seder RA, Gazzinelli R, Sher A, Paul WE. Interleukin 12 acts directly on CD4⁺ T cells to enhance priming for interferon γ production and diminishes interleukin 4 inhibition of such priming. Proc. Natl. Acad. Sci. USA 1993; 90:10188-10192.

151. Schmitt E, Hoehn P, Germann T, Ruede E. T helper type 1 development of naive CD4⁺ T cells requires the coordinate action of interleukin-12 and interferon-γ and is inhibited by transforming growth factor β. Eur. J. Immunol. 1994; 24:793-798.

152. Magram J, Connaughton SE, Warrier RR, Carvajal DM, Wu C-Y, Ferrante J, Stewart C, Sarmiento U, Faherty DA, Gately MK. IL-12-deficient mice are defective in IFN-γ production and type 1 cytokine responses. J. Immunol. 1996; 4:471-481.

153. Manetti R, Parronchi P, Giudizi M-G, Piccinni M-P, Maggi E, Trinchieri G, Romagnani S. Natural killer cell stimulatory factor (interleukin-12) induces T helper type 1 (Th1)-specific immune responses and inhibits the development of IL-4-producing Th cells. J. Exp. Med. 1993; 177:1199-1204.

154. Manetti R, Gerosa F, Giudizi M-G et al. Interleukin 12 induces stable priming for interferon γ (IFN-γ) production during differentiation of human T helper (Th) cells and transient IFN-γ production in established Th2 cell clones. J. Exp. Med. 1994; 179:1273-1283.

155. Hilkens CMU, Snijders A, Vermeulen H, van der Meide P, Wierenga EA, Kapsenberg ML. Accessory cell-derived IL-12 and prostaglandin E₂ determine the IFN-γ levels of activated human CD4⁺ T cells. J. Immunol. 1996; 156:1722-1727.

156. Mocci S, Coffman RL. Induction of a Th2 population from a polarized *Leishmania*-specific Th1 population by in vitro culture with IL-4. J. Immunol. 1995; 154:3779-3787.

157. Bradley LM, Yoshimoto K, Swain SL. The cytokines IL-4, IFN-γ, and IL-12 regulate the development of subsets of memory effector helper T cells in vitro. J. Immunol. 1995; 155:1713-1724.

158. DeKruyff RH, Fang Y, Wolf SF. Umetsu DT. IL-12 inhibits IL-4 synthesis in keyhole limpet hemocyanin-primed CD4⁺ T cells through an effect on antigen-presenting cells. J. Immunol. 1995; 154:2578-2587.

159. Morris SC, Madden KB, Adamovicz JJ, Gause WC, Hubbard BR, Gately MK, Finkelman FD. Effects of IL-12 on in vivo cytokine gene expression and Ig isotype selection. J. Immunol. 1994; 152:1047-1056.

160. Chehimi J, Paganin C, Frank I, Chouaib S, Starr S, Trinchieri G. Interleukin 12 in the pathogenesis and the therapy of HIV infection. Res. Immunol. 1995; 146:605-614.

161. Mingari M-C, Maggi E, Cambiaggi A, Annunziato F, Schiavetti F, Manetti R, Moretta L, Romagnani S. In vitro development of human CD4⁺ thymocytes into functionally mature Th2 cells. Exogenous IL-12 is required for priming thymocytes to the production of both Th1 cytokines and IL-10. Eur. J. Immunol. 1996; 26:1083-1087.

162. O'Garra A, Murphy KM. Role of cytokines in determining T-lymphocyte function. Curr. Opin. Immunol. 1994; 6:458-466.

163. Macatonia SE, Hsieh C-S, Murphy KM, O'Garra A. Dendritic cells and macrophages are required for Th1 development of CD4⁺ T cells from αβ TCR transgenic mice: IL-12 substitution for macrophage to stimulate IFN-γ production is IFN-γ dependent. Intern. Immunol. 1993; 5:1119-1128.

164. Flesch IEA, Hess JH, Huang S, Aguet M, Rothe J, Bluethmann H, Kaufmann SHE. Early interleukin 12 production by macrophages in response to myco-bacterial infection depends on interferon γ and tumor necrosis factor α. J. Exp. Med. 1995; 181:1615-1621.

165. Wang Z-E, Zheng S, Corry DB, Dalton DK, Seder RA, Reiner SL. Locksley RM. Interferon γ-independent effects of interleukin 12 administered during acute or established infection due to *Leishmania major.* Proc. Natl. Acad. Sci. USA 1994; 91:12932-12936.

166. Dighe AS, Campbell D, Hsieh C-S, Clarke S, Greaves DR, Gordon S, Murphy KM, Schreiber RD. Tissue-specific targeting of cytokine unresponsiveness in transgenic mice. Immunity 1995; 3:657-666.

167. McKnight AJ, Zimmer GJ, Folgelman I, Wolf SF, Abbas AK. Effects of IL-12 on helper T cell-dependent immune responses in vivo. J. Immunol. 1994; 152:2172-2179.

168. Via CS, Rus V, Gately MK, Finkelman FD. IL-12 stimulates the develop-ment of acute graft-versus-host disease in mice that normally would develop chronic, autoimmune graft-versus-host-disease. J. Immunol. 1994; 153:4040-4047.

169. Schijns VECJ, Haagmans BL, Rijke EO, Huang S, Aguet M, Horzinek MC. IFN-γ receptor-deficient mice generate antiviral Th1-characteristic cytokine profiles but altered antibody responses. J. Immunol. 1994; 153:2029-2037.

170. Swihart K, Fruth U, Messmer N, Hug K, Behin R, Huang S, Del Giudice G, Aguet M, Louis JA. Mice from a genetically resistant background lacking the interferon γ receptor are susceptible to infection with Leishmania major but mount a polarized T helper cell 1-type CD4⁺ T cell response. J. Exp. Med. 1995; 181:961-971.

171. Wenner C, Guler ML, Macatonia SE, O'Garra A, Murphy KM. Roles of IFN-γ and IFN-α in IL-12-induced Th1 development. J. Immunol. 1996; 156:1442-1447.

172. Swain SL, Huston G, Tonkonogy S, Weinberg AD. Transforming growth factor beta and IL-4 cause helper T cell precursors to develop into distinct effector help cells that differ in lymphokine secretion pattern and cell surface phenotype. J. Immunol. 1991; 147:2991-3000.

173. Nagelkerken L, Gollob KJ, Tielemans M, Coffman RL. Role of transforming growth factor-β in the preferential induction of T helper cells of type 1 by staphylococcal enterotoxin B. Eur. J. Immunol. 1993; 23:2306-2310.

174. Sad S, Mosmann TR. A single IL-2-secreting precursor CD4 T cell can de-velop into either a Th1 or Th2 secreting phenotype. J. Immunol. 1994; 153:3514-3522.

175. Santambrogio L, Hochwald GM, Saxena B et al. Studies on the mechanisms by which transforming growth factor-β (TGF-β) protects against allergic encephalomyelitis. J. Immunol. 1993; 151:1116-1127.

176. Hoehn P, Goedert S, Germann T, Koelsch S, Jin S, Palm N, Ruede E, Schmitt E. Opposing effects of TGF-β2 on the Th1 cell development of naive CD4⁺ T cells isolated from different mouse strains. J. Immunol. 1995; 155:3788-3793.

177. Parronchi P, De Carli M, Manetti R, Simonelli C, Sampognaro S, Piccinni M-P, Macchia D, Maggi E, Del Prete G-F, Romagnani S. Il-4 and IFN(s) (Alpha and Gamma) exert opposite regulatory effects on the development of cytolytic potential by Th1 or Th2 human T cell clones. J. Immunol. 1992; 149:2977-2982.

178. Romagnani S. Induction of T$_H$1 and T$_H$2 response: a key role for the 'natu-ral' immune response? Immunol. Today 1992; 13:379-81.

179. Parronchi P, Mohapatra S, Sampognaro S, Giannarini L, Wahn U, Chong P, Mohapatra SS, Maggi E, Renz H, Romagnani S. Modulation by IFN-α of cytokine profile, T cell receptor repertoire and peptide reactivity of human allergen-specific T cells. Eur. J. Immunol. 1996; 26:697-703.

180. Manetti R, Annunziato F, Tomasevic L, Giannò V, Parronchi P, Romagnani S, Maggi E. Polyinosinic acid: polycytidylic acid promotes T helper type1-specific immune responses by stimulating macrophage production of IFN-α and interleukin-12. Eur. J. Immunol. 1995; 25:2656-2660.

181. Okamura H, Tsutsui H, Komatsu T et al. Cloning of a new cytokine that induces IFN-γ production by T cells. Nature 1995; 378:88-91.

182. Swain SL, Weinberg AD, English M, Huston G. IL-4 directs the development of Th2-like helper effectors. J. Immunol. 1990; 145:3796-3806.

183. Swain SL. IL-4 Dictates T-Cell Differentiation. Res. Immunol. 1993; 144:616-620.

184. Le Gros G, Ben Sasson SZ, Seder R, Finkelman FD, Paul WE. Generation of interleukin-4 (IL-4) producing cells. J. Exp. Med. 1990; 172:921-929.

185. Seder RA, Paul WE, Davis MM, Fazekas de St. Groth B. The presence of interleukin-4 during in vivo priming determines the lymphokine-producing potential of CD4+ T cells from T cell receptor transgenic mice. J. Exp. Med. 1992; 176:1091-1098.

186. Sadick MD, Heinzel FP, Holoday BJ, Pu RT, Dawkins RS, Locksley RM. Cure of murine leishmaniasis with anti-interleukin 4 monoclonal antibody: evidence for a T-cell-dependent, interferon gamma-independent mechanism. J. Exp. Med. 1990; 171:115-127.

187. Coffman RL, Chatelain R, Leal LM, Varkila K. *Leishmania major* infection in mice: a model system for the study of CD4+ T-cell subset differentiation. Res. Immunol. 1991; 142:36-40.

188. Gross A, Ben Sasson SZ, Paul WE. Anti-IL-4 diminishes in vivo priming for antigen-specific IL-4 production by T cells. J. Immunol. 1993; 150:2112-2120.

189. Kopf M, Le Gros G, Bachmann M, Lamers MC, Bluthmann H, Kohler G. Disruption of the murine IL-4 gene blocks Th2 cytokine responses. Nature 1993; 362:245-248.

190. Fargeas C, Wu C-Y, Nakajima T, Cox D, Nutman T, Delespesse G. Differential effect of transforming growth factor β on the synthesis of Th1- and Th2-like lymphokine by human T lymphocytes. Eur. J. Immunol. 1992; 22:2173-2176.

191. Plaut M, Pierce JH, Watson CJ, Hanley HJ, Nordan RP, Paul WE. Mast cell lines produce lymphokines in response to cross-linkage of FcεRI or to calcium ionophores. Nature 1989; 339:64-67.

192. Ben Sasson SZ, Le Gros G, Conrad DH, Finkelman FD, Paul WE. Cross linking Fc receptors stimulates splenic non-B, non-T cells to secrete interleukin 4 and other lymphokines. Proc. Natl. Acad. Sci. USA 1990; 87:1421-1425.

193. Piccinni M-P, Macchia D, Parronchi P, Giudizi M-G, Bani D, Aterini R, Grossi A, Ricci M, Maggi E, Romagnani S. Human bone marrow non-B, non-T cells produce interleukin-4 in response to cross-linkage of Fcε and Fcγ receptors. Proc. Natl. Acad. Sci. USA 1991; 88:8656-8660.

194. Conrad DH, Ben-Sasson S, Le Gros GG, Finkelman FD, Paul WE. Infection with *Nippostrongylus brasiliensis* or injection of anti-IgD antibodies markedly enhances Fc-receptor-mediated interleukin 4 production by non-B, non-T cells. J. Exp. Med. 1990; 171:1497-1508.

195. Aoki I, Kinzer C, Shirai A, Paul WE, Klinman DM. IgE receptor-positive non-B/non-T cells dominate the production of interleukin 4 and interleukin 6 in immunized mice. Proc. Natl. Acad. Sci. USA 1995; 92:2534-2538.

196. Bradding P, Feather IH, Howarth PH et al. Interleukin 4 is localized and released by human mast cells. J. Exp. Med. 1992; 176:1381-1386.

197. Brunner T, Heusser CH, Dahinden CA. Human peripheral blood basophils primed by interleukin 3 (IL-3) produce IL-4 in response to immunoglobulin E receptor stimulation. J. Exp. Med. 1993; 177:605-611.

198. MacGlashan D, White JM, Huang S-K, Ono SJ, Schroeder JT, Lichtenstein LM. Secretion of IL-4 from human basophils. The relationship between IL-4 mRNA and protein in resting and stimulated basophils. J. Immunol. 1994; 152:3006-3016.

199. Okayama Y, Petté Frère C, Kassel O, Semper A, Quint D, Tunon-de-Lara MJ, Bradding P, Holgate ST, Church, MK. IgE-dependent expression of mRNA for IL-4 and IL-5 in human lung mast cells. J. Immunol. 1995; 155:1796-1808.

200. Moqbel R, Ying S, Barkans J, Newman TM, Kimmitt P, Vakelin M, Taborda-Barata L, Meng Q, Corrigan CJ, Durham SR, Kay AB. Identification of mRNA for interleukin-4 in human eosinophils with granule localization and release of the translated product. J. Immunol. 1995; 155:4939-4947.

201. Nonaka M, Nonaka R, Woolley K, Adelroth E, Miura K, Okhawara Y, Glibetic M, Nakano K, O'Byrne P, Dolovich J, Jordana M. Distinct immunohistochemical localization of IL-4 in human inflamed airway tissues. J. Immunol. 1995; 155:3234-3244.

202. Nakajima H, Gleich GJ, Kita H. Constitutive production of IL-4 and IL-10 and stimulated production of IL-8 by normal peripheral blood eosinophils. J. Immunol. 1996; 156:4859-4866.

203. Huels C, Germann T, Goedert S, Hoehn P, Koelsh S, Hultner L, Palm N, Rude E, Schmitt E. Co-activation of naive CD4+ T cells and bone marrow-derived mast cells results in the development of Th2 cells. Int. Immunol. 1995; 7:525-532.

204. Wershil BK, Theodos CM, Galli SJ, Titus RG. Mast cells augment lesion size and persistence during experimental *Leishmania Major* infection in the mouse. J. Immunol. 1994; 152:4563-4571.

205. Schmitz J, Thiel A, Kuhn R, Rajewsky K, Muller W, Assenmacher M, Radbruch A. Induction of interleukin 4 (IL-4) expression In T helper (Th) cells is not dependent on IL-4 from non-T cells. J. Exp. Med. 1994; 179:1349-1353.

206. Finkelman FD, Urban JF. Cytokines: making the right choice. Parasitol. Today 1992; 8:311-314.

207. Oliveira DB, Gillespie K, Wolfreys K, Mathieson PW, Qasim F, Coleman JW. Compounds that induce autoimmunity in the Brown Norway rat sensitize mast cells for mediator release and interleukin-4 expression. Eur. J. Immunol. 1995; 25:2259-2264.

208. Dudler T, Cantarelli Machado D, Kolbe L, Annand RR, Rhodes N, Gelb MH, Koelsch E, Suter M, Helm BA. A link between catalytic activity, IgE-independent mast cell activation, and allergenicity of bee venom phospholipase A_2. J. Immunol. 1995; 155:2605-2613.

209. Ochensberger B, Rihs S, Brunner T, Dahinden CA. IgE-independent interleukin-4 expression and induction of a late phase of leukotriene C4 formation in human blood basophils. Blood 1995; 86:4039-4049.

210. Falcone FH, Dahinden CA, Noll T, Amon U, Hebestreit H, Abrahamsen O, Klaucke J, Schlaak M, Haas H. Human basophils release interleukin-4 after stimulation with *Schistosoma mansoni* egg antigen. Eur. J. Immunol. 1996; 26:1147-1155.

211. Bradley LM, Duncan DD, Tonkonogy S, Swain SL. Characterization of antigen-specific CD4⁺ effector T cells in vivo: immunization results in a transient population of MEL14-, CD45RB- helper cells that secrete interleukin-2 (IL-2), IL-3, IL-4, and interferon-γ. J. Exp. Med. 1991; 174:547-559.

212. Gollob K, Coffman RL. A minority subpopulation of CD4⁺ T cells directs the development of naive CD4⁺ T cells into IL-4-secreting cells. J. Immunol. 1994; 152:5180-5188.

213. Bendelac A, Killeen N, Littman DR, Schwartz RH. A subset of CD4⁺ thymocytes selected by MHC class I molecules. Science 1994; 263:1774-1778.

214. Bendelac A. Mouse NK1⁺ T cells. Curr. Opin. Immunol. 1995; 7:367-374.

215. Arase H, Arase N, Nakagawa K, Good RA, Onoe K. NK1.1⁺ CD4⁺ CD8- thymocytes with specific lymphokine secretion. Eur. J. Immunol. 1993; 23:307-310.

216. Yashimoto T, Paul WE. CD4ᵖᵒˢ, NK1.1ᵖᵒˢ T cells promptly produce interleukin 4 in response to in vivo challenge with anti-CD3. J. Exp. Med. 1994; 179:1285-1295.

217. Bendelac A, Schwartz RH. CD4⁺ and CD8⁺ T cells acquire specific lymphokine secretion potential during thymic maturation. Nature 1991; 365:68-71.

218. Bendelac A, Matzinger P, Seder RA, Paul WE, Schwartz RH. Activation events during thymic selection. J. Exp. Med. 1992; 175:731-742.

219. Yashimoto T, Bendelac A, Watson C, Hu-Li J, Paul WE. CD-1-specific, NK1.1ᵖᵒˢ T cells play a key in vivo role in a Th2 response and in IgE production. Science 1995; 270:1845-1847.

220. Yoshimoto T, Bendelac A, Hu-Li J, Paul WE. Defective IgE production by SJL mice is linked to the absence of a subset of T cells that promptly produce IL-4. Proc. Natl. Acad. Sci. USA 1995; 92:11931-11934.

221. Emoto M, Emoto Y, Kaufmann SHE. Interleukin-4-producing CD4⁺ NK1.1⁺ TCRαβⁱⁿᵗᵉʳᵐᵉᵈⁱᵃᵗᵉ liver lymphocytes are downregulated by *Leisteria monocytogenes*. Eur. J. Immunol. 1995; 25:3321-3325.

222. Launois P, Ohteki T, Swihart K, Robson MacDonald H, Louis JA. In susceptible mice, *Leishmania major* induce very rapid interleukin-4 production by CD4⁺ T cells which are NK1.1⁻. Eur. J. Immunol. 1995; 25:3298-3307.

223. Sieling PA, Chatterjee D, Porcelli SA et al. CD1-restricted T cell recognition of microbial lipoglycan antigens. Science 1995; 269:227-230.

224. Zlotnik A, Bean AGD. Production of IL-4 by non-Th2 T-cell subsets: possible role of CD4-CD8-αβTCR⁺ and CD4 subset T cells in T helper subset regulation. 1993; 144:606-609.

225. do Carmo Leite-de-Moraes M, Herbelin A, Machavoine F, Vicari A, Gombert J-M, Papiernik M, Dy M. MHC class I-selected CD4-CD8-TCR-αβ⁺ T cells are a potential source of IL-4 during primary immune response. J. Immunol. 1995; 155:4544-4550.

226. Croft M, Swain SL. Recently activated naive CD4 T cells can help resting B cells, and can produce sufficient autocrine IL-4 to drive differentiation to secretion of T helper 2-type cytokines. J. Immunol. 1995; 154:4269-4282.

227. Kalinski P, Hilkens CMU, Wierenga EA et al. Functional maturation of human naive T helper cells in the absence of accessory cells. Generation of IL-4-producing T helper cells does not require exogenous IL-4. J. Immunol. 1995; 154:3753-3760.

228. Demeure CE, Yang LP, Byun DG, Ishihara H, Vezzio N, Delespesse G. Human naive CD4 T cells produce interleukin-4 at priming and acquire a Th2 phenotype upon repetitive stimulations in neutral conditions. Eur. J. Immunol. 1995; 25:2722-2725.

229. Yang L-P, Demeure D-G, Vezzio CE, Delespesse G. Default development of cloned human naive CD4 T cells into interleukin-4- and interleukin-5-producing effector cells. Eur. J. Immunol. 1995; 12:3517-3520.

230. D'Andrea A, Aste-Amezaga M, Valiante NM, Ma X, Kubin M, Trinchieri G. Interleukin 10 (IL-10) inhibits human lymphocyte interferon γ production by suppressing natural killer cell stimulatory factor IL-12 synthesis in accessory cells. J. Exp. Med. 1993; 178:1041-1048.

231. Chang T-L, Shea CM, Urioste S, Thompson RC, Boom WH, Abbas AK. Heterogeneity of helper/inducer T lymphocytes. III. Responses of IL-2 and IL-4 producing (Th1 and Th2) clones to antigens presented by different accessory cells. J. Immunol. 1990; 145:280-2808.

232. Williams IR, Unanue ER. Characterization of accessory cell costimulation of Th1 cytokine synthesis. J. Immunol. 1991; 147:3752-3760.

233. Zubiaga AM, Munoz E, Huber BT. Production of IL-1α by activated Th type 2 cells. J. Immunol. 1991; 146:3849-3856.

234. Schmitz J, Radbruch A. Distinct antigen presenting cell-derived signals induce Th cell proliferation and expression of effector cytokines. Int. Immunol. 1992; 4:43-51.

235. Manetti R, Barak V, Piccinni M-P, Sampognaro S, Parronchi P, Maggi E, Dinarello CA, Romagnani S. Interleukin-1 favours the in vitro development of type 2 T helper (Th2) human T-cell clones. Res. Immunol. 1994; 145:93-100.

236. Daynes RA, Araneo BA. Contrasting effects of glucocorticoids on the capacity of T cells to produce the growth factor interleukin 2 and interleukin 4. Eur. J. Immunol. 1989; 19:2319-2325.

237. Ramrez F, Fowell DJ, Puklavec M, Simmonds S, Mason D. Gluocorticoids promote a Th2 cytokine response by CD4⁺ T cells in vitro. J. Immunol. 1996; 156:2406-2412.

238. Snijdewint FG, Kapsenberg ML, Wauben-Penris PJ, Bos JD. Corticosteroids class-dependently inhibit in vitro Th1- and Th2-type cytokine production. Immunopharmacology 1995; 29:93-101.

239. Brinkmann V, Kristofic C. Regulation by corticosteroids of Th1 and Th2 cytokine production in human CD4⁺ effector T cells generated from CD45RO- and CD45RO⁺ subsets. J. Immunol. 1995; 155:3322-3328.

240. Daynes RA, Dudley DJ, Araneo BA. Regulation of murine lymphokine production in vivo - II. Dehydrepiandrosterone is a natural enhancer of interleukin 2 synthesis by helper T cells. J. Immunol. 1990; 20:793-802.

241. Araneo BA, Dowell T, Terui T, Diegel M, Daynes RA. Dihydrotestosterone exerts a depressive influence on the production of IL-4, IL-5 and IFN-γ, but not IL-2 by activated murine cells. Blood 1991; 78:688-699.

242. Araneo BA, Woods ML, Daynes RA. J. Reversal of the immunosenescent phenotype by dehydroepiandrosterone: hormone treatment provides an adjuvant effect on the immunization of aged mice with recombinant hepatitis B surface antigen. Infect. Dis. 1993; 167:830-840.

243. Daynes RA, Araneo BA, Ershler WB, Maloney C, Li GZ, Ryu SY. Altered regulation of IL-6 production with normal aging. Possible linkage to the age-associated decline in dehydroepiandrosterone and its sulfated derivative. J. Immunol. 1993; 150:5219-5230.

244. Daynes RA, Araneo BA, Dowell TA, Huang K, Dudley D. Regulation of murine lymphokine production in vivo. III. The lymphoid tissue microenvironment exerts regulatory influences over T helper cell function. J. Exp. Med. 1990; 171:979-996.

245. Daynes RA, Meikle AW, Araneo BA. Locally active steroid hormones may facilitate compartmentalization of immunity by regulating the types of lymphokines produced by helper T cells. Res. Immunol. 1991; 142:40-44.

246. Rook GAW, Hernandez-Pando R, Lightman SL. Hormones, peripherally activated prohormones and regulation of the Th1/Th2 balance. Immunol. Today 1994; 15:301-303.

247. Rook GAW. The role of vitamin D in tuberculosis. Am. Rev. Resp. Dis. 1988; 138:768-770.

248. Lemire JM, Archer DC, Beck L, Spiegelberg HL. Immunosuppressive actions of 1,25-dihydroxyvitamin D3: preferential inhibition of Th1 functions. J. Nutr. 1995; 125: (6 suppl.)1704-1708.

249. Seymour JF, Gagel RF. Calcitriol: the major humoral mediator of hypercalcemia in Hodgkin's disease and non-Hodgkin's lymphomas. Blood 1993; 82:1383-1394.

250. Rigby WF, Denome S, Fanger MW. Regulation of lymphokine production and human T lymphocyte activation by 1,25-dihydroxyvitamin D3: specific inhibition at the level of messenger RNA. J. Clin. Invest. 1987; 79:1659-1664.

251. Piccinni M-P, Giudizi M-G, Biagiotti R et al. Progesterone favors the development of human T helper (Th) cells producing Th2-type cytokines and promotes both IL-4 production and membrane CD30 expression in established Th1 clones. J. Immunol. 1995; 155:128-133.

252. Wegmann TG, Lin H, Guilbert L, Mosmann TR. Bidirectional cytokine interactions in the maternal-fetal relationship: is successful pregnancy a Th2 phenomenon? Immunol. Today 1993; 14:353-356.

253. Piccinni M-P, Romagnani S. Regulation of fetal allograft survival by hormone-controlled Th1 and Th2-type cytokines. Immunol. Res. 1996; (in press)

254. Renz H, Bradley C, Saloga J, Loader J, Larsen G, Gelfand EW. T cells expressing specific Vβ elements regulate immunoglobulin E production and airways responsiveness in vivo. J. Exp. Med. 1993; 177:1175-11180.

255. Mohapatra SS, Mohapatra S, Yang M, Anari AA, Parronchi P, Maggi E, Romagnani S. Molecular basis of cross-reactivity among allergen-specific human T cells: T-cell receptor Vα gene usage and epitope structure. Immunology 1994; 81:15-20.

256. Snijdewint FGM, Kalinski P, Wierenga EA, Bos JD, Kapsenberg ML. Prostaglandin E_2 differentially modulates cytokine secretion profiles of human T helper lymphocytes. J. Immunol. 1993; 150:5321-5329.

257. Katamura K, Shintaku N, Yamauchi Y, Fukui T, Ohshima Y, Mayumi M, Furusho K. Prostaglandin E_2 at priming of naive CD4[+] T cells inhibits acquisition of ability to produce IFN-γ and IL-2, but not IL-4 and IL-5. J. Immunol. 1995; 155:4604-4612.

258. Taylor-Robinson AW, Liew FY, Severn A, Xu D, McSorley SJ, Garside P, Padron J, Phillips RS. Regulation of the immune response by nitric oxide differentially produced by T helper type 1 and T helper type 2 cells. Eur. J. Immunol. 1994; 24:980-984.

259. Liew FY. Regulation of lymphocyte function by nitric oxide. Curr. Opin. Immunol. 1995; 7:396-399.

260. Bauer H, Jung T, Tsikas D, Stichtenoth DO, Frolich J, Neumann C. Nitric oxide inhibits the secretion of T-helper 1 and T-helper 2 cytokines in activated human T-cells. Eur. J. Immunol. 1996.

261. Brown EL, Rivas JM, Ulrich SE, Young CR, Norris SJ, Kripke ML. Modulation of immunity to Borrelia burgdorferi by ultraviolet irradiation: different effects on Th1 and Th2 immune responses. Eur. J. Immunol. 1995; 25:3017-3022.

262. Yagi H, Tokura Y, Wakita H, Furukawa F, Takigawa M. TCRVbeta7[+] Th2 cells mediate UVB-induced suppression of murine contact photosensitivity by releasing IL-10. J. Immunol. 1996; 156:1824-1831.

263. Enk CD, Sredni D, Blauvelt A, Katz SI. Induction of IL-10 gene expression in human keratinocytes by UVB exposure in vivo and in vitro. J. Immunol. 1995; 154:4851-4856.

264. Schmitt DA, Owen-Schaub L, Ullrich SE. Effect of IL-12 on immune suppression and suppressor cell induction by ultraviolet radiation. J. Immunol. 1995; 154:5114-5120.

265. Prigent P, Saoudi A, Pannetier C, Graber G, Bonnefoy J-Y, Druet P. Mercuric chloride, a chemical responsible for T helper cell (Th2)-mediated autoimmunity in Brown Norways rats, directly triggers T cells to produce interleukin-4. J. Clin. Invest. 1995; 96:1484-1489.

266. Saoudi A, Castedo M, Nochy D, Mandet C, Pasquier R, Druet P, Pelletier L. Self-reactive anti-class II T helper type 2 cell lines derived from gold salt-injected rats trigger B cell polyclonal activation and transfer auotimmunity in CD8-depleted normal syngeneic recipients. Eur. J. Immunol. 1995; 25:1972-1979.

267. McHugh SM, Rifkin IR, Deighton J, Wilson AB, Lachmann PJ, Lockwood CM, Ewan PW. The immunosuppressive drug thalidomide induces T helper cell type 2 (Th2) and concomitantly inhibits Th1 cytokine production in mitogen- and antigen-stimulated humna peripheral blood mononuclear cell cultures. Clin. Exp. Immunol. 1995; 99:160-167.

268. Jeannin P, Delneste Y, Lecoanet-Henchoz S, Gauchat J-F, Life P, Holmes D, Bonnefoy J-Y. Thiols decrease human interleukin (IL)- 4 production and IL-4-induced immunoglobulin synthesis. J. Exp. Med. 1995; 182:1785-1792.

269. Baum CG, Szabo P, Siskind GW, Becker CG, Firpo A, Clarick CJ, Francus T. Cellular control of IgE production by a polyphenol-rich compound. J. Immunol. 1990; 145:779-784.

270. Cantorna MT, Nashold FE, Hayes CE. In vitamin A deficiency multiple mechanisms establish a regulatory T helper cell imbalance with excess Th1 and insufficient Th2 function. J. Immunol. 1994; 152:1515-1522.

271. Cantorna MT, Nashold FE, Chun TY, Hayes CE. Vitamin A down-regulation of IFN-gamma synthesis in cloned mouse Th1 lymphocytes depends on the CD28 costimulatory pathway. J. Immunol. 1996; 156:2674-2679.

272. Cantorna MT, Nashold FE, Hayes CE. Vitamin A deficiency results in a priming environment conducive for Th1 cell development. Eur. J. Immunol. 1995; 25:1673-1679.

273. Haraguchi S, Good RA, James-Yarish M, Cianciolo GJ, Day NK. Differential modulation of Th1-and Th2-related cytokine mRNA expression by a synthetic peptide homologous to a conserved domain within retroviral envelope protein. Proc. Natl. Acad. Sci. USA 1995; 92:3611-3615.

274. Murray JS, Madri J, Tite J, Carding SR, Bottomly K. MHC control of CD4+ T cell subset activation. J. Exp. Med. 1989; 170:2135-2140.

275. Brunner M, Larsen S, Sette A, Mitchison A. Altered Th1/Th2 balance associated with the immunosuppressive/protective effect of the H-2Ab allele on the response to allo-4-hydrxyphenylipyruvate dioxygenase. Eur. J. Immunol. 1995; 25:3285-3289.

276. Hsieh C-H, Macatonia SE, O'Garra A, Murphy KM. T cell genetic background determines default T helper phenotype development in vitro. J. Exp. Med. 1995; 181:713-721.

277. Romani L, Puccetti P, Bistoni F. Biological role of Th cell subsets in candidiasis. Chem. Immunol. 1996; 63:115-137.

278. Daugelat S, Kaufmann SHE. Role of Th1 and Th2 cells in bacterial infections. Chem. Immunol. 1996; 63:66-97.

279. Scott P, Liblau S, Degermann S, Marconi LA, Ogata AJ, Caton HO, McDevitt HO, Lo D. A role for non-MHC genetic polymorphism in susceptibility to spontaneous autoimmunity. Immunity 1994; 1:73-82.

280. Else KJ, Finkelman FD, Maliszewski CR, Grencis RK. Cytokine-mediated regulation of chronic intestinal helminth infection. J. Exp. Med. 1994; 179:347-351.

281. Matyniak JE, Reiner SL. T helper phenotype and genetic susceptibility in experimental Lyme disease. J. Exp. Med. 1995; 181:1251-1254.

282. Romagnani S. Atopic allergy and other hypersensitivities. Editorial overview: technological advances and new insights into pathogenesis prelude novel therapeutic strategies. Curr. Opin. Immunol. 1995; 7:745-750.

283. Guler M, Gorham JD, Hsieh C-S, Mackey AJ, Steen RG, Dietrich WF, Murphy KM. Genetic susceptibility to leishmania: IL-12 responsiveness in Th1 cell development. Science 1996; 271:984-986.

284. Gorham JD, Guler ML, Steen RG, Mackey AJ, Daly MJ, Frederick K, Dietrich WF, Murphy KM. Genetic mapping of a locus controlling development of Th1/Th2 type responses (in press).

285. Novak TJ, Rothenberg EV. cAMP inhibits induction of interleukin-2 but not of interleukin-4 in T cells. Proc. Natl. Acad. Sci. USA 1990; 87:9353-9357.

286. Munoz E, Zubiaga AM, Merrow M, Sauter NP, Huber BT. Cholera toxin discriminates between T helper 1 and 2 cells in T cell receptor-mediated activation: role of cAMP in T cell proliferation. J. Exp. Med. 1990; 172:95-103.

287. Gajewski TF, Fitch FW. Differential activation of murine Th1 and Th2 clones. Res. Immunol. 1991; 142:19-22.

288. Abbas AK, Williams ME, Burstein HJ, Chang TL, Bossu P, Lichtman AH. Activation and functions of CD4$^+$ T cell subsets. Immunol. Rev. 1991; 123:5-22.

289. Barve SS, Cohen DA, De Benedetti A, Rhoads RE, Kaplan AM. Mechanism of differential regulation of IL-2 in murine Th1 and Th2 T cell subsets. J. Immunol. 1994; 152:1171-1181.

290. Lederer JA, Liou JS, Todd MD, Glimcher LH, Lichtman AH. Regulation of cytokine gene expression in T helper cell subsets. J. Immunol. 1994; 152:77-86.

291. Ullman KS, Flanagan WM, Edwards CA, Crabtree GR. Activation of early gene expression in T lymphocytes by Oct-1 and an inducible protein, OAP40. Science 1991; 254:558-562.

292. Schreiber SL, Crabtree GR. The mechanisms of action of cyclosporin A and FK506. Immunol. Today 1992; 13:136-142.

293. Lederer JA, Liou JS, Kim S, Rice N, Lichtman AH. Regulation of NF-κB activation in T helper 1 and T helper 2 cells. J. Immunol. 1996; 156:56-63.

294. Taniguchi T. Cytokine signaling through nonreceptor protein tyrosine kinases. Science 1995; 268:251-256.

295. Darnell JEJr, Kerr IM, Stark GR. Jak-STAT pathways and transcriptional activation in response to IFNs and other extracellular signaling proteins. Science 1994; 264:1415-1421.

296. Ihle JN, Witthuhn BA, Quelle FW, Yamamoto K, Thierfelder WE, Kreider B, Silvennoinen O. Signaling by the cytokine receptor superfamily: JAKs and STATs. Trends Biochem. Sci. 1994; 19:222-227.

297. Schindler U, Penguang W, Rothe M, Brasseur M, McKnight SL. Components of a Stat recognition code: evidence for two layers of meolecular selectivity. Immunity 1995; 2:689-697.

298. Muller M, Briscoe J, Laxton C et al. The protein tyrosine kinase JAK1 complements a mutant cell line defective in the interferon-α/β and γ signal transduction pathways. Nature 1993; 376:337-341.

299. Fu X-Y, Schindler C, Improta T, Aebersold R, Darnell JE. The proteins of ISGF-3, the interferon-α-induced transcriptional activator, defines a gene family

involved in signal transduction. Proc. Natl. Acad. Sci. USA 1992; 89:7840-7843.

300. Schindler C, Fu X-Y, Improta T, Aebersold R, Darnell JE. Proteins of trasncription factor ISGF-3: one gene encodes the 91- and 84-kDa ISGF-3 proteins that are activated by interferon α. Proc. Natl. Acad. Sci. USA 1992; 89:7836-7839.

301. Greenlund AC, Morales MO, Viviano BL, Yan H, Krowleski J, Schreiber RD. Stat recruitment by tyrosine phosphorylated cytokine receptors: an ordered reversible affinity-driven process. Immunity 1995; 2:677-687.

302. Greenlund AC, Farrar MA, Viviano BL, Schreiber RD. Ligand-induced IFN-γ receptor phosporylation couples the receptor to its signal transduction system (p91). EMBO J. 1994; 13:1591-1600.

303. Jacobson NG, Szabo SJ, Weber-Nordt RM, Zhong Z, Schreiber RD, Darnell JE, Murphy KM. Interleukin 12 signaling in T helper type 1 (Th1) cells involves tyrosine phosphorylation of signal transducer and activator of transcription (Stat)3 and Stat 4. J. Exp. Med. 1995; 181:1755-1762.

304. Szabo SJ, Jacobson NG, Dighe AS, Gubler U, Murphy KM. Developmental commitment to the Th2 lineage by extinction of IL-12 signaling. Immunity 1995; 2:666-675.

305. Bacon CM, McVicar DW, Ortaldo JR, Rees RC, O'Shea JJ, Johnston JA. Interleukin 12 (IL-12) induces tyrosine phosphorylation of JAK2 and TYK2: differential use of Janus family tyrosine kinases by IL-2 and IL-12. J. Exp. Med. 1995; 181:399-404.

306. Bacon CM, Petricoin EF, Ortaldo JE, Rees RC, Larner AC, Johnston JA, O'Shea JJ. Interleukin 12 induces tyrosine phosphorylation and activation of STAT4 in human lymphocytes. Proc. Natl. Acad. Sci. USA 1995; 92:7307-7311.

307. Hou J, Schindler U, Henzel WJ, Ho T, Brasseur M, McKnight SL. An interleukin-4-induced transcription factor: IL-4 STAT. Science 1994; 265:1701-1706.

308. Takeda K, Tanaka T, Shi W, Matsumoto M, Minami M, Kashiwamura S-I, Nakanishi K, Yoshida N, Kishimoto T, Akira S. Essential role of Stat6 in IL-4 signalling. Nature 1996; 380:627-630.

309. Shimoda K, van Deursen J, Sangster MY et al. Lack of IL-4-induced Th2 response and IgE class switching in mice with disrupted Stat6 gene. Nature 1996; 380:630-632.

310. Abe E, de Waal-Malefyt R, Matsuda I, Arai K, Arai N. An 11-base-pair DNA sequence motif apparently unique to the human interleukin 4 gene confers responsiveness to T-cell activation signals. Proc. Natl. Acad. Sci. 1992; 89:2864-2868.

311. Li-Weber M, Eder A, Ktaf-Czepa H, Krammer PH. T cell-specific negative regulation of transcription of the human cytokine IL-4. J. Immunol. 1992; 148:1913-1918.

312. Matsuda I, Naito Y, Arai K, Arai N. The structure of the IL-4 gene and regulation of its expression. Res. Immunol. 1993; 144:569-574.

313. Murphy KM, Murphy TL, Gold JS, Szabo SJ. Current understanding of IL-4 gene regulation in T cells. Res. Immunol. 1993; 144:575-578.

314. Rooney JW, Hoey T, Glimcher LH. Coordinate and cooperative roles for NF-AT and AP-1 in the regulation of the murine IL-4 gene. Immunity 1995; 2:473-483.

315. Hodge MR, Rooney JW, Glimcher LH. The proximal promoter of the IL-4 gene is composed of multiple essential regulatory sites that bind at least two distinct factors. J. Immunol. 1995; 154:6397-6405.

316. Hodge MR, Ranger AM, Charles de la Brousse F, Hoey T, Grusby MJ, Glimcher LH. Hyperproliferation and dysregulation of IL-4 expression in NF-ATp-deficient mice. Immunity 1996; 4:397-405.

317. Davydov IV, Krammer PH, Li-Weber M. Nuclear factor-IL-6 activates the human IL-4 promoter in T cells. J. Immunol. 1995; 155:5273-5279.

318. Song Z, Casolaro V, Chen R, Georas SN, Monos D, Ono SJ. Polymorphic nucleotides within the human IL-4 promoter that mediate overexpression of the gene. J. Immunol. 1996; 156:424-429.

319. Tanaka T, Hu-Li J, Seder RA, de St. Groth BF, Paul WE. Interleukin 4 suppresses interleukin 2 and interferon gamma production by naive T cells stimulated by accessory cell-dependent receptor engagement. Proc. Natl. Acad. Sci. USA 1993; 90:5914-5918.

320. Seder RA. The role of IL-12 in the regulation of Th1 and Th2 differentiation. Res. Immunol. 1995; 146:473-476.

321. Chensue SW, Ruth JH, Warmington K, Lincoln P, Kunkel SL. In vivo regulation of macrophage IL-12 production during type 1 and type 2 cytokine-mediated granuloma formation. J. Immunol. 1995; 155:3546-3551.

322. Fiorentino DF, Zlotnik A, Vieira P, Mosmann TR, Howard M, Moore KW, O'Garra A. IL-10 acts on the antigen-presenting cell to inhibit cytokine production by Th1 cells. J. Immunol. 1991; 146:3444-3451.

323. Hino A, Nariuchi H. Negative feedback mechanism suppresses interleukin-12 production by antigen-presenting cells interacting with T helper 2 cells. Eur. J. Immunol. 1996; 26:623-628.

324. Trinchieri G, Scott P. Interleukin-12: a pro-inflammatory cytokine with immunoregulatory functions. Res. Immunol. 1995; 146:423-431.

325. Fitch FW, McKisic MD, Lancki DW, Gajewski TF. Differential regulation of murine T lymphocyte subsets. Annu. Rev. Immunol. 1993; 11:29-48.

326. Zurawski G, de Vries JE. Interleukin 13, an interleukin 4-like cytokine that acts on monocytes and B cells, but not on T cells. Immunol. Today 1994; 15:19-26.

327. de Vries JE. Molecular and biological characteristics of interleukin 13. Chem. Immunol. 1996; 63:204-218.

328. Gajewski TF, Fitch FW. Anti-proliferative effect of IFN-γ in immune regulation. I. IFN-γ inhibits the proliferation of Th2 but not Th1 murine helper T lymphocyte clones. J. Immunol. 140:4245-4252.

329. Gajewski TF, Joyce J, Fitch FW. Anti-proliferative effect of IFN-γ in immune regulation. III. Differential selection of Th1 and Th2 murine helper T lymphocyte clones using recombinant IL-2 and recombinant IFN-γ. J. Immunol. 1989; 143:15-22.

330. Gajewski TF, Fitch FW. Anti-proliferative effect of IFN-gamma in immune regulation. IV. Murine CTL clones produce IL-3 and GM-CSF, the activity of which is masked by the inhibitory action of secreted IFN-gamma. J. Immunol. 1990; 144:548-556.

331. Abed NS, Chace JH, Cowdery JS. T cell-independent and T cell-dependent B cell activation increases IFN-gamma receptor expression and renders B cells sensitive to IFN-gamma-mediated inhibition. J. Immunol. 1994; 153: 3369-3377.

332. Finkelman FD, Svetic A, Gresser I, Snapper C, Holmes J, Trotta PP, Katona IM, Gause WC. Regulation by interferon of immunoglobulin isotype selection and lymphokine production in mice. J. Exp. Med. 1991; 174:1179-1188.

333. Urban JF Jr, Madden KB, Cheever AW, Trotta PP, Katona IM, Finkelman FD. IFN inhibits inflammatory responses and protective immunity in mice infected with the nematode parasite, *Nippostrongylus brasiliensis*. J. Immunol. 1993; 151:7086-7094.

334. Wynn TA, Jankovic D, Hieny S, Zioncheck K, Jardieu P, Cheever AW, Sher A. IL-12 exacerbates rather than suppresses T helper 2-dependent pathology in the absence of endogenous IFN-γ. J. Immunol. 1995; 154:3999-4009.

335. Morris SC, Madden KB, Adamovicz JJ, Gause WC, Hubbard BR, Gately MK, Finkelman FD. Effects of IL-12 on in vivo cytokine gene expression and Ig isotype selection. J. Immunol. 1994; 152:1047-1056.

336. Kiniwa M, Gately M, Gubler U, Chizzonite R, Fargeas C, Delespesse G. Recombinant interleukin-12 suppresses the synthesis of immunoglobulin E by interleukin-4 stimulated human lymphocytes. J. Clin. Invest. 1992; 90:262-266.

337. Bliss J, Van Cleave V, Murray K, Wiencis A, Katchum M, Maylor R, Haire T, Resmini C, Abbas AK, Wolf SF. IL-12, as an adjuvant, promotes a T helper 1 cell, but does not suppress a T helper 2 cell recall response. J. Immunol. 1996; 156:887-894.

338. Meyaard L, Hovenkamp E, Otto SA, Miedema F. IL-12-induced IL-10 production by human T cells as a negative feedback for IL-12-induced immune responses. J. Immunol. 1996; 156:2776-2782.

336. Kabelitz D, Pohl T, Pechhold K. Activation-induced cell death (apoptosis) of mature peripheral T lymphocytes. Immunol. Today 1993; 14:338-339.

337. Beutler B, van Huffel C. Unraveling function in the TNF ligand and receptor families. Science 1994; 264:667-668.

338. Brunner T, Mogil RJ, LaFace D et al. Cell-autonomous Fas (CD95)/Fas-ligand interaction mediates activation-induced apoptosis in T-cell hybrydomas. Nature 1995; 373:441-444.

339. Dhein J, Walczak H, Baumler C, Debatin K-M, Krammer PH. Autocrine T-cell suicide mediated by APO-1(Fas/CD95). Nature 1995; 373:438-441.

340. Ju S-T, Cui H, Panka DJ, Ettinger R, Marshak-Rothstein A. Participation of target Fas protein in apoptosis pathways induced by CD4+ Th1 and CD8+ cytotoxic T cells. Proc. Natl. Acad. Sci. USA 1994; 91:4185-4189.

341. Kagi D, Vignaux F, Ledermann B, Burki K, Depraetere V, Nagata S, Hengartner H, Golstein P. Fas and perforin pathways as major mechanisms of T cell-mediated cytotoxicity. Science 1994; 265:528-530.

342. Stalder T, Hahn S, Erb P. J. Fas antigen is the major target molecule for CD4+ T cell-mediated cytotoxicity. Immunol. 1994; 152:1127-1233.

343. Ramsdell F, Seaman MS, Miller RE, Picha KS, Kennedy MK, Lynch DH. Differential ability of T(h)1 and T(h)2 T cells to express fas ligand and to undergo activation-induced cell death. Int. Immunol. 1994; 6:1545-1553.

344. Suda T, Okazaki T, Naito Y, Yokota T, Arai N, Ozaki S, Nakao K, Nagata S. Expression of the Fas ligand in cells of T cell lineage. J. Immunol. 1995; 154:3806-3813.

345. Lynch DH, Ramsdell F, Alderson MR. Fas and FasL in the homeostatic regulation of immune responses. Immunol. Today 1995; 16:569-574.

346. Ashany D, Song X, Lacy E, Nikolic-Zugic J, Friedman SM, Elkon BK. Th1 CD4+ lymphocytes delete activated macrophages through the Fas/APO-1 antigen pathway. Proc. Natl. Acad. Sci. USA 1995; 92:11225-11229.

347. Sloan-Lancaster J, Evavold BD, Allen PM. Th2 cell clonal anergy as a consequence of partial inactivation. J. Exp. Med. 1994; 180:1195-1205.

348. Gilbert KM, Hoang KD, Weigle WO. Th1 and Th2 clones differ in their response to a tolerogenic signal. J. Immunol. 1990; 144:2063-2071.

349. Jenkins MK, Chen C, Jung G, Mueller DL, Schwartz RH. Inhibition of antigen-specific proliferation of type 1 murine T cell clones after stimulation with immobilized anti-CD3 monoclonal antibody. J. Immunol. 1990; 144:16-22.

350. Williams ME, Lichtman AH, Abbas AK. Anti-CD3 antibody induces unresponsiveness to IL-2 in Th1 clones but not in Th2 clones. J. Immunol. 1990; 144:1208-1214.

351. Williams ME, Shea CM, Lichtman AH, Abbas AK. Antigen receptor-mediated anergy in resting T lymphocytes and T cell clones. Correlation with lymphokine secretion patterns. J. Immunol. 1992; 149:1921-1926.

352. Gilbert KM, Weigle WO. Th1 cell anergy and blockade in G1a phase of the cell cycle. J. Immunol. 1993; 151:1245-1254.

353. Cho EA, Riley MP, Sillman AL, Quill H. Altered thyrosine phosphorylation in anergic Th1 cells. J. Immunol. 1993; 151:20-28.

354. Gajewski TF, Lancki DW, Stack R, Fitch FW. "Anergy" of Th0 helper T lymphocytes induces downregulation of Th1 characteristics and a transition to a Th2-like phenotype. J. Exp. Med. 1994; 179:481-491.

355. Burstein HJ, Shea CM, Abbas AK. Aqueous antigens induce in vivo tolerance selectively in IL-2- and IFN-γ-producing (Th1) cells. J. Immunol. 1992; 148:3687-3691.

356. De Wit D, Van Mechelen M, Ryelandt M, Figueiredo AC, Abramowicz D, Goldman M, Bazin H, Urbain J, Leo O. The injection of deaggregated gamma globulins in adult mice induces antigen-specific unresponsiveness of T helper type 1 but not type 2 lymphocytes. J. Exp. Med. 1992; 175:9-14.

357. Romball CG, Weigle WO. In vivo induction of tolerance in murine CD4+ cell subsets. J. Exp. Med. 1993; 178:1637-1644.

358. Chen Y, Inobe J-I, Marks R, Gonnella P, Kuchroo VK, Weiner HL. Peripheral deletion of antigen-reactive T cells in oral tolerance. Nature 1995; 376:177-180.

359. Melamed D, Fishman-Lovell J, Uni Z, Weiner HL, Friedman A. Peripheral tolerance of Th2 lymphocytes induced by continuous feeding of ovalbumin. Int. Immunol. 1966; 8:717-724.

360. Garside P, Steel M, Worthey EA, Satoskar A, Alexander J, Bluethmann H, Liew FY, Mowat AM. T helper 2 cells are subject to high dose oral tolerance and are not essential for its induction. J. Immunol. 1995; 154:5649-5655.

361. Locksley RM, Heinzel FP, Sadick MD, Holaday BJ, Gardner KD. Murine cutaneous leishmaniasis. Susceptibility correlates with differential expansion of helper T cell subsets. Ann. Inst. Pasteur/Immunol. 1987; 138:744-749.

362. Scott P, Natovitz P, Coffman RL, Pearce E, Sher A. Immunoregulation of cutaneous leishmaniasis. T cell lines that transfer protective immunity or exacerbation belong to different T helper subsets and respond to distinct parasite antigens. J. Exp. Med. 1988; 168:1675-1684.

363. Holaday BJ, Sadick MD, Wang Z-E, Reiner SL, Heinzel FP, Parslow TG, Locksley RM. Reconstitution of Leishmania immunity in severe combined immunodeficient mice using Th1- and Th2-like cell lines. J. Immunol. 1991; 147:1653-1658.

364. Jardim A, Alexander J, Teh HS, Ou D, Olafson RW. Immunoprotective *Leishmania major* synthetic T cell epitopes. J. Exp. Med. 1990; 172:645-648.

365. Murray PJ, Handman E, Glaser TA, Spithill TW. *Leishmania major*: expression and gene structure of the glycoprotein 63 molecule in virulent and avirulent clones and strains. Exp. Parasitol. 1990; 71:294-304.

366. Reiner SL, Locksley RM. The regulation of immunity to *Leishmania Major*. Annu. Rev. Immunol. 1995; 13:151-177.

367. Handman E, Symons FM, Baldwin TM, Curtis JM, Scheerlink J-PY. Protective vaccination with promastigote surface antigen 2 from Leishmania major is mediated by a Th1 type of immune response. Infect. Immunity 1995; 63:4261-4267.

368. Noben-Trauth N, Kropf P, Muller I. Susceptibility to *Leishmania major* infection in interleukin-4-deficient mice. Science 1996; 271:987-990.

369. Satoskar A, Bluethmann H, Alexander J. Disruption of the murine interleukin-4 gene inhibits disease progression during *Leishmania mexicana* infection but does not increase control of *Leishmania donovani* infection. Infect. Immunity 1995; 63:4894-4899.

370. Scott P. IFN-γ modulates the early development of Th1 and Th2 responses in a murine model of cutaneous leishmaniasis. J. Immunol. 1991; 147:3149-3155.

371. Sharton TM, Scott P. Natural killer cells are a source of interferon-γ that drives differentiation of CD4⁺ T cell subsets and induces early resistance to *Leishmania major* in mice. J. Exp. Med. 1993; 178:567-577.

372. Sypek JP, Chung CL, Mayor SEH, Subramanyam JM, Goldman SJ, Sieburth DS, Wolf SF, Schaub RG. Resolution of cutaneous leishmaniasis: interleukin 12 initiates a proteictive T helper type 1 immune response. J. Exp. Med. 1993; 177:1797-1802.

373. Heinzel FP, Schoenhaut DS, Rerko RM, Rosser LE, Gately MK. Recombinant interleukin 12 cures mice infected with *Leishmania major*. J. Exp. Med. 1993; 177:1505-1509.

374. Chatelain R, Varkila K, Coffman RL. IL-4 induces a Th2 response in *Leishmania major*-infected mice. J. Immunol. 1992; 148:1182-1187.

375. Nabors GS, Afonso LCC, Farrell JP, Scott P. Switch from a type 2 to a type 1 T helper cell response and cure of established *Leishmania major* infection in mice is induced by combined therapy with interleukin 12 and pentostam. Proc. Natl. Acad. Sci. USA 1995; 91:3142-3146.

376. Reiner SL, Zheng S, Wang Z-E, Stowring L, Locksley RM. *Leishmania* promastigotes evade interleukin 12 (IL-12) induction by macrophages and stimulate a broad range of cytokines from CD4⁺ T cells during initiation of infection. J. Exp. Med. 1994; 179:447-456.

377. Shankar AH, Titus RG. T cell and non-T cell compartments can independently determine resistance to *Leishmania major*. J. Exp. Med. 1995; 181:845-855.

378. Zwingerberger K, Harms G, Pedrosa C, Omena S, Sandkamp B, Neifer S. Determinants of the immune response in visceral leishmaniasis: evidence for predominance of endogenous interleukin 4 over interferon-gamma production. Clin. Immunol. Immunopathol. 1990; 57:242-249.

379. Ghalib HW, Piuvezam MR, Skeiky YA, Siddig M, Hashim FA, el-Hassan AM, Russo DM, Reed SG. Interleukin 10 production correlates with pathology in human *Leishmania donovani* infections. J. Clin. Invest. 1993; 92:324-329.

380. Holaday BJ, Pompeu MM, Jeronimo S et al. Potential role for interleukin-10 in the immunosuppression associated with kala-azar. J. Clin. Invest. 1993; 92; 2626-2632.

381. Carvalho EM, Bacellar O, Brownell C, Regis T, Coffman RL, Reed SG. Restoration of IFN-γ production and lymphocyte proliferation in visceral leishmaniasis. J. Immunol. 1994; 152:5949-5956.

382. Kemp M, Theander TG, Kharazmi A. The contrasting roles of CD4⁺ T cells in intracellular infections in humans: leishmaniasis as an example. Immunol. Today 1996; 17:13-16.

383. Pirmez C, Cooper C, Paes-OLiveira M, Schubach A, Torigian VK, Modlin RL. Immunologic responsiveness in American cutaneous leishmaniasis lesions. J. Immunol. 1990; 145:3100-3104.

384. Caceres-Dittmar G, Tapia FJ, Sanchez MA, Yamamura M, Uyemura K, Modlin RL, Bloom BR, Convit, J. Determination of the cytokine profile in American cutaneous leishmaniasis using the polymerase chain reaction. Clin. Exp. Immunol. 1993; 91:500-05.

385. Karp CL, El-Safi SH, Wynn TA, Satti MH, Kordofani AM, Hashim FA, Hag-Ali M, Neva FA, Nutman TB, Sacks DL. In vivo cytokine profiles in patients with Kala-azar. Marked elevation of both interleukin-10 and interferon-gamma. J. Clin. Invest. 1993; 91:1644-48.

386. Pirmez C, Yamamura M, Uyemura K, Paes-Oliveira M, Conceicao-Silva F, Modlin RL. Cytokine patterns in the pathogenesis of human leishmaniasis. J. Clin. Invest. 1993; 91:1390-95.

387. Gaafar A, Kharazmi A, Ismail A et al. Dichotomy of the T cell response to Leishmania antigens in patients suffering from cutaneous leishmaniasis; absence or scarcity of Th1 activity is associated with severe infections. Clin. Exp. Immunol. 1995; 100:239-145.

388. Cillari E, Vitale G, Arcoleo F, D'Agostino P, Mocciaro C, Gambino G, Malta R, Stassi G, Giordano C, Milano S. In vivo and in vitro cytokine profiles and mononuclear cells subsets in Sicilian patients with active visceral leishmaniasis. Cytokine 1995; 7:740-745.

389. Badarò R, Johnson WD. The role of interferon-γ in the treatment of visceral and diffuse cutaneous leishmaniasis. J. Infect. Dis. 1993; 167(suppl 1):S13-17.

390. Mougneau E, Altare F, Wakil AE, Zheng S, Coppola T, Wang ZE, Waldmann R, Locksley RM, Glaichenhaus N. Expression cloning of a protective leishmania antigen. Science 1995; 268:563-566.

391. Suzuki Y, Remington JS. Toxoplasmic enecphalitis in AIDS patients and experimental models for the study of the disease and its treatment. Res. Immunol. 1993; 144:66-67.

392. Jankovic D, Sher A. Initiation and regulation of CD4⁺ T-cell function in host-parasite models. Chem. Immunol. 1996; 63:51-65.

393. Gazzinelli RT, Hakim FT, Hieny S, Shearer GM, Sher A. Synergistic role of CD4⁺ and CD8⁺ T lymphocytes in IFN-γ production and protective immunity induced by an attenuated *Toxoplasma gondii* vaccine. J. Immunol. 1991; 146:286-292.

394. Denkers EY, Gazzinelli RT, Martin D, Sher A. Emergence of NK1.1⁺ cells as effectors of immunity to *Toxoplasma gondii* in MHC class I-deficient mice. J. Exp. Med. 1993; 178:1465-1472.

395. Sher A, Oswald IO, Hieny S, Gazzinelli RT. *Toxoplasma gondii* induces a T-independent IFN-γ response in NK cells which requires both adherent acessory cells and TNF-α. J. Immunol. 1993; 150:3982-3989.

396. Hunter CA, Subauste CS, Remington JS. The role of cytokines in toxoplasmosis. Biotherapy 1994; 7:237-247.

397. Hunter CA, Chizzonite R, Remington JS. Interleukin-1β is required for the ability of IL-12 to induce production of IFN-γ by NK cells: a role for IL-1β in the T cell independent mechanism of resistance against intracellular pathogens. J. Immunol. 1995; 155:4347-4354.

398. Gazzinelli RT, Wysocka M, Hayashi S, Denkers EY, Hieny S, Caspar P, Trinchieri G, Sher A. Parasite-induced IL-12 stimulates early IFN-γ synthesis and resistance during acute infection with *Toxoplasma gondii*. J. Immunol. 1994; 153:2533-2543.

399. Scharton-Kersten T, Denkers EY, Gazzinelli R, Sher A. Role of IL-12 in induction of cell-mediated immunity to *Toxoplasma gondii*. Res. Immunol. 1995; 146:539-545.

400. Hunter CA, Bermudez L, Beernink H, Waegell W, Remington JS. Transforming growth factor-β inhibits interleukin-12-induced production of inter-

feron by natural killer cells: a role for transforming growth factor-β in the regulation of T cell-independent resistance to *Toxoplasma gondii*. Eur. J. Immunol. 1995; 25:994-1000.

401. Gazzinelli RT, Wysocka M, Hieny S, Scharton-Kersten T, Cheever A, Kuhn R, Muller W, Trinchieri G, Sher A. In the absence of endogenous IL-10, mice acutely infected with *Toxoplasma gondii* succumb to a lethal immune response dependent on CD4+ T cells and accompanied by overproduction of IL-12, IFN-gamma, and TNF-alpha. J. Immunol. 1996; 157:798-805.

402. Taylor-Robinson AW, Philips RS, Severn A, Moncada S, Liew FJ. The role of Th1 and Th2 cells in a rodent malaria infection. Science 1993; 260:1931-1934.

403. Stevenson MM, Tam MF. Differential induction of helper T-cell subsets during blood-stage *Plasmodium chabaudii* AS infection in resistant and susceptible mice. Clin. Exp. Immunol. 1993; 92:77-83.

404. Taylor-Robinson AW, Philips RS. Th1 and Th2 CD4+ T cell clones specific for Plasmodium chabaudi but not for an unrelated antigen protect against blood stage *P. Chabaudi* infection. Eur. J. Immunol. 1994; 24:158-164.

405. Mellouk S, Hoffman SL, Liu Z, de la Vega P, Billiar TR, Nussler AK. Nitric oxide-mediated antiplasmodial activity in human and murine hepatocytes induced by gamma interferon and the parasite itself: enhancement by exogenous tetrahydrobiopterin. Infect. Immun. 1994; 62:4043-4046.

406. Yap GS, Jacobs P, Stevenson MM. Th cell regulation of host resistance to blood-stage *Plasmodium chabaudi* AS. Res. Immunol. 1994; 145:419-422.

407. Taylor-Robinson AW, Phillips RS. Reconstitution of B-cell-depleted mice with B cells restores Th2-type immune responses during *Plasmodium chabaudi chabaudi* infection. Infect. Immunity 1996; 64:366-370.

408. Sedegah M, Finkelman F, Hoffman SL. Interleukin 12 induction of interferon-γ-dependent protection against malaria. Proc. Natl. Acad. Sci. USA 1994; 91:10700-10702.

409. Stevenson MM, Tam MF, Wolf SF, Sher A. IL-12-induced protection against blood-stage *Plasmodium chabaudi* AS requires IFN-γ and TNF-α and occurs via a nitric oxide-dependent mechanism. J. Immunol. 1995; 155:2545-2556.

410. Crutcher JM, Stevenson MM, Sedegah M, Hoffman SL. Interleukin 12 and malaria. Res. Immunol. 1995; 146:552-559.

411. de Kossodo S, Grau GE. Profiles of cytokine production in relation with susceptibility to cerebral malaria. J. Immunol. 1993; 151:4811-4820.

412. Chizzolini C, Grau GE, Geinoz A, Schrijvers D. Lymphocyte-T interferon-gamma production induced by *Plasmodium falciparum* antigen is high in recently infected non-immune and low in immune subjects. Clin. Exp. Immunol. 1990; 79:95-99.

413. Harpaz R, Edelman R, Wasserman SS, Levine MM, Davis JR. Sztein MB. Serum cytokine profiles in experimental human malaria. Relationship to protection and disease course after challenge. J. Clin. Invest. 1992; 90:515-23.

414. Mshana RN, Boulandi J, Mshana MN, Mayombo J, Mendome G. Cytokines in the pathogenesis of malaria: levels of IL-1β, IL-4, IL-6, TNF-α and IFN-γ in plasma of healthy individuals and malaria patients in a holoendemic area. J. Lab. Clin. Immunol. 1994; 34:131-139.

415. Grau GE, Tacchini-Cottier F, Vesin C, Milon G, Lou J, Piguet PF, Juillard P. An active role for platelets in microvascular pathology of severe malaria. Eur. Cytokine Netw. 1993; 4:415-419.

416. Grau GE, Behr C. T cells and malaria: is Th1 cell activation a prerequisite for pathology? Res. Immunol. 1994; 145:441-454.

417. Ungar BLP, Kao TC, Burris JA, Finkelman FD. *Cryptosporidium* infection in an adult mouse model: independent roles for IFN-gamma and CD4 T lymphocytes in protective immunity. J. Immunol. 1991; 147:1014-

418. Tilley M, McDonald V, Bancroft GJ. Resolution of cryptosporidial infection in mice correlates with parasite-specific lymphocyte proliferation associated with both Th1 and Th2 cytokine secretion. Parasite Immunol. 1995; 17:459-464.

419. Urban JF, Fayer R, Chen S-J, Gause WC, Gately MK, Finkelman FD. IL-12 protects immunocompetent and immunodeficient neonatal mice against infection with *Cryprosporidium parvum*. J. Immunol. 1996; 156:163-268.

420. Daugelat S, Ladel CH, Schoel B, Kaufmann SHE. Antigen-specific T-cell responses during primary and secondary *Leisteria monocytogenes* infection. Infect. Immun. 1994; 62:1881-1888.

421. Tripp CS et al. Interleukin 12 and tumor necrosis factor are costimulators of interferon production by natural killer cells in severe combined immunodeficiency mice with leisteriosis, and interleukin 10 is a physiologic antagonist. Proc. Natl. Acad. Sci. USA 1994; 90:3725-3729.

422. Skeen MJ, Miller MA, Shinnick TM, Ziegler HK. Regulation of murine macrophages IL-12 production. Activation of macrophages in vivo, restimulation in vitro and modulation by other cytokines. J. Immunol. 1996; 156:1196-1206.

423. Tripp CS et al. Immune complexes inhibit antimicrobial responses through interleukin-10 production. J. Clin. Invest. 1995; 95:1628-1634.

424. Strassman G et al. Evidence for the involvement of interleukin 10 in the differential deactivation of murine peritoneal macrophages by prostglandin E_2. J. Exp. Med. 1994; 180:2365-2370.

425. Tripp CS, Kanagawa O, Unanue ER. Secondary response to *Leisteria* infection requires IFN-γ but is partially independent of IL-12. J. Immunol. 1995; 155:3427-3432.

426. Rogers HW, Callery MP, Deck B, Unanue ER. Different stages in the natural and acquired resistance to an intracellular pathogen. Immunology 1995; 3:152-156.

427. Rogers HW, Sheehan KCF, Brunt LM, Dower SK, Unanue ER, Schriber RD. Interleukin 1 participates in the development of anti-*Leisteria* responses in normal and SCID mice. Proc. Natl. Acad. Sci. USA 1992; 89:1011-1015.

428. Haak-Frendscho M, Brown JF, Izawa Y, Wagner RD, Czuprynski CJ. Administration of anti-IL-4 antibody 11B11 increases the resistance of mice to *Leisteria monocytogenes* infection. J. Immunol. 1992; 148:3978-3985.

429. Izawa Y, Wagner RD, Czuprincski CJ. Analysis of cytokine mRNA expression in *Leisteria*-resistant C57BL/6 and *Leisteria*-susceptible A/J mice during *Leisteria monocytogenes* infection. Infect. Immun. 1993; 61:3739-3744.

430. Wagner RD, Czuprinski CJ. Cytokine mRNA expression in livers of mice infected with *Leisteria monocytogenes*. J. Leuc. Biol. 1993; 53:525-531.

431. Izawa Y, Brown JF, Czuprynski CJ. Early expression of cytokine mRNA in mice infected with *Leisteria monocytogenes*. Infect. Immun. 1992; 60:4068-4073.

432. Wagner RD, Maroushek NM, Brown JF, Czuprinski CJ. Treatment with anti-interleukin-10 monoclonal antibody enhances early resistance but impairs complete clearance of *Leisteria monocytogenes* infection in mice. Infect. Immun. 1994; 62:2345-2353.

433. Orme IM. The kinetics of emergence and loss of mediator T lymphocytes acquired in response to infection with *Mycobacterium tuberculosis*. J. Immunol. 1987; 138:293-298.

434. Kaufmann SHE. Tuberculosis. The role of the immune response. Immunologist 1993; 1:109-114.

435. Modlin RL, Melancon-Kaplan J, Primez C, Young SMM, Kino H, Convit J, Rea TH, Bloom BR. Learning from lesions: patterns of tissue inflammation in leprosy. Proc. Natl. Acad. Sci. USA 1988; 85:1213-1217.

436. Ladel CH, Hess J, Daugelat S, Kaufmann SHE. Contribution of α/β and γ/δ T lymphocytes to immunity against *Mycobacterium bovis* BCG infection: studies with T cell receptor deficient knockout mice. Eur. J. Immunol. 1995; 25:838-846.

437. Ladel CH, Blum C, Dreher A, Reifenberg K, Kaufmann SEH. Protective role of γ/δ T cells and α/β T cells in tuberculosis. Eur. J. Immunol. 1995; 25:2877-2881.

438. Kawamura I, Tsukada H, Yoshikawa H, Fujita M, Nomoto K, Mitsuyama M. INF-γ producing ability as a possible marker for the protective T cells against *Mycobacterium bovis* BCG in mice. J. Immunol. 1992; 148:2997-2803.

439. Flynn JL, Chan J, Triebold KJ, Dalton DK, Stewart TA, Bloom BR. An essential role for interferon γ in resistance to *Mycobacterium tuberculosis* infection. J. Exp. Med. 1993; 178:2249-2254.

440. Cooper AM, Dalton DK, Stewart TA, Griffin JP, Russell DG, Orme IM. Disseminated tuberculosis in interferon-γ gene-disrupted mice. J. Exp. Med. 1993; 178:2243-2247.

441. Flynn JL, Goldstein MM, Chan J, Triebold KJ, Pfeffer K, Lowenstein CJ, Schreiber R, Mak TW, Bloom BR. Tumor necrosis factor-alpha is required in the protective immune response against *Mycobacterium tuberculosis* in mice. Immunity 1995; 2:561-572.

442. Kamijo R, Le J, Shapiro D, Havell EA, Huang S, Aguet M, Bosland M, Vilcek J. Mice that lack the interferon-γ receptor have profoundly altered response to infection with bacillus Calmette Guérin and subsequent challenge with lipopolysaccharide. J. Exp. Med. 1993; 178:1435-1440.

443. Huygen K, Abrammowicz D, Vandenbussche P, Jacobs F, De Bruyn J, Kentos A, Drowart A, Van Vooren JP, Goldman M. Spleen cell cytokine secretion in *Mycobacterium bovis* BCG-infected mice. Infect. Immun. 1992; 60:2880-2886.

444. Holland SM, Eisenstein EM, Kuhns DP, Turner ML, Fleisher TA, Strober W, Gallin JI. Treatment of refractory disseminated nontuberculous mycobacterial infection with interferon gamma. N. Engl. J. Med. 1994; 330:1349-1355.

445. Cohn ZA, Kaplan G. Hansen's disease, cell-mediated immunity and recombinant lymphokines. J. Infect. Dis. 1991; 163:1195-1200.

446. Hook S, Griffin F, Mackintosh C, Buchan G. Activation of an interleukin-4 mRNA-producing population of peripheral blood mononuclear cells after infection with *Mycobacterium bovis* or vaccination with killed, but not live, BCG. Immunology 1996; 88:269-274.

447. Tsicopoulos A, Hamid Q, Varney V, Ying S, Moqbel R, Durham SR, Kay AB. Preferential messenger RNA expression of the Th1-type cells (IFN-γ'IL-2$^+$) in classical delayed-type (tuberculin) hypersensitivity reactions in human skin. J. Immunol. 1992; 148:2058-2061.

448. Sander B, Skansen-Saphir U, Damm O, Hakansson L, Andersson J, Andersson U. Sequential production of Th1 and Th2 cytokines in response to live bacillus Calmette-Guerin. Immunology 1995; 86:512-518.

449. Zhang M, Gately MK, Wang E, Gong J, Wolf SF, Lu S, Modlin RL, Barnes PF. Interleukin 12 at the site of disease in tuberculosis. J. Clin. Invest. 1994; 93:1733-1739.

450. Barnes PF, Fong S-J, Brennan PJ, Twomey PE, Mazumder A, Modlin RL. Local production of tumor necrosis factor and IFN-γ in tuberculous pleuritis. J. Immunol. 1990; 145:149-154.

451. Flesch IEA, Kaugfmann SEH. Activation of tuberculostatic macrophage function by gamma-interferon, interleukin-4 and tumor necrosis factor production. Infect. Immun. 1990; 58:2675-2677.

452. Surcel HM, Troye-Blomberg M, Paulic S, Andersson G, Moreno C, Pasvol G, Ivanyi J. Th1/Th2 profiles in tuberculosis based on the proliferation and cytokine response of blood lymphocytes to mycobacterial antigens. Immunology 1994; 81:171-176.

453. Sanchez FO, Rodriguez JI, Agudelo G, Garcia LF. Immune responsiveness and lymphokine production in patients with tuberculosis and healthy controls. Infect. Immun. 1994; 62:5673-5678.

454. Denis M, Ghadirian E. IL-10 neutralization augments mouse resistance to systemic *Mycobacterium avium* infections. J. Immunol. 1993; 151:5425-5430.

455. Zhang M, Lin Y, Iyer DV, Gong J, Abrams JS. T-cell cytokine responses in human infection with *Mycobacterium tuberculosis*. Infect. Immun. 1995; 63:3231-3234.

456. Toossi Z, Gogate P, Shiratsuchi H, Young T, Ellner JJ. Enhanced production of TGF-β by blood monocytes from patients with active tuberculosis and presence of TGF-β in tuberculous granulomatous lung lesions. J. Immunol. 1995; 154:465-473.

457. Sampaio EP, Moreira AL, Kaplan G, Alvin AMS, Duppre NC, Miranda CF, Sarno EN. *Mycobacterium leprae*-induced interferon-γ production by household contacts of leprosy patients: associates with the development of active disease. J. Infect. Dis. 1991; 164:990-993.

458. Misra N, Murtaza A, Walker B, Narayan NP, Misra RS, Ramesh V, Singh S, Colston MJ, Nath I. Cytokine profile of circulating T cells of leprosy patients reflects both indiscriminate and polarized T-helper subsets: T helper phenotype is stable and uninfluenced by related antigens of *Mycobacterium leprae*. Immunology 1995; 86:97-103.

459. Sieling PA, Modlin RL. Cytokine patterns at the site of mycobacterial infection. Immunobiology 1994; 191:378-387.

460. Gil Castro A, Silva RA, Appelberg R. Endogenously produced IL-12 is required for the induction of protective T cells during *Mycobacterium avium* infections in mice. J. Immunol. 1995; 155:2013-2019.

461. Modlin RL, Barnes PF. IL-12 and the human immune response to mycobacteria. Res. Immunol. 1995; 146:526-530.

462. Flynn JL, Goldstein MM, Triebold KJ, Sypek J, Wolf S, Bloom BR. IL-12 increases resistance of BALB/c mice to *Mycobacterium tuberculosis* infection. J. Immunol. 1995; 155:2515-2524.

463. Keane-Myers A, Nickell SP. Role of IL-4 and IFN-γ in modulation of immunity to *Borrelia burgdorferi* in mice. J. Immunol. 1995; 155:2020-2028.

464. Keane-Myers A, Maliszewski CR, Finkelman FD, Nickell SP. Recombinant IL-4 treatment augments resistance to *Borrelia burgdorferi* infections in both normal susceptible and antibody-deficient susceptible mice. J. Immunol. 1996; 156:2488-2494.

465. Matyniak JE, Reiner SL. T helper phenotype and genetic susceptibility in experimental Lyme disease. J. Exp. Med. 1995; 181:1251-1254.

466. Bohn E, Heesemann J, Elhers S, Autenrieth IB. Early gamma interferon mRNA expression is associated with resistance of mice against *Yersinia enterocolitica*. Infect. Immun. 1994; 62:3027-3032.

467. Autenrieth IB, Beer M, Bohn E, Kaufmann SHE, Heesemann J. Immune responses to *Yersinia enterocolitica* in susceptible BALB/c and resistant C57BL/6 mice: an essential role for gamma interferon. Infect. Immun. 1994; 62:2590-2599.

468. Schlaack J, Hermann E, Ringhoffer M, Probst P, Gallati H, Meyer zum Buschenfelde K-H, Fleischer B. Predominance of Th1-type T cells in synovial fluid of patients with *Yersinia*-induced reactive arthritis. Eur. J. Immunol. 1992; 22:2771-2776.

469. Bohn E, Autenrieth IB. IL-12 is essential for resistance against *Yersinia enetrocolitica* by triggering IFN-γ production in NK cells and CD4+ T cells. J. Immunol. 1996; 156:1458-1468.

470. Lahesmaa R, Yssel H, Batsford S, Luukkainen R, Mootonen T, Steinman L, Peltz G. *Yersinia enterocolitica* activates a T helper type 1-like T cell subset in reactive arthritis. J. Immunol. 1992; 148:3079-3085.

471. Igietseme JU, Ramsey KH, Magee DM, Williams DM, Theus SA, Kincy TJ, Rank RG. Resolution of murine chlamydial genital infection by the adoptive transfer of a CD4+, Th1 lymphocyte clone. Reg. Immunol. 1993; 5:311-317.

472. Magee DM, Williams DM, Smith JG, Bleicker CA, Grubbs BG, Schacker J, Rank RG. Role of CD8+ T cells in primary *Chlamydia* infection. Infect. Immun. 1995; 63:516-521.

473. Simon AK, Seipelt E, Wu P, Wenzel B, Braun J, Sieper J. Analysis of cytokine profile in synovial T cell clones from chlamydial-reactive arthritis patients: predominance of the Th1 subset. Clin. Exp. Immunol. 1993; 94:122-126.

474. Petersen JW, Ibsen PH, Haslov K, Heron I. Proliferative responses and gamma interferon and tumor necrosis factor production by lymphocytes isolated from tracheobronchial lymph nodes and spleens of mice aerosol infected with *Bordetella pertussis*. Infect. Immun. 1992; 60:4563-4570.

475. Mills KHG, Barnard A, Wakins J, Redhead K. Cell-mediated immunity to Bordetella pertussis: role of Th1 cells in bacterial clearence in a murine respiratory infection model. Infect. Immun. 1993; 61:399-410.

476. Peppoloni S, Nencioni L, Di Tommaso A, Tagliabue A, Parronchi P, Romagnani S, Rappuoli R, De magistris MT. Lymphokine secretion and cytotoxic activity of human CD4+ T-cell clones against *Bordetella pertussis*. Infect. Immun. 1991; 59:3768-3773.

477. Redhead K, Waktins J, Barnard A, Mills KHG. Effective immunization against *Bordetella pertussis* respiratory infection in mice is dependent on induction of cell-mediated immunity. Infect. Immun. 1993; 61:3190-3198.

478. Barnard A, Mahon BP, Watkins J, Redhead K, Mills KHG. Th1/Th2 dichotomy in acquired immunity to *Bordetella pertussis*: variables in the in vivo priming and in vitro cytokine detection techniques affect the classification of T-cell subsets as Th1, Th2 or Th0. Immunology 1996; 87:372-380.

479. Munoz JJ, Peacock MG. Action of pertussigen (pertussis toxin) on serum IgE and on Fcε receptors on lymphocytes. Cell. Immunol. 1990; 127:327-336.

480. Kamradt T, Soloway PD, Perkins DL, Gefter ML. Pertussis toxin prevents the induction of peripheral T cell anergy and enhances the T cell response to an encephalitogenic peptide of myelin basic protein. J. Immunol. 1991; 147:327-336.

481. Mu HH, Sewell WA. Regulation of DTH and IgE responses by IL-4 and IFN-γ in immunized mice given pertussis toxin. Immunology 1994; 83:639-645.

482. Mielke MEA. T cell subsets in granulomatous inflammation and immunity to *L. Monocytogenes* and *B. abortus*. Behring Inst. Mitt. 1991; 88:99-111.

483. Jones SM, Winter AJ. Survival of virulent and attenuated strains of *Brucella abortus* in normal and gamma-interferon-activated murine peritoneal macrophages. Infect. Immun. 1992; 60:3011-3014.

484. Stevens MG, Plugh GW, Tabatabal LB. Effects of gamma interferon and indomethacine in preventing *Brucella abortus* infections in mice. Infect. Immun. 1992; 60:4407-4409.

485. Zhan Y, Yang J, Cheers C. Differential activation of *Brucella*-reactive CD4[+] T cells by *Brucella* infection or immunization with antigenic extracts. Infect. Immun. 1995; 63:969-975.

486. Oliveira SC, Zhu Y, Splitter GA. Recombinant L7/L12 ribosomal protein and gamma-irradiated *Brucella abortus* induce a T-helper 1 subset response from murine CD4[+] T cells. Immunology 1994; 83:659-664.

487. Sulitzeanu D. Passive protection experiments with *Brucella* antisera. J. Hyg. 1995; 53:133-142.

488. Montaraz JA, Winter AJ, Hunter MD, Sowa BA, Wu AM, Adams LG. Protection against *Brucella abortus* in mice with O-polysaccharide-specific monoclonal antibodies. Infect. Immun. 1986; 51:961-963.

489. Winter AJ, Duncan JR, Santisteban CG, Douglas JT, Adams LG. Capacity of passively administered antibody to prevent establishment of *Brucella abortus* infection in mice. Infect. Immun. 1989; 57:3438-3444.

490. Nauciel C. Role of CD4[+] T cells and T-cell-independent mechanisms in acquired resistance to *Salmonella thypimurium* infection. J. Immunol. 1990; 145:1265-1269.

491. Muotiala A, Makela PH. The role of IFN-γ in murine *Salmonella thyphimurium* infection. Microbial Pathogen 1990; 8:135-141.

492. Nakano Y, Onozuka K, Terada Y, Shinomiya H, Nakano M. Protective effect of recombinant TNF-α in murine salmonellosis. J. Immunol. 1990; 144:1935-1941.

493. Nauciel C, Espinasse-Maes F. Role of gamma-interferon and tumor necrosis factor alpha in resistance to *Salmonella thyphimurium* infection. Infect. Immun. 1992; 60:450-454.

494. Ramarathinam L, Shaban RA, Niesel DW, Klimpel GR. Interferon gamma (IFN-γ) production by gut-associated lymphoid tissue and spleen following oral *Salmonella thyphimurium* challenge. Microbial Pathogen 1991; 11:347-356.

495. Bost KL, Clements JD. In vivo induction of interleukin-12 mRNA expression after oral immunization with *Salmonella dublin* or the B subunit of *Escherichia coli* heat-labile enterotoxin. Infect. Immun. 1995; 63:1976-1803.

496. Mastroeni P, Harrison JA, Chabalgoity JA, Hormaeche CE. Effect of interleukin 12 neutralization on host resistance and gamma-interferon production in mouse typhoid. Infect. Immunity 1996; 64:189-196.

497. Yang DM, Fairweather N, Button LL, McMaster WR, Kahl LP, Liew FY. Oral *Salmonella thyphimurium* (AroA-) vaccine expressing a major leishmanial surface protein (gp63) preferentially induces T helper 1 cells and protective immunity against leishmaniasis. J. Immunol. 1990; 145:2281-2285.

498. VanCott JL, Staats HF, Pascual DW et al. Regulation of mucosal and systemic antibody responses by T helper cell subsets, macrophages, and derived cytokines following oral immunization with live recombinant *Salmonella*. J. Immunol. 1996; 156:1504-1514.

499. Klein TW, Yamamoto Y, Brown HK, Friedman H. Interferon-gamma induced resistance to *Legionella pneumophila* in susceptible A/J mouse macrophages. J. Leuk. Biol. 1991; 49:98-103.

500. Yamamoto Y, Klein TW, Newton CA, Friedman H. Differing macrophage and lymphocyte roles in resistance to *Legionella pneumophila* infection. J. Immunol. 1992; 148:584-589.

501. Klein TW, Newton C, Friedman H. Resistance to *Legionella pneumophila* suppressed by the marijuana component, tetrahydrocannabitol. J. Infect. Dis. 1994; 169:1177-1179.

502. Newton CA, Klein TW, Friedman H. Secondary immunity to *Legionella pneumophila* and Th1 activity are suppressed by delta-9-tetrahydrocannabitol injection. Infect. Immun. 1994; 62:4015-4020.

503. Kartunnen R, Surcel HM, Andersson G, Ekre HPT, Herva E. *Francisella tularensis*-induced in vitro gamma-interferon, tumor necrosis factor alpha, and interleukin-2 responses appear within 2 weeks of tularemia vaccination in human beings. J. Clin. Microbiol. 1991; 29:753-756.

504. Sjostedt A, Erksson M, Sandstrom G, Tarnvik A. Various membrane proteins of *Francisella tularensis* induce interferon-γ production on both CD4⁺ and CD8⁺ T cells of primed humans. Immunology 1992; 76:584-592.

505. Fortier AH, Slayter MV, Ziemba R, Meltzer MS, Nacy CA. Live vaccine strain of *Francisella tularensis:* infection and immunity in mice. Infect. Immun. 1991; 59:2922-2928.

506. Leiby DA, Fortier AH, Crawford RM, Schreiber RD, Nacy CA. In vivo modulation of the murine immune response to *Francisella tularensis* LSV infection in mice. Infect. Immun. 1992; 60:84-89.

507. Golovliov I, Sandstrom G, Ericsson M, Sjostedt A, Tarnvik A. Cytokine expression in the liver during the early phase of murine tularemia. Infect. Immun. 1995; 63:534-538.

508. Nacy CA, Meltzer MS. Macrophages in resistance to rickettsial infection: macrophage activation in vitro for killing of *Rickettsia tsutsugamushi*. J. Immunol. 1979; 123:2544-2549.

509. Li H, Jerrels TR, Spitalny GL, Walker DH. Interferon gamma as a crucial host defense against *Rickettsia conorii* in vivo. Infect. Immun. 1986; 55:1252-1255.

510. Hickman CJ, Stover CK, Joseph SW, Oaks EV. Murine T-cell response to native and recombinant protein antigens of *Rickettsia tsutsugamushi*. Infect. Immun. 1993; 61:1674-1681.

511. Van Voorhis WC, Barrett LK, Koelle DM, Nasio JM, Plummer FA, Lukehart SA. Primary and secondary syphilis lesions contain mRNA for Th1 cytokines. J. Infect. Dis. 1996; 173:491-495.

512. Fitzgerald TJ. The Th1/Th2-like switch in syphilitic infection: is it detrimental? Infect. Immun. 1992; 60:3475-3479.

513. Cleveland MG, Gorham JD, Murphy TL, Tuomanen E, Murphy KM. Lipoteichoic acid preparations of gram-positive bacteria induce interleukin-12 through a CD14-dependent pathway. Infect. Immunity 1996; 064:1906-1912.

514. Bistoni F, Cenci E, Mencacci A, Schiaffella E, Mosci P, Puccetti P, Romani L. Mucosal and systemic T helper cell function after intragastric colonization of adult mice with *Candida albicans*. J. Infect. Dis. 1993; 168:1449-1457.

515. Fidel PL, Lynch ME, Sobel JD. *Candida*-specific Th1-type responsiveness in mice with experimental vaginal candidiasis. Infect. Immun. 1993; 61:4202-4207.

516. Cenci E, Mencacci A, Spaccapelo R, Tonnetti L, Mosci P, Enssle K-H, Puccetti P, Romani L, Bistoni F. T helper cell type 1 (Th1)- and Th2-like responses are present in mice with gastric candidiasis but protective immunity is associated with Th1 development. J. Infect. Dis. 1995; 171:1279-1288.

517. Romani L, Mencacci A, Grohmann U, Mocci S, Mosci P, Puccetti P, Bistoni F. Neutralizing antibody to interleukin 4 induces systemic protection of T helper type 1-associated immunity in murine candidiasis. J. Exp. Med. 1992; 176:19-25.

518. Romani L, Puccetti P, Mencacci A, Cenci E, Spaccapelo R, Tonnetti L, Grohmann U, Bistoni F. Neutralization of IL-10 up-regulates nitric oxide production and protects susceptible mice from challenge with *Candida albicans*. J. Immunol. 1994; 152:3514-3521.

519. Spaccapelo R, Romani L, Tonnetti L, Cenci E, Mencacci A, Del Sero G, Tognellini R, Reed S, Puccetti P, Bistoni F. TGF-β is important in determining the in vivo patterns of susceptibility or resistance in mice infected with *Candida albicans*. J. Immunol. 1995; 155:1349-1360.

520. Romani L, Bistoni F, Mencacci A, Cenci E, Spaccapelo R, Puccetti P. IL-12 in *Candida albicans* infection. Res. Immunol. 1995; 146:532-538.

521. Romani L, Howard DH. Mechanisms of resistance to fungal infections. Curr. Opin. Immunol. 1995; 7:517-523.

522. Kurup VP, Seymour BWP, Choi H, Coffman RL. Particulate *Aspergillus fumigatus* antigens elicit a Th2 response in BALB/c mice. J. Allergy Clin. Immunol. 1994; 93:1013-1020.

523. Knutsen AP, Mueller KR, Levine AD, Choudan B, Hutcheson PS, Slavin RG. Asp f I CD4+ Th2-like T-cell lines in allergic bronchopulmonary aspergillosis. J. Allergy Clin. Immunol. 1994; 94:215-221.

524. Walker C, Bauer W, Braun RK, Menz G, Braun P, Schwartz F, Hansel TT, Villiger B. Activated T cells and cytokines in bronchoalveolar lavage from patients with lung diseases associated with eosinophilia. Am. J. Respir. Crit. Med. Care 1994; 150:1038-1048.

525. Biron CA. Cytokines in the generation of immune responses to, and resolution of, virus infection. Curr. Opin. Immunol. 1994; 6:530-538.

526. Pestka S, Langer JA, Zoon KC, Samuel CE. Interferons and their actions. Ann. Rev. Biochem. 1987; 56:727-777.

527. Lee S, Aggarwal BB, Rinderknecht C, Assisi F, Chiu H. The synergistic antiproliferative effect of γ-interferon and human lymphotoxin. J. Immunol. 1984; 133:1083-1086.

528. Coutelier J-P, van der Logt JRM, Heessen FWA, Warnier G, Snick JV. IgG2a restriction of murine antibodies elicited by viral infections. J. Exp. Med. 1987; 165:64-69.

529. Skeen MJ, Miller MA, Shinnick TM, Ziegler HK. Regulation of murine macrophage IL-12 production. Activation of macrophages in vivo, restimulation in vitro, and modulation by other cytokines. J. Immunol. 1996; 156:1196-1206.

530. Bi Z, Quandt P, Komatsu T, Barna M, Reiss CS. IL-12 promotes enhanced recovery from vescicular stomatitis virus infection of the central nervous system. J. Immunol. 1995; 155:5684-5689.

531. Orange JS, Biron CA. An absolute and restricted requirement for IL-12 in natural killer cell IFN-γ production and antiviral defense. J. Immunol. 1996; 156:1138-1142.

532. Wesselingh SL, Levine B, Fox JR, Choi S, Griffin DE. Intracerebral cytokine mRNA expression during fatal and nonfatal alphavirus encephalitis suggests a predominant type 2 T cell response. J. Immunol. 1994; 152:1289-1297.

533. Jonjic S, Mutter W, Wieland F, Reddehase MJ, Koszinowski UH. Site-restricted persistent cytomegalovirus infection after selective long-term depletion of CD4+ T lymphocytes. J. Exp. Med. 1989; 169:1199-1212.

534. Leist TP, Eppler M, Zinkernagel RM. Enhanced virus replication and inhibition of lymphocytic choriomeningitis virus disease in antigamma-interferon-treated mice. J. Virol. 1989; 63:2813-2819.

535. Orange JS, Wolf SF, Biron CA. Effects of IL-12 on the response and susceptibility to experimental viral infections. J. Immunol. 1994; 152:1253-1264.

536. Orange JS, Salazar-Mather TP, Opal SM, Spencer RL, Miller AH, McEwen BS, Biron CA. Mechanism of interleukin-12-mediated toxicities during experimental viral infections: role of tumor necrosis factor and glucocorticoids. J. Exp. Med. 1995; 181:901-914.

537. Biron AC, Orange JS. IL-12 in acute viral infectious disease. Res. Immunol. 1995; 146:590-597.

538. Newell CK, Martin S, Sendele C, Merchadal M, Rouse BT. Herpes simplex virus-induced stromal keratitis: role of T lymphocyte subsets in immunopathology. J. Virol. 1989; 2:769-775.

539. Niematolski MG, Rouse BT. Phenotypic and functional studies on ocular T cells during herpetic infections of the eyes. J. Immunol. 1992; 148:1864-1870.

540. Niematolski MG, Rouse BT. Predominance of Th1 cells in ocular tissues during herpetic stromal keratitis. J. Immunol. 1992; 149:3035-3039.

541. Hendricks RL, Tumpey TM, Finnegan A. IFN-γ and IL-2 are protective in the skin but pathologic in the corneas of HSV-1-infected mice. J. Immunol. 1992; 149:3023-3028.

542. Jayaraman S, Heiligenhaus A, Rodriguez A, Soukiasan S, Dorf ME, Foster CS. Exacerbation of murine herpes simplex virus-mediated stromal keratitis by Th2 type T cells. J. Immunol. 1993; 151:5777-5789.

543. Babu JS, Kanangat S, Rouse BT. T cell cytokine mRNA expression during the course of the immunopathologic ocular disease herpetic stromal keratitis. J. Immunol. 1995; 154:4822-4829.

544. Kanangat S, Thomas J, Gangappa S, Babu JS, Rouse BT. Herpes simplex virus type 1-mediated up-regulation of IL-12 (p40) mRNA expression. J. Immunol. 1996; 156:1110-1116.

545. Spruance SL, Evans TG, McKeough MB, Thai L, Araneo BA, Daynes RA, Mishkin EM, Abramovitz AS. Th1/Th2-like immunity and resistance to herpes simplex labialis. Antiviral Res. 1995; 28:39-55.

546. Allan W, Tabi Z, Cleary A, Doherty PC. Cellular events in the lymph node and lung of mice with influenza: consequences of depleting CD4+ T cells. J. Immunol. 1990; 144:3980-3986.

547. Eichelberger M, Allan W, Zijstra M, Jaenisch R, Doherty PC. Clearance of influenza virus respiratory infection in mice lacking class I major histocompatibility complex-restricted T cells have delayed viral clearance and increased mortality after influenza virus challenge. J. Exp. Med. 1991; 174:875-880.

548. Allan W, Carding SR, Eichelberger M, Doherty PC. Hsp65 mRNA+ macrophages and γδT cells in influenza virus-infected mice depleted of the CD4+ lymphocyte subsets. Microb. Pathog. 1993; 14; 75-84.

549. Carding SR, Allan W, McMickle A, Doherty P. Activation of cytokine genes in T cells during primary and secondary murine influenza pneumonia. J. Exp. Med. 1993; 177:475-482.

550. Sarawar SR, Sangster M, Coffman RL, Doherty PC. Administration of anti-IFN-γ antibody to β2-microglobulin-deficient mice delays influenza virus clearance but does not switch the response to a T helper cell 2 phenotype. J. Immunol. 1994; 153:1246-1253.

551. Graham MB, Dalton DK, Giltinan D, Braciale VL, Stewart TA, Braciale TJ. Response to influenza infection in mice with a targeted disruption in the interferon γ gene. J. Exp. Med. 1993; 178:1725-1732.

552. Graham MB, Braciale VL, Braciale TJ. Influenza virus-specific CD4+ T helper type 2 T lymphocytes do not promote recovery from experimental virus infection. J. Exp. Med. 1994; 180:1273-1282.

553. Tamura S-i, Miyata K, Matsuo K, Asanuma H, Tekahashi H, Nakajima K, Suzuki Y, Aizawa C, Kurata T. Acceleration of influenza virus clearance by Th1 cells in the nasal site of mice immunized intranasally with adjuvant-combined recombinant nucleoprotein. J. Immunol. 1996; 156:3892-3900.

554. Graham BS, Bunton LA, Wright PF, Karzon DT. Role of T lymphocyte subsets in the pathogenesis of primary infection and rechallenge with respiratory synctytial virus in mice. J. Clin. Invest. 1991; 88:1026-1033.

555. Graham BS, Henderson GS, Tang Y-W, Lu X, Neuzil KM, Colley DC. Priming immunization determines T helper cytokine mRNA expression patterns in lungs of mice challenged with respiratory synctytial virus. J. Immunol. 1993; 151:2032-2040.

556. Alwan WH, Record FM, Openshaw JM. Phenotypic and functional characterization of T cell lines specific for individual respiratory synctytial virus proteins. J. Exp. Med. 1993; 150:5211-5218.

557. Alwan WH, Kozlowska WJ, Openshaw PJM. Distinct types of lung disease caused by functional subsets of antiviral T cells. J. Exp. Med. 1994; 179:81-89.

558. Tang Y-W, Graham BS. Anti-IL-4 treatment at immunization modulates cytokine expression, reduces illness, and increases cytotoxic T lymphocyte activity in mice challenged with respiratory synctytial virus. J. Clin. Invest. 1994; 94:1953-1958.

559. Connors M, Giese NA, Kulkarni AB, Firestone C-Y, Morse HC, Murphy BR. Enhanced pulmonary histopathology induced by respiratory synctytial virus (RSV) challenge of formalin-inactivated RSV-immunized BALB/c mice is abrogated by depletion of interleukin-4 (IL-4) and IL-10. J. Virol. 1994; 68:5321-5325.

560. Panuska JR, Merolla R, Rebert NA, Hoffmann SP, Tsivitse P, Cirino NM, Silverman RH, Rankin JA. Respiratory synctytial virus induces interleukin-10 by human alveolar macrophages. Suppression of early cytokine production and implications for incomplete immunity. J. Clin. Invest. 1995; 96:2445-2453.

561. Finke D, Brinckmann UG, ter Meulen V, Liebert UG. Gamma interferon is a major mediator of antiviral defense in experimental measles virus-induced encephalitis. J. Virol. 1995; 69:5469-5474.

562. Von Pirquet C. Verhalten der kutanen Tuberkulin-Rektion während der Masern. Dtsch. Med. Wochenschr. 1908; 34:1297-1300.

563. Tamashiro VG, Perez HH, Griffin DE. Prospective study of the magnitude and duration of changes in tuberculin reactivity during complicated and uncomplicated measles. Pediatr. Infect. Dis. J. 1987; 6:451-454.

564. Brody JA, McAlister R. Depression of the tuberculin sensitivity following measles vaccination. Am. Rev. Resp. Dis. 1964; 90:607-611.

565. Munyer TP, Mangi RJ, Dolan T, Kantor FS. Depressed lymphocyte function after measles-mumps-rubella vaccination. J. Infect. Dis. 1975; 132:75-78.

566. Hirsch RL, Mokhtarian F, Griffin DE, Brooks BR, Hess J, Johnson RT. Measles virus vaccination of measles seropositive individuals suppress lymphocyte proliferation and chemotactic factor production. Clin Immunol. Immunopathol. 1981; 21:341-350.

567. Fireman P, Friday G, Kumate J. Effect of measles virus vaccine on immunologic responsiveness. Pediatrics 1969; 43:264-272.

568. Van Binnendijk RS, Poelen MCM, Kuijpers KC, Osterhaus ADME, Uytdehaag FGCM. The predominance of CD8+ T cells after infection with measles virus suggests a role for CD8+ class I MHC-restricted cytotoxic T lymphocytes (CTL) in recovery from measles. J. Immunol. 1990; 144:2394-2399.

569. Griffin DE, Cooper SJ, Hirsch RL, Johnson RT, Lindo de Soriano I, Roedenbeck S, Vaisberg A. Changes in plasma IgE levels during complicated and uncomplicated measles virus infection. J. Allergy Clin. Immunol. 1985; 76:206-213.

570. Ward BJ, Johnson RT, Vaisberg A, Jauregui E, Griffin DE. Cytokine production in vitro and the lymphoproliferative defect of natural measles virus infection. Clin. Immunol. Immunopathol. 1991; 61:236-248.

571. Nelson JD, Sandusky G, Peck FB. Measles skin test and serologic response to intradermal measles antigen. JAMA 1966; 198:185-186.

572. Greenstein JI, McFarland HF. Response of human lymphocytes to measles virus after natural infection. Infect. Immun. 1983; 40:198-204.

573. Griffin DE, Ward BJ. Differential CD4 T cell activation in measles. J. Infect. Dis. 1993; 168:275-281.

574. Romagnani S, Del Prete GF, Maggi E, Chilosi M, Caligaris-Cappio F, Pizzolo G. CD30 and type 2 helper (Th2) responses. J. Leukoc. Biol. 1995; 57:726-730.

575. Ward BJ, Griffin DE. Changes in cytokine production after measles virus vaccination: predominant production of IL-4 suggests induction of a Th2 response. Clin. Immunol. Immunopathol. 1993; 2:171-177.

576. Trinchieri G. Interleukin-12. Proc. IV Intern. Conf. on Cytokines. Florence 1996 (Abstr.).

577. Chisari FV, Ferrari C. Hepatitis B virus immunopathogenesis. Annu. Rev. Immunol. 1995; 13:29-60.

578. Simmonds P. Variability of hepatitis C virus. Hepatology 1995; 21:570-581.

579. Milich DR, Peterson DL, Schodel F, Jones JE, Hughes JL. Preferential recognition of hepatitis nucleocapside antigens by Th1 or Th2 cells is epitope and major histocompatibility complex dependent. J. Virol. 1995; 69:2776-2785.

580. Milich DR, Schodel F, Peterson DL, Jones JE, Hughes JL. Characterization of self-reactive T cells that evade tolerance in hepatitis B e antigen transgenic mice. Eur. J. Immunol. 1995; 25:1663-1672.

581. Milich DR, Wolf SF, Hughes JL, Jones JE. Interleukin 12 suppresses autoantibody production by reversing helper T-cell phenotype in hepatitis B e antigen transgenic mice. Proc. Natl. Acad. Sci. USA 1995; 92:6847-6851.

582. Maruyama T, McLachlan A, Iino S, Koike K, Kurokawa K, Milich DR. The serology of chronic hepatitis B infection revisited. J. Clin. Invest. 1993; 91:2586-2595.

583. Maruyama T, Schodel F, Iino S, Koike K, Yasuka K, Peterson D, Milich DR. Distinguishing between acute and symptomatic chronic hepatitis B virus infection. Gastroenterology 1994; 106:1006-1015.

584. Barnaba V, Franco A, Paroli M, Benvenuto R, De Petrillo G, Burgio VL, Santilio I, Balsano C, Bonavita MS, Cappelli G, Colizzi G, Cutrona G, Ferrarini M. Selective expansion of cytotoxic T lymphocytes with a CD4⁺CD56⁺ surface phenotype and a T helper type 1 profile of cytokine secretion in the liver of patients chronically infected with hepatitis B virus. J. Immunol. 1994; 152:3074-3087.

585. Bertoletti A, D'Elios MM, De Carli M, Zignego AL, Durazzo M, Boni C, Missale G, Penna A, Fiaccadori F, Del Prete G-F, Ferrari C. Different cytokine profiles of liver-derived T cell clones in chronic hepatitis B and hepatitis C virus infection. Gastroenterology 1996; (in press).

586. Morse HC, Chattopadhyay SK, Makin M, Fredrikson TN, Hugin AW, Hartley JW. Retrovirus-induced immunodeficiency in the mouse: MAIDS as a model for AIDS. AIDS 1992; 6:607-621.

587. Gazzinelli RT, Makino M, Chattopadhyay SK, Snapper CM, Sher A, Hugin AW, Morse HC. CD4⁺ subset regulation in viral infection: preferential activation of Th2 cells during progression of retrovirus-induced immunodeficiency in mice. J. Immunol. 1992; 148:182-188.

588. Uheara S, Hitoshi Y, Numata F, Makino M, Howard M, Mizuochi T, Takatsu K. An IFN-γ-dependent pathway plays a critical role in the pathogenesis of

murine immunodeficiency syndrome induced by LP-BM5 murine leukemia virus. Int. Immunol. 1994; 6:1937-1947.

589. Morawetz RA, Doherty TM, Giese NA, Hartley JW, Muller W, Kuhn R, Rajewski K, Coffman RL, Morse HC. Resistance to murine acquired immunodeficiency syndrome (MAIDS). Science 1994; 265:265-267.

590. Morse HC, Giese N, Morawetz R, Gazzinelli R, Tang Y, Kim WK, Chattopadhyay S, Hartley JW. Cells and cytokines in the pathogenesis of MAIDS, a retrovirus-induced immunodeficiency syndrome of mice. Springer Semin. Immunopathol. 1995; 17:231-245.

591. Giese NA, Gazzinelli RT, Morawetz RA, Morse HC. Role of IL-12 in MAIDS. Res. Immunol. 1995; 146:600-604.

592. Gazzinelli RT, Giese NA, Morse HC. In vivo treatment with interleukin 12 protects mice from immune abnormalities observed during murine acquired immunodeficiency syndrome (MAIDS). J. Exp. Med. 1994; 180:2199-2208.

593. Faxvaag A, Espevik T, Dalen A. An immunosuppressive murine leukaemia virus induces a Th1—Th2 switch and abrogates the IgM antibody response to sheep erythrocytes by suppressing the production of IL-2. Clin. Exp. Immunol. 1995; 102:487-495.

594. Pantaleo G, Graziosi C, Fauci AS. The immunopathogenesis of human immunodeficiency virus infection. N. Engl. J. Med. 1993; 328:327-335.

595. Clerici M, Shearer GM. A Th1/Th2 switch is a critical step in the etiology of HIV infection. Immunol. Today 1993; 14:107-111.

596. Clerici M, Giogi JV, Chou C-C, Gudeman VK, Zack JA, Gupta P, Ho H-N, Nishanian PG, Berzofski JA, Shearer GM. Cell-mediated immune response to human immunodeficiency virus (HIV) type 1 in seronegative homosexual men with recent exposure to HIV. J. Infect. Dis. 1992; 165:1012-1019.

597. Clerici M, Hakim FT, Venzon DJ, Blatt S, Hendrix CV, Wynn TA, Shearer GM. Changes in interleukin-2 and interleukin-4 production in asymptomatic, human immunodeficiency virus-seropositive individuals. J. Clin. Invest. 1993; 91:759-765.

598. Clerici M, Lucey DR, Berzofsky JA, Pinto LA, Wynn TA, Blatt SP, Dolan MJ, Hendrix CW, Wolf SF, Shearer GM. Restoration of HIV-specific cell-mediated immune responses by interleukin-12 in vitro. Science 1993; 262:1721-1724.

599. Clerici M, Wynn TA, Berzofsky JA, Blatt SP, Hendrix CV, Sher CW, Coffman RL, Shearer GM. Role of interleukin-10 in T helper cell dysfunction in asymptomatic individuals infected with the human immunodeficiency virus. J. Clin. Invest. 1994; 93:768-775.

600. Collette Y, Chang H-L, Cerdan C, Chambost H, Algarte M, Mawas C, Imbert J, Burny A, Olive D. Specific Th1 cytokine down-regulation associated with primary clinically derived human immunodeficiency virus type 1 Nef gene-induced expression. J. Immunol. 1996; 156:360-370.

601. Graziosi C, Pantaleo G, Gantt KR, Fortin J-P, Demarest JF, Cohen OJ, Sekaly RP, Fauci AS. Lack of evidence for the dichotomy of Th1 and Th2 predominance in HIV-infected individuals. Science 1994; 265:248-252.

602. Fan J, Bass HZ, Fahey JL. Elevated IFN-γ and decreased IL-2 gene expression are associated with HIV infection. J. Immunol. 1993; 151:5031-5040.

603. Emilie D, Fior R, Llorente L et al. Cytokines from lymphoid organs of HIV-infected patients: production and role in the immune disequilibrium of the disease and in the development of B lymphomas. Immunol. Rev. 1994; 140:5-28.

604. Maggi E, Macchia D, Parronchi P, Mazzetti M, Ravina A, Milo D, Romagnani S. Reduced production of interleukin-2 and interferon-gamma and enhanced

helper activity for IgG synthesis by cloned CD4+ T cells from patients with AIDS. Eur. J. Immunol. 1987; 17:1685-1690.

605. Maggi E, Mazzetti M, Ravina A et al. Ability of HIV to promote a Th1 to Th0 shift and to replicate preferentially in Th2 and Th0 cells. Science 1994; 265:248-252.

606. Seder RA, Grabstein KH, Berzofsky JA, McDyer JF. Cytokine interactions in human immunodeficiency virus-infected individuals: roles of interleukin (IL)-2, IL-12, and IL-15. J. Exp. Med. 1995; 182:1067-1078.

607. Estaquier J, Idziorek T, Zou W, Emilie D, Farber C-M, Bourez J-M, Ameisen JC. T helper type 1/T helper type 2 cytokines and T cell death: preventive effects of interleukin 12 on activation-induced and CD95 (FAS/APO 1)-mediated apoptosis of CD4+ T cells from human immunodeficiency virus-infected persons. J. Exp. Med. 1995; 182:1759-1767.

608. Hyjek E, Lischner HW, Hyslop T, Bartkowiak J, Kubin M, Trinchieri G, Kozbor D. Cytokine patterns during progression to AIDS in children with perinatal HIV infection. J. Immunol. 1995; 155:4060-4071.

609. Meyaard L, Otto SA, Keet IPM, van Lier RAW, Miedema F. Changes in cytokine secretion patterns of CD4+ T cell clones in human immunodeficiency virus infection. Blood 1994; 34:4262-4268.

610. Romagnani S, Maggi E, Del Prete G-F et al. Role for Th1/Th2 cytokines in HIV infection. Immunol. Rev. 1994; 140:73-92.

611. Romagnani S, Maggi E. Th1 versus Th2 responses in AIDS. Curr. Opin. Immunol. 1994; 6:616-622.

612. Romagnani S, Maggi E, Del Prete GF. An alternative view of the Th1/Th2 switch hypothesis in HIV infection. AIDS Res. Human Retrov. 1994; 10:iii-ix.

613. Poli G, Fauci AS. The effect of cytokines and pharmacologic agents on chronic HIV infection. AIDS Res. Human Retrov. 1992; 8:191-197.

614. Chehimi J, Star SE, Frank I, D'Andrea A, Ma X, MacGregor RR, Sonnelier J, Trinchieri G. Impaired interleukin-12 production in human immunodeficiency virus-infected patients. J. Exp. Med. 1994; 179:1361-1366.

615. Paganin C, Frank I, Trinchieri G. Priming for high interferon-γ production induced by interleukin-12 in both CD4+ and CD8+ T cell clones from HIV-infected patients. J. Clin. Invest. 1995; 96:1677-1682.

616. Gendelman HE, Friedman RM, Joe S, Baca LM, Turpin JA, Dvekster G, Meltzer MS, Dieffenbach C. A selective defect of interferon-α production in human immunodeficiency virus-infected monocytes. J. Exp. Med. 1990; 172:1433-1438.

617. Vyakarnam A. Mechanisms for an opposite role for Th1/Th2 cells in AIDS. Res. Immunol. 1994; 145:618-624.

618. Israel-Biet D, Labrousse F, Tourani J-M, Sors H, Andrieu J-M, Even P. Elevation of IgE in HIV-infected subjects: a marker of poor prognosis. J. Allergy Clin. Immunol. 1992; 89:68-75.

619. Viganò A, Principi N, Crupi L, Onorato J, Vincenzo ZG, Salvaggio A. Elevation of IgE in HIV-infected children and its correlation with the progression of disease. J. Allergy Clin. Immunol. 1995; 95:627-632.

620. Bentwich Z, Kalinkovic A, Weisman Z. Immune activation is a dominant factor in the pathogenesis of African AIDS. Immunol. Today 1995; 16:187-191.

621. Poli G, Kinter AL, Justement JS, Kerhl JH, Bressler P, Stanley S, Fauci AS. Tumor necrosis factor alpha functions in an autocrine manner in the induction of human immunodeficiency virus expression. Proc. Natl. Acad. Sci. USA 1990; 87:782-786.

622. Montaner LJ, Doyle AG, Collin M, Georges H, James W, Minty A, Caput D, Ferrara P, Gordon S. Interleukin 13 inhibits human immunodeficiency virus type 1 production in primary blood-derived human macrophages in vitro. J. Exp. Med. 1993; 178:743-747.

623. Kinter AL, Poli G, Fox L, Hardy E, Fauci AS. HIV replication in IL-2-stimulated peripheral blood mononuclear cells is driven in an autocrine/paracrine manner by endogenous cytokines. J. Immunol. 1995; 154:2448-2459.

624. Biswas P, Poli G, Kinter AL, Justement JS, Stanley SK, Maury WJ, Bressler P, Orenstein JM, Fauci AS. Interferon-gamma induces the expression of human immunodeficiency virus in persistently infected promonocytic cells (U1) and redirects the production of virions to intracytoplasmic vacuoles in phorbol myristate acetate-differentiated U1 cells. J. Exp. Med. 1992; 176:739-750.

625. Schuitemaker H, Koostra NA, Koppelman MH, Bruisten SM, Huisman HG, Tersmette M, Miedema F. Proliferation-dependent HIV-1 infection of monocytes occurs during differentiation into macrophages. J. Clin. Invest. 1992; 89:1154-1160.

626. Foli A, Saville MW, Baseler MW, Yarchoan R. Effects of the Th1 and Th2 stimulatory cytokines interleukin-12 and interleukin-4 on human immunodeficiency virus replication. Blood 1995; 85:2114-2123.

627. Weissman D, Poli G, Fauci AS. Interleukin-10 blocks HIV replication in macrophages by inhibiting the autocrine loop of tumor necrosis factor α and interleukin 6 induction of virus. AIDS Res. Human Retrov. 1994; 10:1199-1206.

628. Barker E, Mackewicz CE, Levy JA. Effects of Th1 and Th2 cytokines on CD8+ cell response against human immunodeficiency virus: implications for long-term survival. Proc. Natl. Acad. Sci. USA 1995; 92:11135-11139.

629. Pizzolo G, Vinante F, Morosato L et al. High serum levels of the soluble form of CD30 molecule in the early phase of HIV-1 infection as an independent predictor of progression to AIDS. AIDS 1994; 8:741-745.

630. Biswas P, Smith CA, Goletti D, Hardy EC, Jackson RW, Fauci AS. Cross-linking of CD30 induces HIV expression in chronically infected T cells. Immunity 1995; 2:587-596.

631. Maggi E, Annunziato F, Manetti R, Biagiotti R, Giudizi M-G, Ravina A, Almerigogna F, Boiani N, Anderson M, Romagnani S. Activation of HIV expression by CD30 triggering in CD4+ cells from HIV-infected individuals. Immunity 1995; 3:251-255.

632. Groux H, Torpier G, Monthé D, Mounton Y, Capron A, Ameisen JC. Activation-induced death by apoptosis in CD4+ T cells from human immunodeficiency virus-infected asymptomatic individuals. J. Exp. Med. 1992; 175:331-340.

633. Meyaard L, Otto SA, Jonker RR, Mijnster MJ, Keet RPM, Miedema F. Programmed death of T cells in HIV-1 infection. Science 1992; 257:217-219.

634. Lewis DE, Ng Tang DS, Adu-Oppong A, Schober W, Rodgers JR. Anergy and apoptosis in CD8+ T cells from HIV-infected persons. J. Immunol. 1994; 153:412-420.

635. Meyaard L, Otto SA, Keet IPM, Roos MTL, Miedema F. Programmed death of T cells in human immunodeficiency virus infection. J. Clin. Invest. 1994; 93:982-988.

636. Katsikis PD, Wunderlich ES, Smith CA, Herzenberg LA, Herzenberg LA. Fas antigen stimulation induces marked apoptosis of T lymphocytes in human immunodeficiency virus-infected individuals. J. Exp. Med. 1995; 181:2029-2036.

637. Hahn S, Stalder T, Wernli M, Burgin D, Tschopp J, Nagata S, Erb P. Down-modulation of CD4⁺ T helper type 2 and type 0 cells by T helper type 1 via Fas/Fas-ligand interaction. Eur. J. Immunol. 1995; 25:2679-2685.

638. Clerici M, Sarin A, Coffman RL, Wynn TA, Blatt SP, Hendrix CW, Wolf SF, Shearer GM, Henkart PA. Type1/type2 cytokine modulation of T-cell programmed death as a model for HIV pathogenesis. Proc. Natl. Acad. Sci. USA 1994; 91:11811-11815.

639. Oyaizu N, Pahwa S. Role of apoptosis in HIV disease pathogenesis. J. Clin. Immunol. 1995; 15:217-231.

640. Finkelman FD, Pearce EJ, Urban JFJr, Sher A. Regulation and biological function of helminth-induced cytokine responses. Immunoparasitol. Today 1991; 12: A62-66.

641. Butterwoth AE. Cell-mediated damage to helminths. Adv. Parasitol. 1984; 23:143-235.

642. Capron A, Dessaint JP, Capron M, Ouma JH, Butterwoth AE. Immunity to schistosomes: progress toward vaccine. Science 1987; 238:1965-1972.

643. Capron M, Capron A. Immunoglobulin E and effector cells in Schistosomiasis. Science 1994; 264:1876-1877.

644. Sher A, Gazzinelli RT, Oswald IP et al. Role of T cell derived cytokines in the downregulation of immune responses in parasitic and retroviral infection. Immunol. Rev. 1992; 127:183-204.

645. Urban JF, Maliszewski CR, Madden KB, Katona IM, Finkelman FD. IL-4 treatment can cure established gastrointestinal nematode infections in immunocompetent and immunodeficient mice. J. Immunol. 1995; 154:4675-4684.

646. Sher A, Coffman RL, Hieny S, Cheever AW. Ablation of eosinophil and IgE responses with anti-IL-5 or anti-IL-4 antibodies fails to affect immunity against *Schistosoma mansonii* in the mouse. J. Immunol. 1990; 145:3911-3916.

647. Sher A, Coffman RL. Regulation of immunity to parasites by T cells and T cell-derived cytokines. Ann. Rev. Immunol. 1992; 10:385-409.

648. Grzych JM, Pierce EJ, Cheever A, Caulada ZA, Caspar P, Hieny S, Lewis F, Sher A. Egg deposition is the major stimulus for the production of Th2 cytokines in murine schistosomiasis mansoni. J. Immunol. 1991; 146:1322-1327.

649. Pierce EJ, Caspar P, Grzych J-M, Lewis FA, Sher A. Downregulation of Th1 cytokine production accompanies induction of Th2 responses by a parasitic helminth, *Schistosoma mansoni*. J. Exp. Med. 1991; 173:159-166.

650. Wynn TA, Eltoum I, Cheever AW, Lewis FA, Gause WC, Sher A. Analysis of cytokine mRNA expression during primary granuloma formation induced by eggs of *Schistosoma mansoni*. J. Immunol. 1993; 151:1430-1440.

651. Chensue SW, Terebuh PD, Warmington KS, Hershey SD, Evanoff HL, Kunkel SL, Higashi GI. Role of interleukin 4 and gamma-interferon in *Schistosoma mansoni* egg-induced hypersensitivity granuloma formation: orchestration, relative contribution and relationshp to macrophage function. J. Immunol. 1992; 148:900-906.

652. Cheever AW, Williams ME, Wynn TA, Finkelman FD, Seder RA, Cox TM, Hieny S, Caspar P, Sher A. Anti-IL-4 treatment of *Schistosoma mansoni*-infected mice inhibits development of T cells and non-B, non-T cells expressing Th2 cytokines while decreasing egg-induced hepatic fibrosis. J. Immunol. 1994; 153:753-759.

653. Amiri P, Locksley RM, Parslow TG, Sadick M, Rector E, Ritter D, McKerrow JH. Tumor necrosis alpha restores granulomas and induces parasite egg-laying in schistosome-infected SCID mice. Nature 1992; 365:604-607.

654. Joseph AL, Boros DL. Tumor necrosis factor plays a role in *Schistosoma mansoni* egg-induced granulomatous inflammation. J. Immunol. 1993; 151:5461-5471.

655. Cheever AW, Finkelman FD, Caspar P, Heiny S, Macedonia JG, Sher A. Treatment with anti-IL-2 antibodies reduces hepatic pathology and eosinophilia in *Schistosoma mansoni*-infected mice while selectively inhibiting T cell IL-5 production. J. Immunol. 1992; 148:3244-3248.

656. Cheever AW, Xu Y, Sher A, Finkelman FD, Cox TM, Macedonia JG. *Schistosoma japonicum*-infected mice show reduced hepatic fibrosis and eosinophilia and selective inhibition of interleukin 5 secretion by CD4⁺ cells after treatment with anti-IL-2 antibodies. Infect. Immun. 1993; 61:1288-1292.

657. Chensue SW, Warmington KS, Ruth J, Lincoln OM, Kunkel SL. Cross-regulatory role of interferon-gamma (IFN-γ), IL-4 and IL-10 in schistosome egg granuloma formation: in vivo regulation of Th activity and inflammation. Clin. Exp. Immunol. 1994; 98:395-400.

658. Wynn TA, Eltoum I, Oswald IP, Cheever AW, Sher A. Endogenous interleukin 12 (IL-12) regulates granuloma formation induced by eggs of *Schistosoma mansoni* and exogenous IL-12 both inhibits and prophylactically immunizes against egg pathology. J. Exp. Med. 1994; 179:1551-1561.

659. Wynn TA, Cheever AW, Jankovic D, Pointdexter RW, Caspar P, Lewis FA, Sher A. An IL-12-based vaccination method for preventing fibrosis induced by schistosome infection. Nature 1995; 376:594-596.

660. Wynn TA, Jankovic D, Hieny S, Cheever AW, Sher A. IL-12 enhances vaccine-induced immunity to *Schistosoma mansoni* in mice and decreases T helper 2 cytokine expression, IgE production, and tissue eosinophilia. J. Immunol. 1995; 154:4701-4709.

661. Chensue SW, Bienkowski M, Eessalu TE, Warmington KS, Hershey SD, Lukacs NW, Kunkel SL. Endogenous IL-1 receptor antagonist protein (IRAP) regulates schistosome egg granuloma formation and the regional lymphoid response. J. Immunol. 1993; 151:3654-3662.

662. Sabin EA, Pearce EJ. Early IL-4 production by non-CD4⁺ cells at the site of antigen deposition predicts the development of a T helper 2 cell response to *Schistosoma mansoni* eggs. J. Immunol. 1995; 155:4844-4853.

663. Velupillai P, Harn DA. Oligosaccharide-specific induction of interleukin-10 production by B220⁺ cells from *Schistosoma*-infected mice: a mechanism for regulation of CD4⁺ T-cell subsets. Proc. Natl. Acad. Sci. USA 1994; 91:18-22.

664. Jankovic D, Aslund L, Oswald IP, Caspar P, Champion C, Pearce E, Colligan JE, Strand M, Sher A, James SL. Calpain is the target antigen of a Th1 clone that transfers protective immunity against *Schistosoma mansoni*. J. Immunol. 1996; 157:806-814.

665. Hagan P, Blumenthal UJ, Dunne D, Simpson AJG, Wilkins HA. Human IgE, IgG4 and resistance to reinfection with *Schistosoma haematobium*. Nature 1991:349:243-245.

666. Rihet P, Demeure C, Burgois A, Prata A, Dessein AJ. Evidence for an association between human resistance to *Schistosoma mansoni* and high anti-larval IgE levels. Eur. J. Immunol. 1991; 21:2679-2686.

667. Dunne DW, Butterworth EE, Fulford JC, Kariuki HC, Langley JG, Ouma JH, Capron A, Pierce RJ, Sturrock RF. Immunity after treatment of human schistosomiasis: association between IgE antibodies to adult worm antigens and resistance to reinfection. Eur. J. Immunol. 1992; 22:1483-1494.

668. Roberts M, Butterworth AE, Kimani G, Kamau T, Fulford AJ, Dunne DW, Ouma JH, Sturrock RF. Immunity after treatment of human schistosomiasis: association between cellular responses and resistance to reinfection. Infect. Immunity 1993; 61:4984-4993.

669. Cuissinier-Paris P, Dessein AJ. *Schistosoma*-specific helper T cell clones from subjects resistant to infection by *Schistosoma mansoni* are Th0/2. Eur. J. Immunol. 1995; 25:2295-2302.

670. Svetic A, Madden KB, Zhou XD, Lu P, Katona IM, Finkelman FD, Urban JF, Gause WC. A primary intestinal helminthic infection rapidly induces a gut-associated elevation of Th2-associated cytokines and IL-3. J. Immunol. 1993; 150:3434-3441.

671. Urban JF, Katona IM, Paul WE, Finkelman FD. Interleukin 4 is important in protective immunity to a gastrointestinal nematode infection in mice. Proc. Natl. Acad. Sci. USA 1991; 88:5513-5517.

672. Finkelman FD, Madden KB, Cheever AW, Katona IM, Morris SC, Gately MK, Hubbard BR, Gause WC, Urban JF. Effects of interleukin 12 on immune responses and host protection in mice infected with intestinal nematose parasites. J. Exp. Med. 1994; 179:1563-1572.

673. Matsuda S, Uchikawa R, Yamada M, Arizono N. Cytokine mRNA expression profiles in rats infected with the intestinal nematode *Nippostrongylus brasiliensis*. Infect. Immunity 1995; 63:4653-4660.

674. Urban JF, Madden KB, Cheever AW, Trotta PP, Katona IM, Finkelman FD. IFN inhibits inflammatory responses and protective immunity in mice infected with the nematode parasite, *Nyppostrongylus brasiliensis*. J. Immunol. 1993; 151:7086-7094.

675. Germann T, Gately MK, Schoenhaut DS, Lohoff M, Mattner F, Fischer S, Jin SC, Schmitt E, Rude E. Interleukin-12/T cell stimulating factor, a cytokine with multiple effects on T helper type 1 (Th1) but not on Th2 cells. Eur. J. Immunol. 1993; 23:1762-1770.

676. King CL, Kumaraswami V, Pointdexter RW, Kumari S, Yayaraman K, Aling DW, Ottesen EA, Nutman TB. Immunologic tolerance in lymphatic filariasis. Diminished parasite-specific T and B lymphocyte precursor frequency in the microfilaremic state. J. Clin. Ivest. 1992; 89:1403-1410.

677. Pearlman E, Kazura JW, Hazlett FE, Boom WH. Modulation of murine cytokine responses to mycobacterial antigens by helminth-induced T helper 2 cell responses. J. Immunol. 1993; 151:4857-4864.

678. Lawrence RA, Allen JE, Osborne J, Maizels RM. Adult and microfilarial stages of the filarial parasite *Brugia malayi* stimulate contrasting cytokine and Ig isotype responses in BALB/c mice. J. Immunol. 1994; 153:1216-1224.

679. Lawrence RA, Allen JE, Gregory WF, Kopf M, Maizels RM. Infection of IL-4-deficient mice with the parasitic nematode *Brugia malayi* demonstrates that host resistance is not dependent on a T helper 2-dominated immune response. J. Immunol. 1995; 154:5995-6001.

680. Mahanthy S, King CL, Kumaraswami V et al. IL-4- and IL-5-secreting lymphocyte populations are preferentially stimulated by parasite-derived antigens in human tissue invasive nematode infections. J. Immunol. 1993; 151:3704-3711.

681. Sanderson CJ. Interleukin-5, eosinophils, and disease. Blood 1992; 79:3101-3109.

682. Lange AM, Yutanawiboonchai W, Scott P, Abraham D. IL-4- and IL-5-dependent protective immunity to *Onchocerca volvulus* infective larvae in BALB/cBYJ mice. J. Immunol. 1994; 153:205-211.

683. Ogilvie BM, De Savigny D. Immune responses to nematodes. In: Cohen S, Warren KS, eds. Immunology of Parasitic Infections. 2nd ed. Oxford: Blackwell Scientific Publications, 1982:715-757.

684. Maizels RM, Kennedy MW, Robertson BD, Smith HV. Shared carbohydrate epitopes of distinct surface and secreted antigens of the parasitic nematode *Toxocara canis*. J. Immunol. 1987; 139:207-214.

685. Mahanthy S, Abrams JS, King CL, Limaye AP, Nutman TB. Parallel regulation of IL-4 and IL-5 in human helminth infections. J. Immunol. 1992; 148:3567-3571.

686. Limaye AP, Abrams JS, Silver JE, Ottesen EA, Nutman TB. Regulation of parasite-induced eosinophilia: selectively increased interleukin-5 production in helminth-infected patients. J. Exp. Med. 1990; 172:399-402.

687. De Carli M, Romagnani S, Del Prete G-F. Human T-cell response to excretory/secretory antigens of *Toxocara canis*. A model of preferential in vitro and in vivo activation of Th2 cells. In: Lewis JW, Maizels RM, eds. *Toxocara* and Toxocariasis: Clinical, Epidemiological and Molecular Perspectives. London, 1993.

688. Ribeiro de Jesus AM, Almeida RP, Bacellar O, Araujo MI, Demeure C, Bina JC, Dessein AJ, Carvalho EM. Correlation between cell-mediated immunity and degreee of infection in subjects living in an endemic area of schistosomiasis. Eur. J. Immunol. 1993; 23:152-158.

689. Hodes RJ. Molecular alterations in the aging immune system. J. Exp. Med. 1995; 182:1-3.

690. Gabriel H, Schmitt B, Kindermann W. Age-related increase of CD45RO⁺ lymphocytes in physically active adults. Eur. J. Immunol. 1993; 23:2704-2706.

691. Dobber R, Tielemans M, Weerd HD, Negelkerken L. Mel14⁺ CD4⁺ T cells from aged mice display functional and phenotypic characteristics of memory cells. Int. Immunol. 1994; 6:1227-1234.

692. Hobbs MV, Weigle WO, Noonan DJ, Torbett BE, McEvilly RJ, Koch RJ, Cardenas GJ, Ernst DN. Patterns of cytokine gene expression by CD4⁺ T cells from young and old mice. J. Immunol. 1993; 150:3602-3614.

693. Ernst DE, Weigle WO, Noonan DJ, McQuitty DN, Hobbs MV. The age-associated increase in IFN-γ synthesis by mouse CD8⁺ T cells correlates with shifts in the frequencies of cell subsets defined by membrane CD44, CD45RB, 3G11, and Mel-14 expression. J. Immunol. 1993; 151:575-587.

694. Engwerda CR, Fox BS, Handwerger BS. Cytokine production by T lymphocytes from young and aged mice. J. Immunol. 1996; 156:3621-3630.

695. Chen N, Gao Q, Field EH. Expansion of memory Th2 cells over Th1 cells in neonatal primed mice. Transplantation 1995; 60:1187-1193.

696. Dobber R, Tielemans M, Nagelkerken L. Enrichment for Th1 cells in the Mel-14⁺ CD4⁺ T cell fraction in aged mice. Cell. Immunol. 1995; 162:321-325.

697. Albright JW, Zuniga-Pflucker JC, Albright JF. Transcriptional control of IL-2 and IL-4 in T cells of young and old mice. Cell. Immunol. 1995; 164:170-175.

698. Danzer R, Kelley KW. Stress and immunity: an integrated view of relationship between the brain and the immune system. Life Sci. 1989; 44:1995-2008.

699. Khansari DN, Murgo JA, Faith RE. Effects of stress on the immune system. Immunol. Today 1990; 11:170-175.

700. Harbuz MS, Chalmers J, De Souza L, Lightman SL. Stress-induced activation of CRF and c-fos mRNAs in the paraventricular nucleus are not affected by serotonin depletion. Brain Res. 1993; 609:167-173.

701. Dhabhar F, Miller AH, McEwen BS, Spencer RL. Effects of stress on immune cell distribution. Dynamics and hormonal mechanisms. J. Immunol. 1994; 154:5511-5527.

702. Sanders VM, Street NE, Fuchs BA. Differential expression of the β2-adrenoreceptor by subsets of T-helper lymphocytes. FASEB J. 1994; 8:A114.

703. Kruszewska B, Felten SY, Moynihan JA. Alterations in cytokine and antibody production following clemical sympathectomy in two strains of mice. J. Immunol. 1995; 155:4613-4620.

704. Maestroni GJ. T-helper-2 lymphocytes as a peripheral target of melatonin. J. Pineal Res. 1995; 18:84-89.

705. Zwilling BS, Brown D, Pearl D. Induction of major histocompatibility complex class II glycoproteins by interferon-gamma: attenuation of the effects of restraint stress. J. Neuroimmunol. 1992; 37:115-122.

706. Bulmer NJ, Johnson PM. Immunohistological characterization of the decidual leucocytic infiltrate related to endometrial gland epithelium in early human pregnancy. Immunology 1885; 55:35-44.

707. Chaouat G, Menu E, Athanassakis I, Wegmann TG. Maternal T cells regulate placental size and fetal survival. Regional Immunol. 1988; 1:143-148.

708. Chaouat G, Menu E, Clark DA, Dy M, Minkovski M, Wegmann TG. Control of survival in CBA X DBA/2 mice by lymphokine therapy. J Reprod Fertil 1990; 89:447-458.

709. Chaouat G. Synergy of lipopolysaccharide and inflammatory cytokines in murine pregnancy. Alloimmunization prevents abortion but does not affect the induction of preterm delivery. Cell Immunol. 1994; 157:328-340.

710. Chaouat G, Assal-Meliani A, Martal J, Raghupathy R, Elliott J, Mosmann T, Wegmann TG. IL-10 prevents naturally occuring fetal loss in the CBA X DBA/2 mating combination and local defect in IL-10 production in this abortion-prone combination is corrected by in vivo injection of IFN t. J. Immunol. 1995; 154:4261-4268.

711. Hill JA, Haimovici F, Anderson DJ. Products of activated lymphocytes and macrophages inhibit mouse embryo development in vitro. J. Immunol. 1987; 132:2250-2254.

712. Haimovici F, Hill JA, Anderson DJ. The effects of soluble products of activated lymphocytes and macrophages on blastocyst implantation events in vitro. Biol. Reprod. 1991; 44:69-75.

713. Berkowitz RS, hill JA, Kurtz CB, Anderson DJ. Effects of products of activated leukocytes (lymphokines and monokines) on the growth of malignant trophoblast cells in vitro. Am. J. Obstet. Gynecol. 1988; 158:199-203.

714. Lin H, Mosmann TR, Guilbert L, Tuntipopipat S, Wegmann TG. Synthesis of T helper 2-type cytokines at maternal-fetal interface. J. Immunol. 1993; 151:4562-4573.

715. Wegmann TG, Lin H, Guilbert L, Mossmann TR. Bidirectional cytokine interactions in the maternal-fetal relationship: is successful pregnancy a Th2 phenomenon? Immunology Today 1993; 14:353-356.

716. Formby B. Immunologic response in pregnancy. Its role in endocrine disorders of pregnancy and influence on the course of maternal auotimmune diseases. Endocrinol. Metab. Clin. North Am. 1995; 24:187-205.

717. Athanassakis I, Vassiliadis S. Effect of IFN-gamma administration in virgin and pregnant mice: distribution of lymphoid and myeloid cells in the spleen. Eur. Cytokine Netw. 1995; 6:167-176.

718. Delassus S, Continho GC, Saucier C, Darche S, Kourilsky P. Differential cytokine expression in maternal blood and placenta during murine gestation. J. Immunol. 1994; 152:2411-2420.

719. Krishnan L, Guilbert LJ, Russell AS, Wegmann TG, Mosmann TR, Belosevic M. Pregnancy impairs resistance of C57BL/6 mice to *Leishmania major* infection and causes decreased antigen-specific IFN-γ responses and increased production of T helper 2 cytokines. J. Immunol. 1996; 156:644-652.

720. Krishnan L, Guilbert LJ, Wegmann T, Belosevic M, Mosmann TR. T helper 1 response against *Leishmania major* in pregnant C57BL/6 mice increases implantation failure and fetal resorptions: correlation with increased IFN-γ and TNF and reduced IL-10 production by placental cells. J. Immunol. 1996; 156:653-662.

721. Mowbry JF. Immunoregulation and fetal survival. In: Gill TJ, Wegmann TG, Nisbet-Brown E, eds. Oxford University Press, 1987:300-308.

722. Da Silva JA, Spector TD. The role of pregnancy in the course and aetiology of rheumatoid arthritis. Clin. Rheumatol. 1992; 11:189-194.

723. Minkoff H, Nanda D, Menez R, Fikrig S. Pregnancies resulting in infants with acquired immunodeficience syndrome or AIDS complex: follow-up of mothers, children and subsequently born siblings. Obstet. Gynecol. 69:288-291.

724. Weber DJ, Wolfson JS, Swartz MN, Hooper DC. Pasteurella multocida infectious. Report of 34 cases and review of the litterature; Medicine Baltimore 1984; 63:133-154.

725. Drutz DJ, Huppert M. Coccidioidomycosis. factors affecting the host-parasite interaction. J. Infect. Dis. 1983; 147:372-390.

726. Watkinson M, Rushton DI. Plasmodial pigmentation of placenta and outcome of pregnancy in West African mothers. Br. Med. J. Clin. Res. 1983; 287:251-254.

727. Jameson EM. Gynecologycal and Obstetrical Tuberculosis. Lea and Febiger 1935.

728. Hill JA, Polgar K, Anderson DJ. T-helper 1-type immunity to trophoblast in women with recurrent spontaneous abortion. JAMA 1995; 2/3:1933-1936.

729. Ito K, Watanebe T, Horie R, Horie M, Shiota S, Wakamura S, Mori S. High expression of the CD30 molecule in human decidual cells. Am. J. Pathol. 1994; 145:276-280.

730. Szekeres-Bartho J. Immunosuppression by progesterone in pregnancy. Bocca Ratton, Ann Arbor, London, Tokyo: CRC Press, 1992.

731. Szekeres-Bartho J, Reznikoff Etievant MF, Varga P, Pichon MF, Varga Z, Chaouat G. Lymphocyte progesterone receptors in normal and pathological human pregnancy. J. Reprod. Immunol. 1989; 16:239-247.

732. White A, Wang MW, King IS, Heap RB. Biotinylated anti-progesterone monoclonal antibodies specifically target the uterine epithelium and block implantation in the mouse. J. Reprod. Immunol. 1992; 21:127-138.

733. Chaouat G, Menu R, Kinski R, David F, Wegmann TG. Immunoregulatory role of the placenta; J. Immunol. Immunopharmacol. 1990; 10:45-50.

734. Bryant-Greenwood GD, Schwabe C. Human relaxins: chemistry and biology. Endocrine Reviews 1994; 15:5-26.

735. Del Prete GF, Tiri A, Maggi E et al. Defective in vitro production of γ-interferon and tumor necrosis factor-α by circulating T cells from patients with the hyper-immunoglobulin E syndrome. J. Clin. Invest. 1989; 84:1830-35.

736. Paganelli R, Scala E, Capobianchi MR, Fanales-Belasio E, D'Offizi G, Fiorilli M, Aiuti F. Selective deficiency of interferon-gamma production in the hyper-IgE syndrome. Relationship to in vitro IgE synthesis. Clin. Exp. Immunol. 1991; 84:28-33.

737. King CL, Gallin JL, Malech HL, Abramson SL, Nutman TB. Regulation of immunoglobulin production in hyperimmunoglobulin E recurrent-infection syndrome by interferon γ. Proc. Natl. Acad. Sci. USA 1989; 86:10085-89.

738. Souillet G, Rousset F, de Vries JE. Alpha-interferon treatment of patient with hyper-IgE syndrome. Lancet 1989; 2:1384-85.

739. Paganelli R, Capobianchi MR, Ensoli B, D'Offizi GP, Facchini J, Dianzani F, Aiuti F. Evidence that defective gamma interferon production in patients with primary immunodeficiencies is due to intrinsic incompetence of lymphocytes. Clin. Exp. Immunol. 1988; 72:124-29.

740. Pastorelli G, Roncarolo M-G, Touraine JL, Peronne G, Tovo PA, de Vries JE. Peripheral blood lymphocytes of patients with common variable immunodeficiency (CVI) produce reduced levels of IL-4, IL-2, and interferon-gamma,

but proliferate normally upon activation with mitogens. Clin. Exp. Immunol. 1989; 78:334-40.

741. Romagnani S. Cytokine action on B cells in disease. In: Callard RE, ed. Cytokines and B Lymphocytes. London: Academic Press, 1990:215-51.

742. Del Prete GF, Maggi E, Parronchi P et al. IL-4 is an essential factor for the IgE synthesis induced in vitro by human T cell clones and their supernatants. J. Immunol. 1988; 140:4193-4198.

743. Jabara HH, Fu SM, Geha RS, Vercelli D. CD40 and IgE: synergism between anti-CD40 monoclonal antibody and interleukin 4 in the induction of IgE synthesis by highly purified human B cells. J. Exp. Med. 1990; 172:1861-1864.

744. Kay AB, Ying S, Varney V, Gaga M, Durham SR, Moqbel R, Wardlaw AJ, Hamid Q. Messenger RNA expression of the cytokine gene cluster interleukin-3 (IL-3), IL-4, IL-5, and granulocyte/macrophage colony-stimulating factor, in allergen-induced late-phase reactions in atopic subjects. J. Exp. Med. 1991; 173:775-778.

745. van der Heijden FL, Wierenga EA, Bos JD, Kapsenberg ML. High frequency of IL-4-producing CD4+ allergen-specific T lymphocytes in atopic dermatitis lesional skin. J. Invest. Dermatol. 1991; 97:389-394.

746. Van Reijsen FC, Bruijnzeel-Koomen CAFM, Kalthoff FS et al. Skin-derived aeroallergen-specific T-cell clones of Th2 phenotype in patients with atopic dermatitis. J. Allergy Clin. Immunol. 1992; 90:184-192.

747. Hamid Q, Azzawi M, Ying S, Moqbel R, Wardlaw AJ, Corrigan CJ, Bradley B, Durham SR, Collins JV, Jeffery PK, Quint DJ, Kay AB. Expression of mRNA for interleukin-5 in mucosal bronchial biopsies from asthma. J. Clin. Invest. 1991; 87:1541-1546.

748. Robinson DS, Hamid Q, Ying S, Tsicopoulos A, Barkans J, Bentley AM, Corrigan CJ, Durham SR, Kay AB. Predominant Th2-like bronchoalveolar T-lymphocyte population in atopic asthma. New Engl. J. Med. 1992; 326:295-304.

749. Del Prete GF, De Carli M, D'Elios MM, Maestrelli P, Ricci M, Fabbri L, Romagnani S: Allergen exposure induces the activation of allergen-specific Th2 cells in the airway mucosa of patients with allergic respiratory disorders. Eur. J. Immunol. 1993; 23:1445-1449.

750. Robinson D, Hamid Q, Bentley A, Ying S, Kay AB, Durham SR. Activation of CD4+ T cells, increased Th2-type cytokine mRNA expression, and eosinophil recruitment in bronchoalveolar lavage after allergen inhalation challenge in patients with atopic asthma. J. Allergy Clin. Immunol. 1993; 92:313-324.

751. Varney VA, Hamid Q, Gaga M, Ying S, Jacobson M, Frew AJ, Kay AB, Durham SR. Influence of grass pollen immunotherapy on cellular infiltration and cytokine mRNA expression during allergen-induced late-phase cutaneous responses. J. Clin. Invest. 1993; 92:644-651.

752. Secrist H, Chelen CJ, Wen Y, Marshall JD, Umetsu DT. Allergen immunotherapy decreases interleukin 4 production in CD4+ T cells from allergic individuals. J. Exp. Med. 1993; 178:2123-2130.

753. Jutel M, Pichler WJ, Skrbic D, Urwyler A, Dahinden C, Muller UR. Bee venom immunotherapy results in decrease of IL-4 and IL-5 and increase of IFN-γ secretion in specific allergen-stimulated T cell cultures. J. Immunol. 1995; 154:4187-4194.

754. McHugh SM, Deighton J, Stewart AG, Lachmann PJ, Ewan PW. Bee venom immunotherapy induces a shift in cytokine responses from a Th2 to a Th1 dominant pattern: comparison of rush and conventional immunotherapy. Clin. Exper. Allergy 1995; 25:828-838.

755. Holt PG, Oliver J, McMenamin C, Bilik N, Kraal G, Thepen T. The antigen presentation functions of lung dendritic cells are downmodulated in situ by soluble mediators from pulmonary alvelolar macrophages J. Exp. Med. 1993. 177:397-402.

756. Parronchi P, De Carli M, Manetti R et al. Aberrant interleukin (IL)-4 and IL-5 production in vitro by CD4⁺ helper T cells from atopic subjects. Eur. J. Immunol. 1992. 22:1615-1620.

757. Piccinni M-P, Beloni L, Giannarini L, Livi C, Scarselli G, Romagnani S, Maggi E. Abnormal production of Th2-type cytokines (IL-4 and IL-5) by T cells from newborns with atopic parents. Eur. J. Immunol. 1996 (in press).

758. Marsh DG, Lockhart A, Holgate ST. The Genetics of Asthma. Oxford: Blackwell Scientific Publications, 1993.

759. Moffatt MF, Hill MR, Cornelis F et al. Genetic linkage of T-cell receptor α/δ complex to specific IgE response. Lancet 1994; 343:1597-1600.

760. Marsh DG, Neely JD, Breazeale DR, Ghosh B, Freidhoff LR, Ehrlich-Kautzky E, Schou C, Krishnaswamy G, Beaty TH. Linkage analysis of IL-4 and other chromosome 5q31.1 markers and total serum immunoglobulin E concentrations. Science 1994. 264:1152-1156.

761. Kemeny M. The role of CD8⁺ T cells in the regulation of IgE. Clin. Exper. Allergy 1993; 23:466-470.

762. McMenamin C, Holt PG. The natural immune response to inhaled soluble protein antigens involves Major Histocompatibility Complex (MHC) class I-restricted CD8⁺ T cell-mediated but MHC class-II-restricted CD4⁺ T cell-dependent immune deviation resulting in selective suppression of immunoglobulin E production. J. Exp. Med. 1993; 178:889-899.

763. McMenamin C, McKersey M, Kuhnlein P, Hunig T, Holt PG. γδ T Cells down-regulate primary IgE responses in rats to inhaled soluble protein antigens. J. Immunol. 1995; 154:4390-4394.

764. Romagnani S. Regulation of the development of type 2 T-helper cells in allergy. Curr. Opin. Immunol. 1994; 6:838-846.

765. Tepper RI, Levinson DA, Stonger BL, Campos-Torres J, Abbas AK, Leder P. IL-4 induces allergic-like inflammatory disease and alters T cell development in transgenic mice. Cell 1990; 62:457-467.

766. Varney VA, Jacobson R, Sudderinck MR et al. Immunohistology of the nasal mucosa following allergen-induced rhinitis: identification of activated T lymphocytes, eosinophils and neutrophils. Am. Rev. Respir. Dis. 1992; 146:170-176.

767. Nagai H, Yamaguchi S, Inagaki N, Tsuruoka N, Hitoshi Y, Takatsu K. Effect of anti-IL-5 monoclonal antibody on allergic bronchial eosinophilia and airway hyperresponsiveness in mice. Life Sci. 1993; 53:143-247.

768. Iwamoto I, Tomeo S, Tomioka H, Takatsu K, Yoshida S. Role of CD4⁺ T lymphocytes and interleukin 5 in antigen-induced eosinophil recruitment into the site of cutaneous late-phase reaction in mice. J. Leuk. Biol. 1992; 52:572-578.

769. Garlisi CG, Falcone A, Kung TT, Stelts D, Pennlike KG, Beavis AJ, Smith SR, Egan RW, Umland SP. T cells are necessary for Th2 cytokine production and eosinophil accumulation in airways of antigen-challenged allergic mice. Clin. Immunol. Immunopathol. 1995; 75:75-83.

770. Gavett SH, O'Hearn DJ, Li X, Huang S-K, Finkelman FD, Wills-Karp M. Interleukin 12 inhibits antigen-induced airway hyperresponsiveness, inflammation, and Th2 cytokine expression in mice. J. Exp. Med. 1995; 182:1527-1536.

771. Snapper CM, Finkelman FD, Paul WE. Differential regulation of IgG1 and IgE synthesis by interleukin 4. J. Exp. Med. 1988; 167:183-196.

772. Renz H, Enssle K, Lauffer L, Kurrle R, Gelfand EW. Inhibition of allergen-induced IgE and IgG1 production by soluble IL-4 receptor. Int. Arch. Allergy Immunol. 1995; 106:46-54.

773. Corry DB, Folkesson HG, Warnock ML, Erle DJ, Matthay MA, Wiener-Kronish JP, Locksley RM. Interleukin-4, but not interleukin 5 or eosinophils is required in a murine model of acute airway hyperreactivity. J. Exp. Med. 1996; 183:109-117.

774. Muller KM, Jaunin F, Masouyé I, Saurat J-H, Hauser C. Th2 cells mediate IL-4-dependent local tissue inflammation. J. Immunol. 1993; 150:5576-5584.

775. Egan RW, Athwahl D, Chou C-C, Emtage S, Jehn C-H, Kung TT, Mauser PJ, Murgolo NJ, Bodmer MW. Inhibition of pulmonary eosinophilia and hyperreactivity by antibodies to interleukin 5. Int. Arch. Allergy Immunol. 1995; 107:321-322.

776. Foster PS, Hogan SP, Ramsay AJ, Matthaei KI, Young IG. Interleukin 5 deficiency abolishes eosinophilia, airways hyperreactivity, and lung damage in a mouse asthma model. J. Exp. Med. 1996; 183:195-201.

777. Nakaijima H, Nakao A, Watanabe Y, Yoshida S, Iwamoto I. IFN-γ inhibits antigen-induced eosinophil and CD4$^+$ T cell recruitment into tissue. J. Immunol. 1994; 153:1264-1270.

778. Lack G, Renz H, Saloga J, Bradley K, Loader J, Leung DYM, Gelfand EW. Nebulized but not parenteral IFN-γ decreases IgE production and normalizes airways function in a murine model of allergen sensitization. J. Immunol. 1994; 152:2546-2554.

779. Renz H, Lack G, Saloga J, Schwinzer R, Bradley K, Loader J, Kupfer A, Larsen GL, Gelfand EW. Inhibition of IgE production and normalization of airways responsiveness by sensitized CD8 T cells in a mouse model of allergen-induced sensitization. J. Immunol. 1994; 152:351-360.

780. Coyle AJ, Tsuyuki S, Bertrand C, Huang S, Aguet M, Alkan SS, Anderson GP. Mice lacking the IFN-gamma receptor have an impaired ability to resolve a lung eosinophilic inflammatory response associated with a prolonged capacity of T cells to exhibit a Th2 cytokine profile. J. Immunol. 1996; 156:2680-2685.

781. Mauser PJ, Pitman A, Witt A et al. Inhibitory effect of the TRFK-5 anti-IL-5 antibody in a guinea pig model of asthma. Am. Rev. Respir. Dis. 1993; 148:1623-1627.

782. Iwama T, Nagai H, Koda A. Effects of murine recombinant interleukin-5 on the cell population in guinea pig airways. Br. J. Pharmacol. 1992; 105:19-22.

783. Mauser PJ, Pitman AM, Fernandez X, Foran SK, Adams GK, Kreutner W, Egan RW, Chapman RW. Effects of an antibody to interleukin 5 in a monkey model of asthma. Am. J. Respir. Crit. Care Med. 1995; 152:467-472.

784. Drazen JM, Arm JP, Austen KF. Sorting out the cytokines of asthma. J. Exp. Med. 1996; 183:1-5.

785. Wardlaw AJ, Dunnette S, Gleich GJ, Collins JV, Kay, AB. Eosinophils and mast cells in bronchoalveolar lavage in mild asthma. Relationship to bronchial hyperreactivity. Am. Rev. Respir. Dis. 1988; 137:62-69.

786. Azzawi M, Bradley B, Jeffery PK et al. Identification of activated T lymphocytes and eosinophils in bronchial biopsies in stable atopic asthma. Am. Rev. Respir. Dis. 1990; 142:1407-1413.

787. Robinson D, Hamid Q, Ying S, Bentley A, Assoufi B, Durham SR, Kay AB. Prednisolone treatment in asthma is associated with modulation of bronchoalveolar lavage cell interleukin-4, interleukin-5, and interferon-γ cytokine gene expression. Am. Rev. Respir. Dis. 1993; 148:401-406.

788. Mori A, Suko M, Nishizaki Y, Kaminuma O, Kobayashi S, Matsuzaki G, Yamamoto K, Ito K, Tsuruoka N, Okudaira H. IL-5 production by CD4+ T cells of asthmatic patients is suppressed by gluocorticoids and the immunosuppressants FK506 and cyclosporin A. Intern. Immunol. 1995; 7:449-457.

789. Leung DYM, Martin RJ, Szefler SJ, Sher ER, Kay AB, Hamid Q. Dysregulation of interleukin-4, interleukin-5, and interferon-γ gene expression in steroid-resistant asthma. J. Exp. Med. 1995; 181:33-40.

790. Ying S, Durham SR, Corrigan CJ, Hamid Q, Kay AB. Phenotype of cells expressing mRNA for Th2-type (interleukin-4 and interleukin-5) and Th1-type (interleukin-2 and interferon-γ) cytokines in bronchoalveolar lavage and bronchial biopsies from atopic asthmatic and normal control subjects. Am. J. Respir. Cell Mol. Biol. 1995; 12:477-487.

791. Tang MLK, Coleman J, Kemp AS. Interleukin-4 and interferon-gamma production in atopic and non-atopic children with asthma. Clin. Exp. Allergy 1995; 25:515-521.

792. Corrigan CJ. Elevated interleukin-4 secretion by T lymphocytes: a feature of atopy or asthma? Clin. Exp. Allergy 1995; 25:485-487.

793. Walker C, Bode E, Boer L, Hansel TT, Blaser K, Virchow J-C. Allergic and nonallergic asthmatics have distinct patterns of T-cell activation and cytokine production in peripheral blood and bronchoalveolar lavage. Am. Rev. Respir. Dis. 1992; 146:109-115.

794. Till S, Li B, Durham SR, Humbert, Assoufi B, Huston D, Dickinson R, Jeannin P, Kay AB, Corrigan C. Secretion of the eosinophil-active cytokines interleukin-5, granulocyte/macrophage colony-stimulating factor and interleukin-3 by bronchoalveolar lavage CD4+ and CD8+ T cell lines in atopic asthmatics, and atopic and non-atopic controls. Eur. J. Immunol. 1995; 25:2727-2731.

795. Zachary CB, MacDonald DM. Quantitative analysis of T lymphocyte subsets in atopic eczema, using monoclonal antibodies and flow cytometry. Br. J. Dermatol. 1983; 108:411-422.

796. Sillevis Smitt J, Bos JD, Hulsebosch HJ, Krieg SR. In situ immunophenotyping of antigen presenting cells and T cell subsets in atopic dermatitis. Clin. Exper. Dermatol. 1986; 11:159-168.

797. Tang M, Kemp A. Production and secretion of interferon-gamma in children with atopic dermatitis. Clin. Exp. Immunol. 1994; 95:66-72.

798. Kimata H, Fujimoto M. Furusho K. Involvement of interleukin (IL)-13, but not IL-4, in spontaneous IgE and IgG4 production in nephrotic syndrome. Eur. J. Immunol. 1995; 25:1497-1501.

799. Tang MLK, Varigos G, Kemp AS. Reduced interferon-gamma (IFN-γ) secretion with increased IFN-γ mRNA expression in atopic dermatitis: evidence for a post-transcriptional defect. Clin. Exp. Immunol. 1994; 97:483-490.

800. Lester MR, Hofer MF, Gately M, Trumble A, Leung DYM. Down-regulating effects of IL-4 and IL-10 on the IFN-γ response in atopic dermatitis. J. Immunol. 1995; 154:6174-6181.

801. Reinhold U, Kukel S, Goeden B. Neumann C, Kreysel HW. Functional characterization of skin-infiltrating lymphocytes in atopic dermatitis. Clin. Exp. Immunol. 1991; 86:444-448.

802. Sager N, Feldmann A, Schilling G, Kreitsch P, Neumann C. House dust mite-specific T cells in the skin of subjects with atopic dermatitis: frequency and lymphokine profile in the allergen patch test. J. Allergy Clin. Immunol. 1992; 89:801-810.

803. Gutgesell C, Yssel H, Scheel D, Gerdes J, Neumann C. IL-10 secretion of allergen-specific skin-derived T cells correlates positively with that of the Th2 cytokines IL-4 and IL-5. Exp. Dermatol. 1994; 3:304-313.

804. Virtanen T, Maggi E, Manetti R et al. No relationship between skin-infiltrating Th2-like cells and allergen-specific IgE response in atopic dermatitis. J. Allergy Clin. Immunol. 1995; 96:411-420.

805. Ohmen JD, Hanifin JM. Nickoloff BJ, Rea TH, Wyzykowski R, Kim J, Jullien D, McHugh T, Nassif AS, Chan SC, Modlin RL. Overexpression of IL-10 in atopic dermatitis. Contrasting cytokine patterns with delayed-type hypersensitivity reactions. J. Immunol. 1995; 154:1956-1963.

806. Gocinskin GL, Tigelaar RE. Roles of CD4+ and CD8+ T cells in murine contact sensitivity revealed by in vivo monoclonal antibody depletion. J. Immunol. 1990; 144:4121-4128.

807. Piguet PF, Grau GE, Hauser C, Vassalli P. Tumor necrosis factor is a critical mediator in hapten-induced irritant and contact hypersensitivity reactions. J. Exp. Med. 1991; 173:673-679.

808. Higashi N, Yoshizuka N, Kobayashi Y. Phenotypic properties and cytokine production of skin-infiltrating cells obtained from guinea pigs delayed-type hypersensitivity reaction sites. Cell. Immunol. 1995; 164:28-35.

809. Enk AH, Katz SI. Early molecular events in the induction phase of contact sensitivity. Proc. Natl. Acad. Sci. USA 1992; 39:1398-1402.

810. Muller G, Saloga J, Germann T, Schuler G, Knop J, Enk AH. IL-12 as mediator and adjuvant for the induction of contact sensitivity in vivo. J. Immunol. 1995; 155:4661-4668.

811. Riemann H, Schwartz A, Grabbe S, Aragane Y, Luger TA, Wysocka M, Kubin M, Trinchieri G, Schwarz T. Neutralization of IL-12 in vivo prevents induction of contact hypersensitivity and induces hapten-specific tolerance. J. Immunol. 1996; 156:1799-1803.

812. Ferguson TA, Dube P, Griffith TS. Regulation of contact hypersensitivity by interleukin 10. J. Exp. Med. 1994; 179:1597-1604.

813. Enk AH, Saloga J, Becker D, Mohamadzadeh M, Knop J. Induction of hapten-specific tolerance by interleukin 10 in vivo. J. Exp. Med. 1994; 179:1397-1402.

814. Schwartz A, Grabbe S, Riemann H et al. In vivo effects of interleukin 10 on contact hypersensitivity and delayed-type hypersensitivity reactions. J. Invest. Dermatol. 1994; 103:211-216.

815. Gautam SC, Chikkala NF, Hamilton TA. Antiinflammatory action of IL-4. Negative regulation of contact sensitivity to trinitrochlorobenzene. J. Immunol. 1992; 148:1411-1415.

816. Berg DJ, Leach MW, Kuhn R, Rajewsky K, Muller W, Davidson NJ, Rennick D. Interleukin 10 but not interleukin 4 is a natural suppressant of cutaneous inflammatory responses. J. Exp. Med. 1995; 182:99-108.

817. Tang A, Judge TA, Nickoloff BJ, Turka LA. Suppression of murine allergic contact dermatitis by CTLA4Ig. J. Immunol. 1996; 157:117-125.

818. Xu H, DiIulio NA, Fairchild RL. T cell populations primed by hapten sensitization in contact sensitivity are distinguished by polarized patterns of cytokine production: interferon-γ-producing (Tc1) effector CD8+ T cells and interleukin (IL) 4/10-producing (Th2) negative regulatory CD4+ T cells. J. Exp. Med. 1996; 183:1001-1012.

819. Kapsenberg ML, Wierenga EA, Sriekema FEM, Tiggelman AMBC, Bos JD. Th1 lymphokine production profiles of nickel-specific CD4+ T lymphocyte clones from nickel contact allergic and nonallergic individuals. J. Invest. Dermatol. 1992; 98:59-63.

820. Probst P, Kuntzlin D, Fleischer B. Th2-type infiltrating T cells cells in nickel-induced contact dermatitis. Cell. Immunol. 1995; 165:134-140.

821. Romagnani S, Ricci M, Passaleva A, Biliotti G. Cell-mediated immune responses to heterologous and homologous thyroglobulin in guinea pigs immunized with heterologous thyroid extract. Immunology 1970; 19:599-612.

822. Romball CG, Weigle WO. Transfer of experimental autoimmune thyroiditis with T-cell clones. J. Immunol. 1987. 138:1092-1098.

823. Sugihara S, Fujiwara H, Shearer GM. Autoimmune thyroiditis induced in mice depleted of particular T cell subsets. J. Immunol. 1993; 150:683-694.

824. Sugihara S, Fujiwara H, Niimi H, Shearer GM. Self-thyroid epithelial cell (TEC)-reactive CD8+ T cell lines/clones derived from autoimmune thyroiditis lesions. J. Immunol. 1995; 155:1619-1628.

825. Zipris D, Greiner DL, Malkani S, Whalen B, Mordes JP, Rossini AA. Cytokine gene expression in islets and thyroids of BB rats. IFN-γ and IL-12p40 mRNA increase with age in both diabetic and insulin-treated nondiabetic BB rats. J. Immunol. 1996; 156:1315-1321.

826. Mignon-Godefroy K, Brazillet MP, Rott O, Charreire J. Distinctive modulation by IL-4 and IL-10 of the effector function of murine thyroglobulin-primed cells in "transfer-experimental autoimmune thyroiditis". Cell. Immunol. 1995; 162:171-177.

827. Braley-Mullen H, Sharp GC, Bickel JT, Kyriakos M. Induction of severe granulomatous experimental autoimmune thyroiditis in mice by effector cells activated in the presence of anti-IL-2 receptor antibody. J. Exp. Med. 1991; 173:899-912.

828. Stull SJ, Sharp GC, Kyriakos M, Bickel JT, Braley-Mullen H. Induction of granulomatous autoimmune thyroiditis in mice with in vitro activated effector T-cells and anti-IFN-γ antibody. J. Immunol. 1992; 149:2219-2226.

829. Del Prete GF, Tiri A, De Carli M, Mariotti S, Pinchera A, Chretien I, Romagnani S, Ricci M. High potential to tumor necrosis factor α (TNF-α) production of thyroid infiltrating T lymphocytes in Hashimoto's thyroiditis: a peculiar feature of destructive thyroid autoimmunity. Autoimmunity 1989; 4:267-276.

830. Turner M, Londei M, Feldman M. Human T cells from auotimmune and normal individuals can produce tumor necrosis factor. Eur. J. Immunol. 1987; 17:1807-1814.

831. Margolick JB, Weetman AP, Burman KD. Immunohistochemical analysis of intrathyroidal lymphocytes in Graves' disease: evidence of activated T cells and production of interferon-gamma. Clin. Immunol. Immunopathol. 1988; 47:208-218.

832. Hamilton F, Black M, Farquharson MA, Stewwart C, Foulis AK. Spatial correlation between thyroid epithelial cells expressing class II MHC molecules and interferon-gamma-containing lymphocytes in human thyroid autoimmune disease. Clin. Exp. Immunol. 1991; 83:64-68.

833. Rutenfranz I, Kruse A, Rink L, Wenzel B, Wenzel H, Arnholdt H, Kirchner H. In situ hybridization of the mRNA for interferon-gamma, interferon-alpha E, interferon-beta, interferon-1beta, and interleukin-6 and characterization of infiltrating cells in thyroid tissues. J. Immunol. Methods 1992; 148:233-242.

834. Zheng RQH, Abney ER, Chu CQ, Field M, Maini RN, Lamb JR, Feldmann M. Detection of in vivo production of tumor necrosis factor-alpha by human thyroid epithelial cells. Immunology 1992; 75:456-462.

835. De Carli M, D'Elios MM, Mariotti S, Marcocci C, Pinchera A, Ricci M, Romagnani S, Del Prete GF. Cytolytic T cells with Th1-like cytokine profile predominate in retroorbital lymphocytic infiltrates of Graves' ophtalmopathy. J. Clin. Endocrinol. Metab. 1993; 77:1120-1124.

836. Watson PF, Pickering P, Davies R, Weetman AP. Analysis of cytokine gene expression in Graves' disease and multinodular goiter. J. Clin. Endocrinol. Metab. 1994; 79:355-360.

837. Paschke R, Schuppert E, Taton M, Velu T. Intrathyroidal cytokine gene expression profiles in autoimmune thyroiditis. J. Endocrinol. 1994; 41:309-315.

838. McLachlan SM, Prummel MF, Rapoport B. Cell-mediated or humoral immunity in Graves' ophtalmopathy? Profiles of T-cell cytokines amplified by polymerase chain reaction from orbital tissue. J. Clin. Endocrinol. Metab. 1994; 78:1070-1074.

839. Grubeck-Loebenstein B, Trieb K, Sztankay A, Holter W, Anderl H, Wick G. Retrobulbar T cells from patients with Graves' ophtalmopathy are CD8+ and specifically recognize autologous fibroblasts. J. Clin. Invest. 1994; 93:2738-2743.

840. Roura-Mir C, Catalfamo M, Lucas-Martin A, Sospedra M, Pujol-Borrell R, Jaraquemada D. IL-4/IFN-γ balance in Graves' disease contrasts with IFN-γ dominance in Hashimoto's thyroiditis. Proc. IV Intern. Conf. on Cytokines. Florence 1996 (Abstr.).

841. Mullins RJ, Cohen SBA, Webb LMC, Chernajovsky Y, Dayan CM, Londei M, Feldmann M. Identification of thyroid stimulating hormone receptor-specific T cells in Graves' disease thyroid using autoantigen-transfected Epstein Barr virus-transformed B cell lines. J. Clin. Invest. 1995; 96:30-37.

842. Windhagen A, Nicholson LB, Weiner HL, Kuchroo VK, Hafler DA. Role of Th1 and Th2 cells in neurologic disorders. Chem. Immunol. 1996; 63:181-186.

843. Wekerle H. Experimental autoimmune encephalomyelitis as a model of immune-mediated CNS disease. Curr. Opin. Neurobiol. 1993; 3:779-784.

844. Renno T, Krakowski M, Piccirillo C, Lin JY, Owens T. TNF-alpha expression by resident microglia and infiltrating leukocytes in the central nervous system of mice with experimental allergic encephalomyelitis. Regulation by Th1 cytokines. J. Immunol. 1995; 154:944-953.

845. Kuchroo VK, Sobel RA, Laning JC, Martin CA, Greenfield E, Dorf ME, Less MB. Experimental allergic encephalomyelitis mediated by cloned T cells specific for a synthetic peptide of myelin proteolipid protein. J. Immunol. 1992; 148:3776-3782.

846. Van der Veen RC, Kapp JA, Trotter JL. Fine-specificity differences in the recognition of an encephalitogenic peptide by T helper 1 and 2 cells. J. Neuroimmunol. 1993; 48:221-226.

847. Voskuhl RR, Martin R, Bergman C, Dalal M, Ruddle NH, McFarland HF. T helper 1 (Th1) functional phenotype of human myelic basic protein-specific T lymphocytes. Autoimmunity 1993; 15:137-143.

848. Zamvil SS, Steinman L. The T lymphocyte in experimental allergic encephalomyelitis. Annu. Rev. Immunol. 1990; 8:579-621.

849. Ruddle NH, Bergman CM, McGrath KM, Lingenheld EG, Grunnet ML, Padula SJ, Clark RB. An antibody to lymphotoxin and tumor necrosis factor prevents transfer of experimental allergic encephalomyelitis. J. Exp. Med. 1990; 172:1193-1200.

850. Chung IY, Norris JG, Benveniste EN. Differential tumor necrosis factor-α expression by astrocytes from experimental allergic encephalomyelitis-susceptible and -resistant rat strains. J. Exp. Med. 1991; 173:801-811.

851. Khoury SJ, Akalin E, Chandraker A, Turka LA, Linsley PS, Sayegh MH, Hancock WW. CD28-B7 costimulatory blockade at CTLA4Ig prevents actively induced experimental autoimmune encephalomyelitis and inhibits Th1 but spares Th2 cytokines in the central nervous system. J. Immunol. 1995; 155:4521-4524.

852. Racke MK, Bonomo A, Scott DE, Cannella B, Levine A, Raine CS, Shevach EM, Rocken M. Cytokine-induced immune deviation as a therapy for inflammatory autoimmune disease. J. Exp. Med. 1994; 180:1961-1966.

853. Racke MK, Scott DE, Quigley L, Gray GS, Abe R, June CH, Perrin PJ. Distinct role for B7-1 (CD-80) and B7-2 (CD-86) in the initiation of experimental allergic encephalomyelitis. J. Clin. Invest. 1995; 96:2195-2203.

854. Crisi GM, Santambrogio L, Hochwald GM, Smith SR, Carlino JA, Thorbecke GJ. Staphylococcal enterotoxin B and tumor-necrosis factor-α-induced relapses of experimental allergic encephalomyelitis: protection by transforming growth factor-β and interleukin-10. Eur. J. Immunol. 1995; 25:3035-3040.

855. Rott O, Cash E, Fleischer B. Phosphodiesterase inhibitor pentoxifylline, a selective suppressor of T helper type 1- but not type 2-associated lymphokine production, prevents induction of experimental autoimmune encephalomyelitis in Lewis rats. Eur. J. Immunol. 1993; 23:1745-1751.

856. Acha-Orbea H, Mitchell DJ, Timmerman L, Wraith DC, Tausch GS, Waldor MK, Zamvil SS, McDevitt HO, Steinman, L. Limited heterogeneity of T cell receptors from lymphocytes mediating autoimmune encephalomyelitis allows specific immune intervention. Cell 1988; 54:263-273.

857. Wall M, Southwood S, Sidney J et al. High affinity for class II molecules as a necessary but not sufficient characteristic of encephalitogenic determinants. Int. Immunol. 1992; 4:773-777.

858. Abromson-Leeman S, Alexander J, Bronson R, Carroll J, Southwood S, Dorf M. Experimental autoimmune encephalomyelitis-resistant mice have highly encephalitogenic myelin basic protein (MBP)-specific T-cell clones that recognize a MBP peptide with high affinity for MHC Class II. J. Immunol. 1995; 154:388-398.

859. Cua DJ, Hinton DR, Stohlman SA. Self-antigen-induced Th2 responses in experimental allergic encephalomyelitis (EAE)-resistant mice. J. Immunol. 1995; 155:4052-4059.

860. Perrin PJ, Scott D, Quigley L, Albert PS, Feder O, Gray GS, Abe R, June CH, Racke MK. Role of B7:CD28/CTLA-4 in the induction of chronic relapsing experimental allergic encephalomyelitis. J. Immunol. 1995; 154:1481-1490.

861. Cross AH, Girard TJ, Giacoletto KS, Evans RJ, Keeling RM, Lin RF, Trotter JL, Karr RW. Long term inhibition of murine experimental autoimmune encephalomyelitis. Using CTLA4-Fc supports a key role for CD28 costimulation. J. Clin. Invest. 1995; 95:2783-2789.

862. Khoury SJ, Hancock WW, Weiner HL. Oral tolerance to myelin basic protein and natural recovery from experimental autoimmune encephalomyelitis are associated with downregulation of inflammatory cytokines and differential upregulation of transforming growth factor β, interleukin 4 and prostaglandin E expression in the brain. J. Exp. Med. 1992; 176:1335-1364.

863. Leonard JP, Waldburger KE, Goldman SJ. Prevention of experimental auotimmune encephalomyelitis by antibodies against interleukin 12. J. Exp. Med. 1995; 181:381-386.

864. Whitacre CC, Gienapp IE, Orosz CG, Bitar DM. Oral tolerance in experimental autoimmune encephalomyelitis. III. Evidence for clonal anergy. J. Immunol. 1991; 147:2155-2163.

865. Miller A, Al-Sabbagh A, Santos LMB, Prabhu Das M, Weiner HL. Epitopes of myelin basic protein that trigger TGF-β release after oral tolerization are distinct from encephalitogenic epitopes and mediate epitope-driven bystander suppression. J. Immunol. 1993; 151:7307-7315.

866. Kuchroo VK, Greer JM, Kaul D, Ishioka G, Franco A, Sette A, Sobel RA, Lees MB. A single TCR antagonist peptide inhibits experimental allergic encephalomyelitis mediated by a diverse T cell repertoire. J. Immunol. 1994; 153:3326-3336.

867. Brocke S, Gijbels K, Allegretta M et al. Treatment of experimental encephalomyelitis with a peptide analogue of myelin basic protein. Nature 1996; 379:343-346.

868. Ferber IA, Brocke S, Taylor-Edwards C, Ridgway W, Dinisco C, Steinman L, Dalton D, Garrison Fayhman C. Mice with a disrupted IFN-γ gene are susceptible to the induction of experimental autoimmune encephalomyelitis (EAE). J. Immunol. 1996; 156:5-7.

869. Khoruts A, Miller SD, Jenkins MK. Neuroantigen-specific Th2 cells are inefficient suppressors of experimental autoimmune encephalomyelitis induced by effector Th1 cells. J. Immunol. 1995; 155:5011-5017.

870. Sharief MK, Hentges R. Association between tumor necrosis factor alpha and disease progression in patients with multiple sclerosis. N. Engl. J. Med. 1991; 325:467-472.

871. Tsukada N, Miyagi K, Matsuda M, Yanagisawa N, Yone K. Tumor necrosis factor and interleukin 1 in the CSF and sera of patients with multiple sclerosis. J. Neurol. Sci. 1991; 102:230-234.

872. Chofflon M, Juillard C, Juillard P, Gauthier G, Grau GE. Tumor necrosis factor alpha production as a possible predictor of relapse in patients with multiple sclerosis. Eur. Cytokine Netw. 1992; 3:523-531.

873. Rieckmann P, Albrecht M, Kitze B, Weber T, Tumani H, Broocks A, Luer V Poser S. Cytokine mRNA levels in mononuclear blood cells from patients with multiple sclerosis. Neurology 1994; 44:1523-1526.

874. Rieckmann P, Albrecht M, Kitze B, Weber T, Tumani H, Broocks A, Luer V, Helwig A, Poser S. Tumor necrosis factor alpha messenger RNA expression in patients with relapsing remitting multiple sclerosis is associated with disease activity. Ann. Neurol. 1995; 37:82-88.

875. Brod S, Benjamin D, Hafler DA. Restricted T cell expression of IL2/IFN-γ mRNA in human inflammatory disease. J. Immunol. 1991; 147:810-815.

876. Benvenuto R, Paroli M, Buttinelli C, Franco A, Barnaba V, Fieschi C, Balsano F. Tumor necrosis factor-alpha synthesis by cerebrospinal-fluid-derived T cell clones from patients with multiple sclerosis. Clin. Exp. Immunol. 1991; 84:97-102.

877. Olsson T. Cytokines in neuroinflammatory disease: role of myelin-autoreactive T cell production of interferon-gamma. J. Neuroimmunol. 1993; 40:211-218.

878. Correale J, Gilmore W, McMillan M, Li S, McCarthy K, Le T, Weiner LP. Patterns of cytokine secretion by autoreactive proteolipid protein-specific T cell clones during the course of multiple sclerosis. J. Immunol. 1995; 154:2959-2968.

879. Selmaj K, Raine CS, Cannella B, Brosnan CF. Identification of lymphotoxin and tumor necrosis factor in multiple sclerosis lesions. J. Clin. Invest. 1991; 87:949-954.

880. Windhagen A, Newcombe J, Dangond F, Strand C, Woodroofe MN, Cuzner ML, Hafler DA. Expression of costimulatory molecules B7-1 (CD80), B7-2 (CD86), and interleukin-12 cytokine in multiple sclerosis lesions. J. Exp. Med. 1995; 182:1985-1996.

881. Panitch HS, Hirsch RL, Schindler J, Johnson KP. Treatment of multiple sclerosis with gamma-interferon: exacerbations associated with activation of the immune system. Neurology 1987; 37:1097-1102.

882. The IFNB Multiple Sclerosis Study Group. Interferon beta-1b is effective in relapsing-remitting multiple sclerosis. I. Clinical results of a multicenter, randomized, double-blind, placebo-controlled trial. Neurology 1993; 43:655-661.

883. Gery I, Wiggert B, Redmond TM, Kuwabara T, Crawford MA, Vistica BP, Chader GJ. Uveoretinitis and pinealitis induced by immunization with interphotoreceptor retinoid-binding protein. Invest. Ophtalmol. Vis. Sci. 1986; 27:1296-1300.

884. Hirose S, Singh VK, Donoso LA, Shinohara T, Kotake S, Tanaka T, Kuwabara T, Yamaki K, Gery I, Nussenblatt R. An 18-mer peptide derived from the retinal S antigen induces uveitis and pinealitis in primates. Clin. Exp. Immunol. 1989; 77:106-111.

885. Savion S, Grover S, Kawano Y, Caspi RR. Uveitogenicity of T cell lines in the rat does not correlate with their production of TNF, IFN-γ or IL-3. Invest. Ophtalmol. Vis. Sci. 1992; 33:932-935.

886. Saoudi A, Kuhn J, Huygen K, de Kozak Y, Velu T, Goldman M, Druet P, Bellon B. Th2 activated cells prevent experimental autoimmune uveoretinitis: a Th1-dependent autoimmune disease. Eur. J. Immunol. 1993; 23:3096-3103.

887. Caspi RR, Chan C-C, Grubbs BG, Silve P, Wiggert B, Parsa CF, Bahmaniar S, Billiau A, Heremans H. Endogenous systemic interferon-gamma has a protective effect against ocular autoimmunity in mice. J. Immunol. 1994; 152:890-899.

888. Lehner T, Batchelor JR. Classification and animmunogenic basis of Beçhet's syndrome. In: Lehner T, Barnes CG, eds. Behçet's Syndrome: Clinical and Immunological Features. London: Academic Press, 1989:13.

889. Poulter LW, Lehner T. Immunohistology of oral lesions from patients with recurrent oral ulcers and Behçet's syndrome. Clin. Exp. Immunol. 1989; 78:189-195.

890. Yamamato JH, Fujino Y, Lin C, Nieda M, Juji T, Masuda K. S-antigen specific T cell clones from a patient with Behçet's disease. Br. J. Ophtalmol. 1994; 78:927-932.

891. Fujii N, Minigawa T, Nakane, A. Spontaneous production of interferon-gamma in culture of T lymphocytes obtained from patients with Behçet's disease. J. Immunol. 1983; 130:1683-1686.

892. Bacon TH, Ozbakir F, Elms CA, Denman AM. Interferon-gamma production by peripheral blood mononuclear cells from patients with Behçet's syndrome. Clin. Exp. Immunol. 1984; 58:541-547.

893. Katayama T, Tachinami K, Ishiguro M, Kubota Y. The relation between Behçet's disease and interleukin beta production. Nippon Ganka Gakkai Zasshi 1994; 98:197-201.

894. Eisenbarth GS. Type 1 diabetes mellitus. A chronic autoimmune disease. N. Engl. J. Med. 1986; 314:1360-1368.

895. Marliss EB, Nakhooda AF, Poussier P. Clinical forms and natural history of the diabetic syndrome and insulin and glucagon secretion in the BB rat. Metabolism 1993; 32(suppl.):11-16.

896. Leiter EH, Prochazka M, Coleman DL. The nonbese diabetic (NOD) mouse. Am. J. Pathol. 1987; 128:380-393.

897. Bottazzo GF, Dean BM, McNally JM, Mackay EH, Swift PGF, Gamble DR. In situ characterization of autoimmune phenomena and expression of HLA molecules in the pancreas in diabetic insulitis. N. Engl. J. Med. 1985; 31:353-360.

898. Foulis AK, Farquharson MA. Aberrant expression of HLA-DR antigens by insulin containing beta cells in recent onset type 1 (insulin-dependent) diabetes mellitus. Diabetes 1986; 35:1215-1224.

899. Bach J-F. Mechanisms of autoimmunity in insulin-dependent diabetes mellitus. Clin. Exp. Immunol. 1988; 72:1-8.

900. Lampeter EF, Signore A, Gale EAM, Pozzilli P. Lessons from the NOD mouse for the pathogenesis and immunotherapy of human type 1 (insulin-dependent) diabetes mellitus. Diabetologia 1989; 32:703-708.

901. Wong FS, Visintin I, Wen L, Flavell RA, Janeway CA Jr. CD8 T cell clones from young nonobese diabetic (NOD) islets can transfer rapid onset of diabetes in NOD mice in the absence of CD4 cells. J. Exp. Med. 1996; 183:67-76.

902. Haskins K, Portas M, Bergman B. Lafferty K, Bradley B. Pancreatic islet-specific T cell clones from non-obese diabetic mice. Proc. Natl. Acad. Sci. USA 1989; 86:8000-8004.

903. Bergman B, Haskins K. Islet-specific T-cell clones from the NOD mouse respond to beta-granule antigen. Diabetes 1994; 43:197-203.

904. Healey D, Ozegbe P, Arden S, Chandler P, Hutton J, Cooke A. In vivo activity and in vitro specificity of CD4⁺ Th1 and Th2 cells derived from the spleens of diabetic NOD mice. J. Clin. Invest. 1995; 95:2979-2985.

905. Katz JD, Benoist C, Mathis D. T helper cell subsets in insulin-dependent diabetes. Science, 1995; 268:1185-1188.

906. Kaufmann DL, Clare-Salzler M, Tian J et al. Spontaneous loss of T-cell tolerance to glutamic acid decarboxylase in murine insulin-dependent diabetes. Nature 1993; 366:69-72.

907. Tisch R, Yang X-D, Singer SM. Liblau RS, Fugger L, McDevitt HO. Immune response to glutamic acid decarboxylase correlates with insulitis in non-obese diabetic mice. Nature 1993; 366:72-75.

908. Campbell IL, Kay TW, Oxbrow L, Harrison LC. Essential role for interferon-gamma and interleukin-6 in autoimmune insulin-dependent diabetes in NOD/Wehi mice. J. Clin. Invest. 1991; 87:237-248.

909. Debray-Sachs M, Carnaus C, Boitard C, Cohen H, Gresser I, Bedossa P, Bach J-F. Prevention of diabetes in NOD mice treated with antibody to murine IFN-gamma. J. Autoimmun. 1991; 4:237-248.

910. Stewart TA, Hultgren B, Huang X, Pitts-Meek S, Hully J, MacLachla NJ. Induction of type I diabetes by interferon-alpha in transgenic mice. Science 1993; 260:1942-1946.

911. Rabinovitch A, Suarez-Pinzon WL, Sorensen O, Bleackey RC, Power RF, Rajotte RV. Combined therapy with interleukin-4 and interleukin-10 inhibits autoimmune diabetes recurrence in syngeneic islet-transplanted nonobese diabetic mice. Transplantation 1995; 60:368-374.

912. Shehadeh NN, LaRosa F, Lafferty KJ. Altered cytokine activity in adjuvant inhibition of autoimmune diabetes. J. Autoimmun. 1993; 6:291-300.

913. Trembleau S, Penna G, Bosi E, Mortara A, Gately MK. Adorini L. Interleukin 12 administration induces T helper type 1 cells and accelerates autoimmune diabetes in NOD mice. J. Exp. Med. 1995; 181:817-821.

914. O'Hara RM, Henderson SL. FASEB J. 1995; 9:5938-5938 (Abstr.).

915. Trembleau S et al. Proc. IV Intern. Conf. on Cytokines. Florence 1996 (Abstr.).

916. Rapoport MJ, Jeramillo A, Zipris D. Lazarus AH, Serreze DV, Leiter EH, Cyopick P, Danska JS, Delovitch TL. Interleukin 4 reverses T cell proliferative unresponsiveness and prevents the onset of diabetes in nonobese diabetic mice. J. Exp. Med. 1993; 178:87-99.

917. Scott B, Liblau R, Degermann S, Marconi LA, Ogata L, Caton AJ, McDEvitt HO. A role for non-MHC genetic polymorphism in susceptibility to spontaneous autoimmunity. Immunity 1994; 1:1-20.

918. Liblau RS, Singer SM, McDevitt HO. Th1 and Th2 CD4⁺ T cells in the pathogenesis of organ-specific autoimmune diseases. Immunol. Today 1995; 16:34-38.

919. Rabinovitch A, Suarez-Pinzon WL, Sorensen O, Bleackey RC, Power RF. IFN-gamma gene expression in pancreatic islet-infiltrating mononuclear cells correlates with autoimmune diabetes in nonobese diabetic mice. J. Immunol. 1995a; 154:4874-4882.

920. Wogensen L, Lee MS, Sarvetnick N. Production of interleukin 10 by islet cells accelerates immune-mediated destruction of beta cells in nonobese diabetic mice. J. Exp. Med. 1994; 179:1379-1384.

921. Foulis AK, McGill M, Farquharson, MA. Insulitis in type 1 (insulin-dependent) diabetes mellitus in man. Macrophages, lymphocytes, and interferon-gamma containing cells. J. Pathol. 1991; 165:97-103.

922. Chang JC, Linarelli LG, Laxer JA, Froning KJ, Caralli LL, Brostoff SW, Carlo DJ. Insulin-secretory-granule specific T cell clones in human insulin dependent diabetes mellitus. J. Autoimm. 1995; 8:221-234.

923. Harris ED Jr. Rheumatoid arthritis: pathophysiology and implications for therapy. N. Engl. J. Med. 1990; 322:1277-1289.

924. Ranges GE, Sriram S, Cooper SM. Prevention of type II collagen-induced arthritis by in vivo treatment with anti-L3T4. J. Exp. Med. 1985; 162 1105-1110.

925. Hom JT, Bendele AM, Carlson DG. In vivo administration with IL-1 accelerates the development of collagen-induced arthritis in mice. J. Immunol. 1988; 141:834-841.

926. Goldschmidt TJ, Andersson M, Malmstrom V, Holmdahl R. Activated type II collagen-reactive T cells are not eliminated by in vivo anti-CD4 treatment. Implications for therapeutic approaches on autoimmune arthritis. Immunobiology 1992; 184:359-371.

927. Williams RO, Feldmann M, Maini RN. Anti-tumor necrosis factor ameliorates joint disease in murine collagen-induced arthritis. Proc. Natl. Acad. Sci. USA 1992; 89:9784-9788.

928. Piguet PF, Grau GE, Vesin CE et al. Evolution of collagen arthritis in mice is arrested by treatment with anti-tumor necrosis factor (TNF) antibody or a recombinant soluble TNF receptor. Immunology 1992; 77:510-514.

929. Van den Berg WB, Joosten AB, Helsen M, Van de Loo FA. Amelioration of established murine collagen-induced arthritis. Clin. Exp. Immunol. 1994; 95:237-243.

930. Brandes ME, Allen JB, Ogawa Y et al. Transforming growth factor β1 suppresses acute and chronic arthritis in experimental animals. J. Clin. Invest. 1991; 87:1108-1113.

931. Kuruvilla AP, Shah R, Hochwald GM, Liggitt HD, Palladino MA, Thorbecke GJ. Protective effect of transforming growth factor β1 on experimental autoimmune diseases in mice. Proc. Natl. Acad. Sci. USA 1991; 88:2918-2921.

932. Williams RO, Mason LJ, Feldmann M, Maini RN. Synergy between anti-CD4 and anti-tumor necrosis factor in the amelioration of established collagen-induced arthritis. Proc. Natl. Acad. Sci. USA 1994; 91:2762-2766.

933. Myers LK, Rosloniec EF, Seyer JM, Stuart JM, Kang AH. A synthetic peptide analogue of a determinant of type II collagen prevents the onset of collagen-induced arthritis. J. Immunol. 1993; 150:4652-4658.

934. Germann T, Szeliga J, Hess H, Storkel S, Podlaski FJ, Gately MK, Schmidt E, Rude E. Administration of interleukin 12 in combination with type II collagen induces severe arthritis in DBA/1 mice. Proc. Natl. Acad. Sci. USA 1995a; 92:4823-4827.

935. Germann T, Bogartz M, Dlugonska H, Hess H, Schmitt E, Kolbe L, Kolsch E, Podlaski FJ, Gately MK, Rude E. Interleukin 12 profoundly up-regulates the synthesis of antigen-specific complement-fixing IgG2a, IgG2b and IgG3 antibody subclasses in vivo. Eur. J. Immunol. 1995b; 25:823-829.

936. Khare SD, Krco CJ, Griffiths MM, Luthra HS, David CS. Oral administration of an immunodominant human collagen peptide modulates collagen-induced arthritis. J. Immunol. 1995; 155:3653-3659.

937. Nakajima H, Takamori H, Hiyama Y, Tsukada W. The effect of treatment with interferon-γ on type II collagen-induced arthritis. Clin. Exp. Immunol. 1990; 81:441-445.

938. Hess H, Gately MK, Rude E, Schmidt E, Szeliga J, Germann T. High doses of interleukin 12 inhibit the development of joint disease in DBA/1 mice immunized with type II collagen in complete Freund's adjuvant. Eur. J. Immunol. 1996; 26:187-191.

939. Di Giovine FS, Nuki G, Duff GW. Tumor necrosis factor in synovial exudates. Ann. Rheum. Dis. 1988; 47:768-772.

940. Hirano T, Matsuda T, Turner M et al. Excessive production of interleukin 6/B cell stimulatory factor-2 in rheumatoid arthritis. Eur. J. Immunol. 1988; 18:1797-1801.

941. Haworth C, Brennan FM, Chantry D, Turner M, Maini RN, Feldmann M. Expression of granulocyte-macrophage colony-stimulating factor in rheumatoid arthritis: regulation by tumor necrosis factor-α. Eur. J. Immunol. 1991; 21:2575-2579.

942. Bucala R, Ritchlin C. Winchester R, Cerami A. Constitutive production of inflammatory and mitogenic cytokines by rheumatoid synovial fibroblasts. J. Exp. Med. 1991; 173:569-574.

943. Wood NC, Symons JA, Dickens E, Duff GW. In situ hybridization of IL-6 in rheumatoid arthritis. Clin. Exp. Immunol. 1992; 87:183-189.

944. Deleuran B, Chu C-Q, Field M, Brennan FM, Katsikis P, Fleldmann M, Maini RN. Localization of interleukin 1α (IL-1α), type 1 IL-1 receptor and interleukin 1 receptor antagonist protein in the synovial membrane and cartilage/pannus junction in rheumatoid arthritis. Br. J. Rheum. 1992; 91:801-809.

945. Hosaka S, Akahoshi T, Wada C, Kondo H. Expression of the chemokine superfamily in rheumatoid arthritis. Clin. Exp. Immunol. 1994; 97:451-457.

946. Feldmann M, Brennan FM, Field M, Maini RN. Pathogenesis of rheumatoid arthritis: cellular and cytokine interactions. In: Smolen J, Kalden J, Maini RN, eds. Rheumatoid Arthritis. Heidelberg: Springer-Verlag, 1992:41-54.

947. Firestein GS, Xu W-D, Townsend K, Broide D, Alvaro-Garcia J, Glasebrook A, Zvaifler NJ. Cytokines in chronic inflammatory arthritis. I. Failure to detect T cell lymphokines (interleukin 2 and interleukin 3) and presence of macrophage colony-stimulating factor (CSF-1) and a novel mast cell growth factor in rheumatoid synovitis. J. Exp. Med. 1988; 168:1573-1586.

948. Brennan FM, Chantry D, Turner M, Foxwell B, Maini RN, Feldmann M. Detection of transforming growth factor-beta in rheumatoid arthritis synvial tissue: lack of effect on spontaneous cytokine production in joint cell cultures. Clin. Exp. Immunol. 1990; 81:278-285.

949. Hovdenes J, Gaudernack G, Kvien TK, Egeland T. Expression of activation markers on CD4+ and CD8+ cells from synovial fluid, synovial tissue and peripheral blood of patients with inflammatory arthritis. Scand. J. Immunol. 1989; 29:631-639.

950. Firestein GS, Zvaifler NJ. The role of T cells in rheumatoid arthritis. Ann. Rheum. Dis. 1993; 52:765-765.

951. Panayi GS, Lanchbury JS, Kingsley GH. The importance of the T cell in initiating and maintaning the chronic synovitis of rheumatoid arthritis. Arthritis Rheum. 1992; 35:729-735.

952. Buchan GK, Barrett T, Fujita T, Taniguchi T, Maini RN, Feldmann M. Detection of activated T products in the rheumatoid joint using cDNA probes

to interleukin 2 (IL-2), IL-2 receptor and IFN-gamma. Clin. Exp. Immunol. 1988; 71:295-301.

953. Firestein GS, Alvaro-Garcia JM, Maki R. Quantitative analysis of cytokine gene expression in rheumatoid arthritis. J. Immunol. 1990; 144:3347-3353.

954. Simon AK, Seipelt E, Sieper J. Divergent T-cell cytokines patterns in inflammatory arthritis. Proc. Natl. Acad. Sci. USA 1994; 91:8562-8566.

955. Miltenburg AMM, Van Laar JM, De Kniper R, Daha MR, Breedveld FC. T cell clones from human rheumatoid synovial membrane functionally represent the TH1 subset. Scand. J. Immunol. 1992; 35:603-610.

956. Quayle AJ, Chomarat P, Miossec P. Kjeldsen-Kragh J, Forre O, Natvig JB. Rheumatoid inflammatory T-cell clones express mostly Th1 but also Th2 and mixed (Th0-like) cytokine patterns. Scand. J. Immunol. 1993; 38:75-82.

957. Katsikis PD, Chu C-Q, Brennan FM, Maini R, Feldmann M. Immunoregulatory role of interleukin 10 in rheumatoid arthritis. J. Exp. Med. 1994; 179:1517-1527.

958. Shulze-Koops H, Lipsky PE, Kavanaugh AF, Benefit LS. Elevated Th1- or Th0-like cytokine mRNA in peripheral circulation of patients with rheumatoid arthritis. J. Immunol. 1995; 155:5029-5037.

959. Gerli R, Muscat C, Bistoni O, Falini B, Agea E, Tognellini R. Biagini P, Bertotto A. High levels of the soluble form of CD30 molecule in rheumatoid arthritis (RA) are expression of CD30⁺ T cell involvement in the inflammed joints. Clin. Exp. Immunol. 1995; 102:547-550.

960. Isomaki P, Luukkainen R, Saario R, Toivanen P, Punnonen J. Interleukin-10 functions as an antiinflammatory cytokine in rheumatoid synovium. Arthritis Rheum. 1996; 39:386-395.

961. McInnes IB, Al-Mughales J, Field M, Leung BP, Huang F-P, Dixon R, Sturrock RD, Wilkinson PC, Liew FY. The role of interleukin-15 in T-cell migration and activation in rheumatoid arthritis. Nature Med. 1996; 2:175-182.

962. Skopouli FN, Dorsos AA, Papaioannu T, Moutsopoulos, HM. Preliminary diagnostic criteria for Sjogren's syndrome. Scand. J. Rheumatol. 1986; 61(suppl.):22-25.

963. Fox RI, Kang H-I. Pathogenesis of Sjogren's syndrome. Rheum. Dis. Clin. North Am. 1992; 18:517-538.

964. Roxe D, Griffith M, Stewart J, Novick D, Beverley PCL, Isenberg DA. HLA class I and class II, interferon, interleukin-2, and the interleukin-2 receptor expression on labial biopsy specimens from patients with Sjogren's syndrome. Ann. Rheum. Dis. 1987; 46:580-586.

965. Oxholm P, Daniels TE, Bendtzen K. Cytokine expression in labial salivary glands from patients with primary Sjogren's syndrome. Autoimmunity 1992; 12:185-191.

966. Al-Janadi M, Al-Balla S, Al-Dalaan A, Raziuddin S. Cytokine profile in systemic lupus erythematosus, rheumatoid arthritis, and other rheumatic diseases. J. Clin. Immunol. 1993; 13:58-67.

967. Villareal GM, Alcocer-Varela J, Llorente L. Cytokine gene and CD25 antigen expression by peripheral blood T cells from patients with primary Sjogren's syndrome. Autoimmunity 1995; 20:223-229.

968. Llorente L, Richaud-Patin Y, Fior R, Alcocer-Varela J, Wijdenes J, Morel Fourrier B, Galanaud P, Emilie D. In vivo production of interleukin 10 by non-T cells in rheumatoid arthritis, Sjogren's syndrome, and systemic lupus erythematosus. Arthritis Rheum. 1994; 37:1647-1655.

969. Dang H, Geiser AG, Letterio JJ, Nakabayashi T, Kong L, Fernandes G, Talal N. SLE-like autoantibodies and Sjogren's syndrome-like lymphoproliferation in TGF-β knockout mice. J. Immunol. 1995; 155:3205-3212.

970. Mills JA. Systemic lupus erythematosus. N. Engl. J. Med. 1994; 330:1871-1879.
971. Klinman DM, Steinberg AD. Systemic autoimmune disease arises from polyclonal B cell activation. J. Exp. Med. 1987; 165 1755-1760.
972. Boussiotis VA, Barber DL, Nakarai T et al. Prevention of T cell anergy by signaling through the gamma chain of the IL-2 receptor. Science 1994; 266:1039-1042.
973. Goldman M, Druet P, Gleichmann E. Th2 cells in systemic autoimmunity: insights from allogenic diseases and chemically-induced autoimmunity. Immunol. Today 1991; 12:223-227.
974. de Wit D, Van Mechele M, Zanin C et al. Preferential activation of Th2 cells in chronic graft-versus-host-reaction. J. Immunol. 1993; 150:361-366.
975. Ozmen L, Roman D, Fountoulakis M, Schmid G, Ryffel B, Garotta G. Experimental therapy of systemic lupus erythematosus: the treatment of NZB/W mice with soluble interferon-gamma receptor inhibits the onset of glomerulonephritis. Eur. J. Immunol. 1995; 25:6-12.
976. Ishida H, Muchamuel T, Sakaguchi S, Menon S, Howard M. Continuous administration of anti-interleukin 10 antibodies delays onset of autoimmunity in NZB/W mice. J. Exp. Med. 1994; 179:305-310.
977. Diaz Gallo C, Jevnikar A, Brennan D, Florquin S, Pacheco-Silva A, Rubin Kelley V. Autoreactive kidney-infiltrating T-cell clones in murine lupus nephritis. Kidney Int. 1992; 42:851-859.
978. Finck BK, Chan B, Wofsy D. Interleukin 6 promotes murine lupus in NZB/NZW F1 mice. J. Clin. Invest. 1994; 94:585-591.
979. Mori K, Kobayashi S, Inobe M, Jia W-Y, Tamakoshi M, Miyazaki T, Uede T. In vivo cytokine gene expression in various T cell subsets of the autoimmune MRL:Mp-lpr/lpr mouse. Autoimmunity 1994; 17:49-57.
980. Prud'homme GJ, Kono DH, Theofilopoulos AN. Quantitative polymerase chain reaction reveals marked overexpression of interleukin-1 beta, interleukin-10 and interferon-gamma mRNA in the lymph nodes of lupus-prone mice. Mol. Immunol. 1995; 32:495-503.
981. Takahashi S, Fossati L, Iwamoto M, Merino R, Motta R, Kobayakawa T, Izui S. Imbalance towards Th1 predominance is associated with acceleration of lupus-like autoimmune syndrome in MRL mice. J. Clin. Invest. 1996; 97.
982. Huang F-P, Feng G-, Lindop G, Stott DI, Liew FY. The role of interleukin 12 and nitric oxide in the development of spontaneous autoimmune disease in MRL/MP-lpr/lpr mice. J. Exp. Med. 1996; 183:1447-1460.
983. Klinman DM, Haynes BF, Conover J. Activation of IL-4 and IL-6 secreting cells by HIV-specific peptides. AIDS Res. and Human Retro. 1995; 11:97-105.
984. Hagiwara E, Gourley MF, Lee M, Klinman DM. Disease severity in patients with systemic lupus erythematosus correlates with an increased ratio of interleukin-10/interferon-secreting cells in peripheral blood. Arthritis Rheum. 1996; 39:379-385.
985. Dueymes M, Barrier J, Bescancenot JF et al. Relationship of IL-4 to isotypic distribution of anti-DS DNA antibodies in SLE. Int. Arch. Allergy Appl. Immunol. 1993; 101:408-415.
986. Ogawa N, Itoh M, Goto Y. Abnormal production of B cell growth factor in patients with systemic lupus erythematosus. Clin. Exp. Immunol. 1992; 89:26-31.
987. Caligaris-Cappio F, Bertero MT, Converso M, Stacchini A, Vinante F, Romagnani S, Pizzolo G. Circulating levels of soluble CD30, a marker of cells producing Th2-type cytokines, are increased in patients with systemic lupus erythematosus and correlate with disease activity. Clin. Exp. Rheum. 1995; 13:339-343.

988. Linker-Israeli M, Deans R, Wallace D, Prehn J, Ozeri-Chen T, Klinenburg, J. Elevated levels of endogenous IL-6 in systemic lupus erythematosus. J. Immunol. 1991; 147:117-123.

989. Spronk P, Ter Borg E, Limburg P, Kallenberg C. Plasma concentration of IL-6 in systemic lupus erythematosus; an indicator of disease activity? Clin. Exp. Immunol. 1992; 90:106-110.

990. Nagafuchi H, Suzuki N, Mizushima Y, Sakane T. Constitutive expression of IL-6 receptors and their role in the excessive B cell function in patients with systemic lupus erythematosus. J. Immunol. 1993; 151:6525-6534.

991. Llorente L, Zou W, Levy Y et al. Role of interleukin 10 in the B lymphocyte hyperactivity and autoantibody production of human systemic lupus erythematosus. J. Exp. Med. 1995; 181:839-844.

992. Fleischmajer R, Perlish R, Duncan M. Scleroderma. A model for fibrosis. Arch. Dermatol. 1983; 119:957-962.

993. Roumm AD, Whiteside TL. Medsger TA, Rodnan GP. Lymphocytes in the skin of patients with progressive systemic sclerosis. Quantification, subtyping, and clinical correlations. Arthritis Rheum. 1984; 6:645-653.

994. Kovacs EJ. Fibrogenic cytokines: the role of immune mediators in the development of scar tissue. Immunol. Today 1991; 12:17-23.

995. Postlethwhaite AE, Seyer JM. Fibroblast chemotaxis induction by human recombinant interleukin 4: identification by synthetic peptide analysis of two chemotactic domains residing in aminoacid sequences 70-88 and 89-122. J. Clin. Invest. 1991; 87:2147-2152.

996. Postlethwhaite AE, Holness A, Katai H, Raghow R. Human fibroblasts synthesize elevated levels of extracellular matrix proteins in response to interleukin 4. J. Clin. Invest. 1992; 90:1479-1485.

997. Gillery P, Fertin C, Nicolas JF, Chastang F, Kalis B, Banchereau J, Maquart FX. Interleukin-4 stimulates collagen gene expression in human fibroblast monolayer cultures. Fed. Eur. Biochem. Sci. 1992; 302:231-234.

998. Famularo G, Procopio A, Giacomelli R, Danese C, Sacchetti S, Perego MA. Santoni A, Tonietti G. Soluble interleukin-2 receptor, interleukin-2 and interleukin-4 in sera and supernatants from patients with progressive systemic sclerosis. Clin. Exp. Immunol. 1990; 81:368-372.

999. Needleman BW, Wigley FM, Stair RW. Interleukin 2, interleukin 4, interleukin 6, tumor necrosis factor α, and interferon γ levels in sera from scleroderma patients. Arthritis Rheum. 1992; 35:67-72.

1000. Sato IH, Fujimoto S, Kikuchi M, Takehara K. Demonstration of IL-2, IL-4, IL-6 in sera from patients with scleroderma. Arch. Dermatol. Res. 1995; 287:193-197.

1001. Marshall BJ. Helicobacter pilori. Amer. J. Gastroenterolgy 1994; 89:116-128.

1002. Kreiss C, Blum AL, Malfertheiner P. Peptic ulcer pathogenesis. Curr. Opin. Immunol. 1995; 11:25-31.

1003. Marchetti M, Aricò B, Burroni D, Figura N, Rappuoli R, Ghiara P. Development of a mouse model of Helicobacter pylori infection that mimics human disease. Science 1995; 267:1655-1668.

1004. Mohammadi M, Czinn S, Nedrud J. *Helicobacter*-specific cell-mediated immune responses display a predominant Th1 phenotype and promote a delayed-type hypersensitivity response in the stomachs of mice. J. Immunol. 1996; 156:4729-4736.

1005. Kirsner JB, Shorter RG. Recent developments in "nonspecific" inflammatory bowel disease. N. Engl. J. Med. 1982; 306:775-837.

1006. Mombaerts P, Mizoguchi E, Grusby MJ. Glimcher LH, Bahn AK, Tonegawa S. Spontaneous development of inflammatory bowel disease in T cell receptor mutant mice. Cell 1993; 75:275-282.

1007. Sadlack B, Merz H, Schorle H, Scimpl A, Feller AC. Horvak I. Ulcerative colitis-like disease in mice with a disrupted interleukin-2 gene. Cell 1993; 75:253-261.

1008. Kuhn R, Rajewski K, Muller W. Generation and analysis of interleukin-4 deficient mice. Science 1991; 254:707-710.

1009. Kuhn R, Lohler J, Rennick D, Rajewski K, Muller W. Interleukin-10-deficient mice develop chronic enterocolitis. Cell 1993; 75:263-274.

1010. Kulkarni AB, Huh CG, Becker D et al. Transforming growth factor β1 null mutation in mice causes excessive inflammatory response and early death. Proc. Natl. Acad. Sci. USA 1993; 90:770-774.

1011. Rudolph U, Finegold MJ, Rich SS et al. Ulcerative colitis and adenocarcinoma of the colon in G alpha i2-deficient mice. Nature Genet. 1995; 10:143-150.

1012. Neurath MF, Fuss I, Kelsall BL, Stuber E, Strober W. Antibodies to interleukin 12 abrogate esablished experimental colitis in mice. J. Exp. Med. 1995; 182:1281-1290.

1013. Powrie F. T cells in inflammatory bowel disease: protective and pathogenic roles. Immunity 1995; 3:171-174.

1014. Powrie F, Correa-Oliveira R, Mauze S, Coffman RL. Regulatory interactions between CD45RBhi and CD45RBlo CD4+ T cells are important for the balance between protective and pathogenic cell-mediated immunity. J. Exp. Med. 1994a; 179:589-600.

1015. Powrie F, Leach MW, Mauze S, Menon S, Caddle LB, Coffman RL. Inhibition of Th1 responses prevents inflammatory bowel disease in scid mice reconstituted with CD45RBhi CD4+ T cells. Immunity 1994b; 1:553-562.

1016. Mueller Ch, Knoflach P, Zielinski CC. T-cell activation in Crohn's disease. Increased levels of soluble interleukin-2 receptor in serum and in supernatants of stimulated peripheral blood mononuclear cells. Gastroenterology 1990; 98:639-646.

1017. Mullin E, Lazenby AJ, Harris ML, Bayless TM, James SP. Increased interleukin-2 messenger RNA in the intestinal mucosa lesions of Crohn's disease but not ulcerative colitis. Gastroenterology 1992; 102:1620-1627.

1018. Gross V, Andus T, Caesar I, Roth M, Scholmerick J. Evidence for continuous stimulation of interleukin-6 production in Crohn's disease. Gastroenterology 1992; 102:514-519.

1019. Braegger CP, Nicholis S, Murch SH, Stephens S, MacDonald TT. Tumor necrosis factor alpha in stool as a marker of intestinal inflammation. Lancet 1992; 339:89-91.

1020. Raab Y, Hallegren R, Gerdin B. Enhanced intestinal synthesis of interleukin-6 is related to the disease severity and activity in ulcerative colitis. Digestion 1994; 55:44-49.

1021. Mazlam MZ, Hodgson HJF. Interactions between interleukin-6, interleukin-1β, plasma C-reactive protein values, and in vitro C-reactive protein generation in patients with inflammatory bowel disease. Gut 1994; 35:77-83.

1022. Breese EJ, Michie CA, Nicholls SW, Murch SH, Williams CB, Domizio P, Walker-Smith JA, MacDonald TT. Tumor necrosis factor alpha-producing cells in the intestinal mucosa of children with inflammatory bowel disease. Gastroenterology 1994; 106:1455-1466.

1023. Mitsuyama K, Toyonaga A, Sasaki E et al. Interleukin-8 as an important chemoattractant for neutrophils in ulcerative colitis and Crohn's disease. Clin. Exp. Immunol. 1994; 96:432-436.

1024. Niessner M, Volk BA. Altered Th1/Th2 cytokine profiles in the intestinal mucosa of patients with inflammatory bowel disease as assessed by quantitative transcribed polymerase chain reaction (RT-PCR). Clin. Exp. Immunol. 1995; 101:428-435.

1025. Giri SN, Hyde DM, Marafino BJ. Ameliorating effect of murine interferon gamma on bleomycin-induced lung collagen fibrosis in mice. Biochem. Med. Metab. Biol. 1986; 36:194-197.

1026. Goldring MB, Sandell LJ, Stephenson ML. Immune interferon suppresses levels of procollagen mRNA and type II collagen synthesis in cultured human articular and costal chondrocytes. J. Immunol. 1986; 261:9049-9056.

1027. Baecher-Allan CM, Barth RK. PCR analysis of cytokine induction profiles associated with mouse strain variation in susceptibility to pulmonary fibrosis. Regional Immunol. 1993; 5:207-217.

1028. Sempowski GD, Beckmann MP, Derdak S, Phipps RP. Subsets of murine lung fibroblasts express membrane-bound and soluble IL-4 receptors. J. Immunol. 1994; 152:3606-3614.

1029. Farmer ER. Human cutaneous graft versus host disease. J. Invest. Dermatol. 1985; 85:1249-1252.

1030. Peterson MW, Monick M, Hunninghake GW. Prognostic role of eosinophils in pulmonary fibrosis. Chest 1987; 92:51-56.

1031. Hallgren R, Bjermer L, Lundgren R, Venge P. The eosinophil component of the alveolitis in idiopathic pulmonary fibrosis. Signs of eosinophil activation in the lung is associated with impaired lung function. Am. Rev. Resp. Dis. 1989; 139:373-383.

1032. Birkland TP, Cheavens MD, Pincus SH. Human eosinophils stimulate DNA synthesis and matrix production by dermal fibroblasts. Arch. Dermatol. Res. 1994; 286:312-318.

1033. Wallace WAH, Ramage EA, Lamb D, Howie SEM. A type 2 (Th2-like) pattern of immune response predominates in the pulmonary interstitium of patients with cryptogenic fibrosing alveolitis (CFA). Clin. Exp. Immunol. 1995; 101:436-441.

1034. Moller DR, Forman JD, Liu MC et al. Enhanced expression of IL-12 associaed with Th1 cytokine profiles in active pulmonary sarcoidosis. J. Immunol. 1996; 156:4952-4960.

1035. Uyemura K, Demer LL, Castle SC, Jullien D, Berliner JA, Gately MK, Warrier RR, Pham N, Fogelman AM, Modlin RL. Cross-regulatory roles of interleukin (IL)-12 and IL-10 in atherosclerosis. J. Clin. Invest. 1996; 97:

1036. Nickerson P, Steurer W, Steiger J, Zheng X, Steele AW, Strom TB. Cytokines and the Th1/Th2 paradigm in transplantation. Curr. Opin. Immunol. 1994; 6:757-764.

1037. Suthanthiran M, Strom TB. Immunobiology and immunopharmacology of organ allograft rejection. J. Clin. Immunol. 1995; 15:161-171.

1038. Navry CPJ, Teppo AM. Raised serum levels of cachectin/tumor necrosis factor α in renal allograft rejection. J. Exp. Med. 1987; 166:1132-1137.

1039. Hoffman NW, Wonigeit K, Steinoff G, Behrend H, Flad HD, Pichlmayr R. Tumor necrosis factor alpha and interleukin-1β in rejecting human liver grafts. Transpl. Proc. 1991; 23:1421-1423.

1040. Caillat-Zucman S, van de Broecke C, Legendre C, Noel LH, Kreis H, Bach JF, Tovey MG. Differential in situ expression of cytokine genes in human renal rejection. Transpl. Proc. 1991; 23:229-230.

1041. Benvenuto RA, Bachloni A, Cinti P, Sallusto F, Franco F, Molajoni ER, Barnaba V, Balsano F, Cortesini R. Enhanced production of interferon-γ by T lymphocytes cloned from rejected kidney grafts. Transplantation 1991; 51:887-892.

1042. Kirk AD, Ibrahim MA, Bollinger RR, Dawson DV, Finn OJ. Renal allograft-infiltrating lymphocytes. A prospective analysis of in vitro growth characteristics and clinical relevance. Transplantation 1992; 53:329-338.

1043. Noronha IL, Eberlein-Gonska M, Hartley B, Stephens S, Cameron JS, Waldherr R. In situ expression of tumor necrosis factor alpha, interferon-gamma, and interleukin-2 receptors in renal allograft biopsies. Transplantation 1992; 54:1017-1024.

1044. Dallman MJ. Cytokines as mediators of organ graft rejection and tolerance. Curr. Opin. Immunol. 1993; 5:788-793.

1045. Krams SM, Falco DA, Villanueva JC et al. Cytokine and T cell receptor gene expression at the site of allograft rejection. Transplantation 1992; 53:151-156.

1046. Takeuchi T, Lowry RP, Konieczny B. Heart allografts in murine systems. Transplantation 1992; 53:1281-1294.

1047. Francalancia NA, Wang SC, Thai NL, Aeba R, Simmons RL, Yousem SA, Hardesty RL, Griffith BP. Graft cytokine mRNA activity in rat single lung transplants by reverse transcription-polymerase chain reaction: effect of cyclosporine. J. Heart Lung Transplant. 1992; 11:1041-1045.

1048. Field EH, Rouse TM, Fleming AL, Jamali I, Cowdery JS. Altered IFN-gamma and IL-4 pattern lymphokine secretion in mice partially depleted of CD4 T cells by anti-CD4 monoclonal antibody. J. Immunol. 1992; 149:1131-1137.

1049. Sayegh MH, Akalin E, Hancock WW, Russell ME, Carpenter CB, Linsley PS, Turka LA. CD28-B7 blockade after alloantigenic challenge in vivo inhibits Th1 cytokines but spares Th2. J. Exp. Med. 1995; 181:1869-1874.

1050. Mottram PL, Han WR, Purcell LJ, McKenzie IFC, Hancock WW. Increased expression of IL-4 and IL-10 and decreased expression of IL-2 and interferon-γ in long-surviving mouse heart allografts after brief CD4 monoclonal antibody therapy. Transplantation 1995; 59:559-565.

1051. Maeda H, Takata M, Takahashi S, Ogoshi S, Fujimoto S. Adoptive transfer of Th2-like cell line prolongs MHC class II antigen disparate skin allograft survival in the mouse. Int. Immunol. 1994; 6:855-862.

1052. Ledingham DL, McAlister VC, Ehigiator HN, Giacomantonio C, Theal M, Lee TD. Prolongation of rat kidney allograft survival by nematodes. Transplantation 1996; 61:184-188.

1053. Gorczynski RM, Chen Z, Rossi-Bergman B. A subset of $\gamma\delta$T-cell receptor-positive cells produce T-helper type 2 cytokines and regulate mouse skin graft rejection following portal venous pretransplant preimmunization. Immunology 1996; 87:381-389.

1054. Bugeon L, Cuturi M-C, Hallet M-M, Paineau J, Chabannes D, Soulillou J-P. Peripheral tolerance of an allograft in adult rats - characterization by low interleukin-2 and interferon-gamma mRNA levels and by strong accumulation of major histocompatibility complex transcripts in the graft. Transplantation 1992; 54:219-225.

1055. Josien R, Pannetier C, Douillard P, Cantarovich D, Menoret S, Bugeon L, Kourilsky P, Soulillou J-P, Cuturi M-C. Graft infiltrating T helper cells CD45RC phenotype and Th1/Th2-related cytokines in donor specific transfusion-induced tolerance in adult rats. Transplantation 1995; 60:1131-1139.

1056. Farges O, Morris PJ, Dallman MJ. Spontaneous acceptance of rat liver allografts is associated with an early downregulation of intragraft IL-4 mRNA expression. Hepatology 1995; 21:767-775.

1057. Morris CF, Simeonovic CJ, Fung MC, Wilson JD, Hapel AJ. Intragraft expression of cytokine transcript during pig proislet xenograft rejection and tolerance in mice. J. Immunol. 1995; 154:2470-2482.

1058. Merville P, Lambert C, Durand I, Pouteil-Noble C, Touraine JL, Berthoux F, Banchereau J. High frequency of IL-10-secreting CD4$^+$ graft-infiltrating T lymphocytes in promptly rejected kidney allografts. Transplantation 1995; 59:1113-1119.

1059. Bishop GA, Rokahr KL, Napoli J, McCaughan GW. Intragraft cytokine mRNA levels in human liver allograft rejection analysed by reverse transcription and semiquantitative polymerase chain reaction amplification. Transplant. Immunol. 1993; 1:253-261.

1060. Sun J, McCaughan GW, Matsumoto Y, Sheil AGR, Gallagher ND, Bishop GA. Tolerance to rat liver allograft. Transplantation 1994; 57:1349-1357.

1061. Zheng XX, Steele AW, Nickerson PW, Steurer W, Steiger J, Strom TB. Administration of noncytolytic IL-10/Fc in murine models of lipopolysaccharide-induced septic shock and allogeneic islet transplantation. J. Immunol. 1995; 154:5590-5600.

1062. Lowry RP, Konieczny B, Alexander D, Larsen C, Pearson T, Smith S, Narula S. Interleukin-10 eliminates anti-CD3 monoclonal antibody-induced mortality and prolongs heart allograft survival in inbred mice. Transplant. Proc. 1995; 27:392-394.

1063. Vossen ACTM, Tibbe GJM, Benner R, Savelkoul HFJ. T-lymphocyte and cytokine-directed strategies for inhibiting skin allograft rejection in mice. Transplant. Proc. 1995; 27:380-382.

1064. Dallman MJ. Cytokines and transplantation: Th1/Th2 regulation of the immune response to solid organ transplants in the adult. Curr. Opin. Immunol. 1995; 7:632-638.

1065. Qin L, Chavin KD, Ding Y et al. Multiple vectors effectively achieve gene transfer in a murine cardiac transplantation model. Immunosuppression with TGF-β1 or vIL-10. Transplantation 1995; 59:809-816.

1066. Chan SY, DeBruyne LA, Goodman RE, Eichwald EJ, Bishop DK. *In vivo* depletion of CD8⁺ T cells results in Th2 cytokine production and alternate mechanisms of allograft rejection. Transplantation 1995; 59:1155-1161.

1067. Gleichmann E, Pals ST, Rolink AG, Radaszkiewicz T, Gleichmann H. Graft-versus-host-reactions: clues to the etiopathology of a spectrum of immunological diseases. Immunol. Today 1984; 5:324.

1068. Moser M, Iwazaki T, Shearer GM. Cellular interactions in graft-versus-host induced T cell immune deficiency. Immunol. Rev. 1985; 88:135-151.

1069. Rus V, Svetic A, Nguyen P, Gause WC, Via CS. Kinetics of Th1 and Th2 cytokine production during the early course of acute and chronic murine graft-versus-host disease. J. Immunol. 1995; 155:2396-2406.

1070. Allen RD, Staley TA, Sidman CL. Differential cytokine expression in acute and chronic murine graft-versus-host disease. Eur. J. Immunol. 1993; 23:333-337.

1071. Via CS, Finkelman FD. Critical role of interleukin-2 in the development of acute graft-versus-host disease. Int. Immunol. 1993; 5:565-572.

1072. Ellison CA, MacDonald GC, rector ES, Gartner JG. γδ T cells in the pathobiology of murine acute graft-versus-host disease. Evidence that γδ T cells mediate natural killer-like cytotoxicity in the host and that elimination of these cells from donors significantly reduces mortality. J. Immunol. 1995; 155:4189-4198.

1073. Williamson E, Garside P, Bradley JA, Mowat AMcI. IL-12 is a central mediator of acute graft-versus-host disease. J. Immunol. 1996; 157:689-699.

1074. Krenger W, Snyder KM, Byon JC, Falzarano G, Ferrara JL. Polarized type 2 alloreactive CD4⁺ and CD8⁺ donor T cells fail to induce experimental acute graft-versus-host-disease. J. Immunol. 1995; 155:585-593.

1075. Doutrelepont JM, Moser M, Leo O, Abramowicz D, Vanderhaegen ML, Urbain J, Goldman M. Hyper IgE in stimulatory graft-versus-host disease: role of interleukin-4. Clin. Exp. Immunol. 1991; 83:133-136.

1076. Ushiyama C, Hirano T, Miyajima H, Okumura K, Ovary Z, Hashimoto H. Anti-IL-4 antibody prevents graft-versus-host disease in mice after bone marrow transplantation. J. Immunol. 1995; 154:2687-2696.

1077. Via CS, Rus V, Gately MK, Finkelman FD. IL-12 stimulates the development of acute graft-versus-host disease in mice that normally would develop chronic, autoimmune graft-versus-host disease. J. Immunol. 1994; 153:4040-4047.

1078. Ferrara JLM. Cytokine dysregulation as a mechanism of graft versus host disease. Curr. Opin. Immunol. 1993; 5:794-799.

1079. Borish L, Dishuck J, Cox L, Mascali JJ, Williams J, Rosenwasser LJ. Sézary syndrome with elevated serum IgE and hypereosinophilia: role of dysregulated cytokine production. J. Allergy Clin. Immunol. 1993; 92:123-131.

1080. Rook AH, Lessin SR, Jaworsky C, Singh A, Vowels BR. The immunopathogenesis of cutaneous T cell lymphoma: abnormal cytokine production by Sézary T cells. Arch. Dermatol. 1993; 129:486-489.

1081. Vowels BR, Cassin M, Vonderheid EC, Rook AH. Aberrant cytokine production by Sézary syndrome patients: cytokine secretion pattern resembles murine Th2 cells. J. Invest. Dermatol. 1992; 99:90-94.

1082. Tendler CL, Burton JD, Jaffe J, Danielpour D, Charley M, McCoy JP, Pittelkow MR, Waldmann TA. Abnormal cytokine expression in Sézary and adult T-cell leukemia correlates with the functional diversity between these T-cell malignancies. Cancer Res. 1994; 54:4430-4435.

1083. Vowels BR, Lessin SR, Cassin M, Jaworsky C, Benoit B, Wolfe JT, Rook AH. Th2 cytokine mRNA expression in skin in cutaneous T-cell lymphoma. J. Invest. Dermatol. 1994; 103:669-673.

1084. Rook AH, Kubin M, Cassin M, Vonderheid EC, Vowels BR, Wolfe JT, Wolf SF, Singh A, Trinchieri G, Lessin SR. IL-12 reverses cytokine and immune abnormalities in Sézary syndrome. J. Immunol. 1995; 154:1491-1498.

1085. Saed G, Fivenson DP, Naidu Y, Nickoloff BJ. Mycosis fungoides exhibits a Th1-type cell-mediated cytokine profile whereas Sézary syndrome expresses a Th2-type profile. J. Invest. Dermatol. 1994; 103:29-33.

1086. Yamamoto T, Sasaki G, Sato T, Katayama I, Nishioka K. Cytokine profile of tumor cells in mycosis fungoides: successful treatment with intra-lesional interferon-gamma combined with chemotherapy. J. Dermatol. 1995; 22:650-654.

1087. Cogan E, Schandené L, Crusiaux A, Cochaux P, Velu T, Goldman M. Brief report: clonal proliferation of type 2 helper T cells in a man with the hypereosinophilic syndrome. N. Engl. J. Med. 1994; 330:535-538.

1088. Barth RJ, Mulé JJ, Spiess PJ, Rosenberg SA. Interferon-gamma and tumor necrosis factor have a role in tumor regressions mediated by murine CD8[+] tumor-infiltrating lymphocytes. J. Exp. Med. 1991; 173:647-658.

1089. Forni G, Fujiwara H, Martino F, Hamaoka T, Jemma C, Caretto P, Giovarelli M. Helper strategy in tumor immunology: expansion of helper lymphocytes and utilization of helper lymphocytes for experimental and clinical immunotherapy. Cancer Met. Rev. 1988; 7:289-309.

1090. Nagarkatty M, Clary SR, Nagarkatty PS. Characterization of tumor-infiltrating CD4[+] T cells as Th1 cells based on lymphokine secretion and functional properties. J. Immunol. 1990; 144:4898-4905.

1091. Taylor CW, Grogan TM, Salmon SE. Effects of interleukin 4 on the in vitro growth of human lymphoid and plasma cell neoplasms. Blood 1990; 75:1114-1118.

1092. Tepper RI, Coffman RL, Leder P. An eosinophil-dependent mechanism for the antitumor effect of IL-4. Science 1992; 257:548-551.

1093. Pericle F, Giovarelli M, Colombo MP et al. An efficient Th2-type memory follows CD8+ lymphocyte-driven and eosinophil-mediated rejection of a spontaneous mouse mammary adenocarcinoma engineered to release IL-4. J. Immunol. 1994; 153; 5659-5673.

1094. Ghosh P, Komschlies KL, Cippitelli M et al. Gradual loss of T-helper 1 populations in spleen of mice during progressive tumor growth. J. Natl. Cancer Inst. 1995; 87:1478-1483.

1095. Ruzek MC, Mathur A. Specific decrease of Th1-like activity in mice with plasma cell tumors. Int. Immunol. 1995; 7:1029-1035.

1096. Rohrer JW, Coggin Jr JH. CD8 T cell clones inhibit antitumor T cell function by secreting IL-10. J. Immunol. 1995; 155:5719-5727.

1097. Gorelik L, Prokhorova A, Mokyr MB. Low-dose melphalan-induced shift in the production of a Th2-type cytokine to a Th1-type cytokine in mice bearing a large MOPC-315 tumor. Cancer Immunol. Immunother. 1994; 39:117-126.

1098. Maeda H, Shirashi A. TGF-beta contributes to the shift toward Th2-type responses through direct and IL-10-mediated pathways in tumor-bearing mice. J. Immunol. 1996; 156:73-78.

1099. Yamamura M, Modlin RL, Ohmen JD, Moy RL. Local expression of antiinflammatory cytokines in cancer. J. Clin. Invest. 1993; 91:1005-1010.

1100. Goedegebuure PS, Lee KY, Matory YL, Peoples GE, Yoshino I, Eberlein TJ. Classification of CD4+ T helper cell clones in human melanoma. Cell Immunol. 1994; 156:170-179.

1101. Lee KY, Goedegebuure PS, Linehan DC, Eberlein TJ. Immunoregulatory effects of CD4+ T helper subsets in human melanoma. Surgery 1995; 117:365-372.

1102. Kharkevitch DD, Seito D, Balch GC, Maeda T, Balch CM, Itoh K. Characterization of autologous tumor-specific T-helper 2 cells in tumor-infiltrating lymphocytes from a patient with metastatic melanoma. Int. J. Cancer 1994; 58:317-323.

1103. Ozdemirli M, Akdeniz H, El-Khatib M, Ju S-T. A novel cytotoxicity of CD4+ Th1 clones on heat-shocked tumor targets. I. Implications for internal disintegration model for target death and hyperthermia treatment of cancers. J. Immunol. 1991; 147:4027-4034.

1104. McAdam AJ, Pulaski BA, Harkins SS, Hutter EK, Lord EM, Frelinger JG. Synergistic effects of co-expression of the Th1-cytokines IL-2 and IFN-gamma on generation of murine tumor-reactive cytotoxic cells. Int. J. Cancer 1995; 61:628-634.

1105. McAveney KM, Gomella LG, Lattime EC. Induction of Th1- and Th2-associated cytokine mRNA in mouse bladder following intravesical growth of the murine bladder tumor MB49 and BCG immunotherapy. Cancer Immunol. Immunother. 1994; 39:401-406.

1106. Kuge S, Miura Y, Nakamura Y, Mitomi T, Habu S, Nishimura T. Superantigen-induced human CD4+ helper/killer T cell phenomenon. Selective induction of Th1 helper/killer T cells and application to tumor immunotherapy. J. Immunol. 1995; 154:1777-1785.

1107. Gately MK, Gunler U, Brunda MJ, Nadeau RR, Anderson TD, Lipman JM, Sarmiento U. Interleukin-12: a cytokine with therapeutic potential in oncology and infectious diseases. Ther. Immunol. 1994; 1:187-196.

1108. Brunda MJ, Luistro L, Warrier RR, Wright RB, Hubbard BR, Murphy M, Wolf SF, Gately MK. Antitumor and antimetastatic activity of interleukin-12 against murine tumours. J. Exp. Med. 1994; 178:1223-

1109. Nastala CL, Edington HD, McKinney TG et al. Recombinant interleukin-12 (IL-12) administration induces tumor regression in association with interferon-gamma production. J. Immunol. 1994; 153:1697-1706.

1110. Tannenbaum CS, Wicker N, Armstrong D, Tubbs R, Finke J, Bukowski RM, Hamilton TA. Cytokine and chemokine expression in tumors of mice receiving systemic therapy with IL-12. J. Immunol. 1996; 156:693-699.

1111. Zitvogel L, Mayordomo JI, Tjandrawn T, DeLeo AB, Clarke MR, Lotze MT, Storkus WJ. Therapy of murine tumors with tumor peptide-pulsed dendritic cells: dependence on T cells, B7 costimulation, and T helper cell 1-associated cytokines. J. Exp. Med. 1996; 183:87-97.

1112. Fallarino F, Uyttenhove C, Boon T, Gajewski TF. Endogenous IL-12 is necessary for rejection of P815 tumor variants in vivo. J. Immunol. 1996; 156:1095-1100.

1113. Abdelhak S; Louzir H; Timm J, Blel L, Benlasfar Z, Lagranderie M, Gheorghiu M, Dallagi K, Gicquel B. Recombinant BCG expressing the leishmania surface antigen Gp62 induces protective immunity against *Leishmania major* infection in BALB/c mice. Microbiology 1995; 141:1582-1592.

1114. Murray PJ, Aldovini A, Young RA. Manipulation and potentiation of antimycobacterial immunity using recombinant bacille Calmette-Guérin strains that secrete cytokines. Proc. Natl. Acad. Sci. USA 1996; 93:934-939.

1115. Fennelly GJ, Flynn JL, ter Meulen V, Liebert UG, Bloom BR. Recombinant bacille Calmette-Guérin priming against measles. J. Infect. Dis. 1995; 172:698-705.

1116. Nash AD, Lofthouse SA, Barcham GJ, Jacobs HJ, Ashman K, Meeusen E, Brandon M, Andrews A. Recombinant cytokines as immunological adjuvants. Immunol. Cell Biol. 1993; 71:367-379.

1117. Miller MA, Skeen MJ, Ziegler HK. Nonviable bacterial antigens administered with IL-12 generate antigen-specific T cell responses and protective immunity against *Leisteria monocytogenes*. J. Immunol. 1995; 155:4817-4828.

1118. Mountford AP, Anderson S, Wilson RA. Induction of Th1 cell-mediated protective immunity to *Schistosoma mansoni* by co-administration of larval antigens and IL-12 as an adjuvant. J. Immunol. 1996; 156:4739-4745.

1119. Taylor CE. Cytokines as adjuvants for vaccines: antigen-specific responses differ from polyclonal responses. Infect. Immunity 1995; 63:3241-3244.

1120. Wolff JA, Malone RW, Williams P, Riedy M, DeVit MJ, McElligott SG, Stanford JC. Direct gene transfer into mouse muscle in vitro. Science 1990; 247:1465-1468.

1121. Tang D, DeVit M, Johnston SA. Genetic immunization is a simple method for eliciting an immune response. Nature 1992; 365:152-154.

1122. Hildegund CJ, Xiang Z. Novel vaccine approaches. J. Immunol. 1996; 156:3779-3582.

1123. McDonnell VM, Askari FK. DNA vaccines. New Engl. J. Med. 1996; 334:41-45.

1124. Raz E, Tighe E, Sato Y, Corr M, Dudler JA, Roman M, Swain SL, Spiegelberg HL, Carson DA. Preferential induction of a Th1 immune response and inhibition of specific IgE antibody formation by plasmid DNA immunization. Proc. Natl. Acad. Sci. USA 1996; 93:5141-5145.

1125. Perez VL, Lederer JA, Lichtman AH, Abbas AK. Stability of Th1 and Th2 populations. Int. Immunol. 1995; 7:869-875.

1126. Murphy E, Shibuya K, Hosken N, Openshaw P, Maino V, Davis K, Murphy K, O'Garra A. Reversibility of T helper 1 and 2 populations is lost after long-term stimulation. J. Exp. Med. 1996; 183:901-914.

1127. Aversa G, Punnonen J, Cocks BG, de Waal Malefyt R, Vega FJr, Zurawski SM, Zurawski G, de Vries JE. An interleukin 4 (IL-4) mutant protein inhibits both IL-4 or IL-13-induced human immunoglobulin G4 (IgG4) and IgE synthesis and B cell proliferation: support for a common component shared by IL-4 and IL-13 receptors. J. Exp. Med. 1993; 178:2213-2218.

1128. Carballido JM, Aversa G, Schols D, Punnonen J, de Vries JE. Inhibition of human IgE synthesis in vitro and in SCID-hu mice by an interleukin-4 receptor antagonist. Int. Arch. Allergy Immunol. 1995; 107:304-307.

1129. Kung TT, Stelts DM, Zurcher JA, Adams GK, Egan RW, Kreutner W, Watnick AS, Jones H, Chapman RW. Involvement of IL-5 in a murine model of allergic pulmonary inflammation: prophylactic and theraputic effect of an anti-IL-5 antibody. Am. J. Respir. Cell Mol. Biol. 1995; 13:360-365.

1130. Mori A, Suko M, Kaminuma P et al. Enhanced Production and Gene Expression of IL-5 in Bronchial Asthma. Possible Management of Atopic Diseases with IL-5 Specific Gene Transcription Inhibitor. In: Sehon A, Kraft D, eds. Molecular Biology of Allergens and the Atopic Immune Response. New York: Plenum Press, 1996.

1131. Mitchison A, Sieper J. Immunological basis of oral tolerance. Z. Rheumatol. 1995; 54:141-144.

1132. Friedman A. Induction of anergy in Th1 lymphocytes by oral tolerance. Importance of antigen dosage and frequency of feeding. Ann. N.Y. Acad. Sci. 1996; 778:103-110.

1133. Vischer TL. Oral desensitization in the treatment of human immune diseases. Z. Rheumatol. 1995; 54:155-157.

1134. Withacre CC, Gienapp IE, Meyer A, Cox KL, Javed N. Oral tolerance in experimental autoimmune encephalomyelitis. Ann. N.Y. Acad. Sci. 1996; 778:217-227.

1135. Nussenblatt RB, Withcup SM, de Smet MD, Caspi RR, Kozhich AT, Weiner HL, Vistica B, Gery I. Intraocular inflammatory disease (uveitis) and the use of oral tolerance: a status report. Ann. N.Y. Acad. Sci. 1996; 778:325-337.

1136. Wang ZY, He B, Qiao J, Link H. Suppression of experimental auotimmune myastenia gravis and experimental allergic encephalomyelitis by oral administration of acetylcholine receptor and myelin basic protein: double tolerance. J. Neuroimmunol. 1995; 63:79-86.

1137. Tian JD, Atkinson MA, Salzler MC, Herschenfeld A, Forsthuber T, Lehmann PV, Kaufman DL. Nasal administration of glutamate decarboxylase (GAD65) peptides induces Th2 responses and prevents murine insulin-dependent diabetes. J. Exp. Med. 1996; 183:1561- 1568.

1138. Fukaura H, Kent SC, Pietrusewicz MJ, Khoury SJ, Weiner HL, Hafler DA. Antigen-specific TGF-beta1 secretion within bovine myelin oral tolerization in multiple sclerosis. Ann. N.Y. Acad. Sci. 1996; 778:251-257.

1139. Sieper J, Kary S, Sorensen H et al. Oral type II collagen treatment in early rheumatoid arthritis. A double-blind, placebo-controlled, randomized trial. Arthritis Rheum. 1996; 39:41-51.

1140. Li L, Elliott JF, Mosmann TR. IL-10 inhibits cytokine production, vascular leakage, and swelling during T helper 1 cell-induced delayed type hypersensitivity. J. Immunol. 1994; 153:3967-3978.

1141. Howard M, Muchamuel T, Andrade S, Menon S. Interleukin 10 protects mice from lethal endotoxemia. J. Exp. Med. 1993; 177:1205-1208.

1142. van der Poll T, Marchant A, Buurman WA et al. Endogenous IL-10 protects mice from death during septic peritonitis. J. Immunol. 1995; 155:5397-5401.

1143. van Roon JAG, van Roy JLAM, Gmelig-Meyling FHJ, Lafeber FPJG, Bijlsma WJ. Prevention and reversal of cartilage degradation in rheumatoid arthritis by interleukin-10 and interleukin-4. Arthritis Rheum. 1996; 39:829-835.

1144. Rocken M, Racke M, Shevach E. Interleukin 4-induced immune deviation as antigen-specific therapy for inflammatory auotimmune disease. Immunol. Today 1996; 17:225-231.

1145. Chernoff AE, Granowitz EV, Shapiro L et al. A randomized, controlled trial of IL-10 in humans. Inhibition of inflammatory cytokine production and immune response. J. Immunol. 1995; 154:5492-5499.

1146. Maggi E, Manetti R, Annunziato F, Cosmi L, Guidizi MG, Biagiotti R, Galli G, Zuccati G, Romagnani S. Functional characterization and modulation of cytokine profile of CD8+ T cell clones from HIV-infected individuals. Blood 1997 (in press).

1147. Romagnani S, Annunziato F, Manetti R, Almerigogna F, Biagiotti R, Giudizi MG, Ravina A, Giannò V, Tomasevic L, Maggi E. Role for CD30 in HIV expression. Immunol. Letters 1996; 51:83-88.

1148. D'Elios MM, Manghetti M, De Carli M, Costa F, Baldari CT, Burroni D, Telford JL, Romagnani S, Del Prete GF. Th1 effector cells specific for helicobacter pilori in the gastric antrum of patients with peptic ulcer. J. Immunol. 1997 (in press).

1149. Parronchi P, Romagnani P, Annunziato F, Sampognaro F, Becchio A, Giannarini L, Maggi E, Pupilli C, Tonelli F, Romagnani S. Type 1 helper (Th1)-predominance and IL-12 expression in the gut of patients with Crohn's disease. Amer. J. Pathol. 1997 (in press).

INDEX

Model Th1 cytokines during gestation promoting a Th1 profile in susceptable offspring.